D1317226

Disorders of the Spleen

MPP

38

RICHARD S. NEIMAN, M.D.
Director, Division of Hematopathology
Department of Pathology and Laboratory
  Medicine
Professor of Pathology and Laboratory
  Medicine and of Medicine
Indiana University School of Medicine
Indianapolis, Indiana

**ATTILIO ORAZI, M.D.,
M.R.C.PATH.**
Director, Immunohistology Laboratory
Division of Hematopathology
Department of Pathology and Laboratory
  Medicine
Professor of Pathology and Laboratory
  Medicine
Indiana University School of Medicine
Indianapolis, Indiana

Presently:

Professor of Pathology
Director, Division of Hematopathology
Department of Pathology
College of Physicians and Surgeons of
  Columbia University
New York, New York

Disorders of the Spleen

Volume 38 in the Series

MAJOR PROBLEMS IN PATHOLOGY

second edition

W.B. SAUNDERS COMPANY
A Division of Harcourt Brace & Company
PHILADELPHIA   LONDON   TORONTO   MONTREAL   SYDNEY   TOKYO

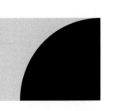

W.B. SAUNDERS COMPANY
A Division of Harcourt Brace & Company

The Curtis Center
Independence Square West
Philadelphia, Pennsylvania 19106

Library of Congress Catalog card number is 99–31814

To: Sandra

and

To: Maria, Giulia and Rita

Preface

Although the gross anatomy and microscopic anatomy of the spleen have been well described and the spleen's functions have been reasonably well elucidated, the organ retains a degree of mystery for most physicians. The relative lack of understanding of the spleen is due in great measure to the fact that the organ is not ideally accessible to comprehensive study. The majority of the pathologic processes involving the spleen are either self-limited or occur in other hematopoietic organs as well. Biopsy of the bone marrow or a lymph node is faster and less risk to the patient than splenectomy, which is not ususally necessary for diagnostic purposes. Because removal of a diseased and often greatly enlarged spleen entails certain risks to the patient, therapeutic splenectomy is usually resorted to only after such other therapeutic modalities as corticosteroids, cytotoxic or immuno-suppressive agents, or radiotherapy have failed to produce the desired effects. The result is that in most therapeutic splenectomy specimens, characteristic diagnostic features are altered or obliterated by previous therapy. In addition, recent advances in therapeutic management of many disorders affecting the spleen, such as hairy cell disease, Hodgkin's disease, and Gaucher disease, have decreased the incidence of splenectomy. Finally, autopsy tissue is often unsatisfactory because of therapeutic changes and rapid postmortem autolysis. It is, therefore, not surprising that pathologists sometimes feel uncomfortable when called upon to interpret pathologic processes in the spleen.

In the 10-year-period since the publication of the first edition of *Disorders of the Spleen* by Wolf and Neiman, there have been more contributions to the literature relating to the spleen than perhaps in any previous decade. The result is a second edition that contains more revisions and additions than might have been expected. Because the literature on the spleen has become so vast, we have confined our discussion of the anatomy, embryology, and physiology of the organ to those studies that relate to humans except in a few specific cases, which we have specifically indicated. In addition, we have arbitrarily limited the number of references in certain topics to those that we believe have made specific and valuable contributions. We have, however, retained many old references, either because they are seminal studies or because they still contribute valuable information. The result is a bibliography with references ranging from 50 or more years ago to the present.

Where possible, we have used the most recent terminology proposed but have referred to other terminology that has been used historically as a basis for reference. We have used the most recent draft of the World Health Organization Classification for the malignant lymphomas, based on its presentation at the European Association for Hematopathology Meeting in the Netherlands in April 1998. Although the final publication of the WHO Classification has not occurred at the time this book has gone to press, we hope that future changes will be minimal.

As in the case of the first edition of this text, we have attempted to provide a clinical and pathologic study of the spleen that relates to splenic pathophysiology, avoiding the approach frequently used that enumerates and describes a long list of individual diseases. We believe our approach is more meaningful to both pathologists and clinical hematologists. We hope our readers agree.

Acknowledgments

We have benefited from the contributions of many people in the writing of this book. Innumerable colleagues have shared their case material with us over the years, either by requesting consultations in puzzling cases or by sharing an unusual or particularly instructive case. Occasionally, others have provided us with excellent gross photographs. Although we cannot acknowledge all of the individuals who provided us with case material, we wish to thank them as a group. We also wish to thank a group of dedicated individuals with whom we work within the Department of Pathology at Indiana University. They include Bradley Johnson and Delilah Colbert for their excellence in providing us with high-quality tissue sections for photography. Members of our departmental photography laboratory include Michael Goheen, who provided us with the excellent scanning and transition electron micrographs; Nancy McGuire; and in particular Susan Cooper, whose meticulous attention to detail has resulted in many photomicrographs of superior quality. Finally, this book could not have been written without the excellence and dedication of our secretary, Regina D. Bennett, along with the additional secretarial support of Cathi Iweriebor.

Contents

Introduction

Study of the normal morphology of and pathologic processes in the spleen is perhaps more dependent upon technical factors than any other organ. Therefore, attention to the techniques of fixation and tissue processing are critical. Because of the nature of the red pulp, the spleen contains a relatively large amount of blood in relation to its total volume. This is particularly true in splenectomy specimens that are removed because of the enlargement of the organ. Fixation is therefore hampered because of slow penetration of the fixative. In addition, the spleen is subject to rapid cellular breakdown because of the large number of enzymes within the macrophages of the organ and because of the numerous polymorphonuclear leukocytes normally sequestered. As a result, the majority of splenectomy specimens suffer from technical artifact. Color Plate 1 is an example of a normal spleen fixed overnight without sectioning of the organ. It is obvious that penetration of the fixative into the organ is not great and that the central portion of the specimen remains unfixed. Histologic examination of this area of the spleen subsequent to processing will show significant tissue artifact.

We believe that all splenectomy specimens should be submitted to the pathology laboratory in the fresh state so that the pathologist can control the processing of the specimen. Surgeons and attending physicians of patients undergoing splenectomy must recognize that even in cases of therapeutic splenectomy or removal of the organ after splenic rupture, there may be unsuspected pathology present that can be appreciated only if the specimen is handled expeditiously. Pathologists must recognize that, even in such cases, detection of possible underlying pathology cannot be achieved if the spleen is not processed properly. In addition, prompt delivery of the splenectomy specimen in the fresh state to the pathology laboratory provides an opportunity to perform ancillary studies that may be critical in the diagnosis. These include touch imprints, which are particularly useful in diagnosing such conditions as myeloproliferative disorders, autoimmune hemolytic anemia, and immune thrombocytopenic purpura; flow cytometry; and molecular and cytogenetic studies, many of which have become standard diagnostic techniques in the workup of many hematologic disorders. We believe that it is mandatory for tissue sections of the spleen to fix overnight. Rapid 1-day turnaround of diagnostic or therapeutic splenectomy specimens is seldom of practical value. There is no reason for an urgent confirmation of a clinical diagnosis in a therapeutic splenectomy specimen; and few, if any, patients are treated for the disease found in diagnostic splenectomy specimens while they are still recuperating from abdominal surgery.

The role of the frozen section in splenic diagnosis is controversial. We believe that frozen section of an enlarged and bloody organ is frequently unsatisfactory because in many cases the diagnosis depends upon the recognition of cytologic detail that cannot be adequately appreciated in frozen sections. Therefore, we believe that frozen sections of spleens should be discouraged in most instances.

However, if diagnostic splenectomy reveals the presence of tumor masses or focal lesions, frozen section may be a valuable procedure.

In our laboratory, we are in the habit of preparing tissue blocks from the spleen that are no more than 3–4 mm thick. We invariably use a volume of at least 10 times as much fixative as the volume of specimen being fixed. In particularly bloody specimens, we usually change the fixative after 1 hour. We believe that the type of fixative used in processing sections of spleen is of less importance than the care taken in fixation. Our own preference is B5 fixative because of the superior cellular detail obtained. However, because many immunohistologic stains are more successfully performed and DNA preservation is better maintained for molecular analysis in formalin-fixed tissue, we invariably fix one tissue block in that fixative.

In addition to the routine hematoxylin and eosin stain, we have found that the periodic acid–Schiff stain is of particular value in studying sections of the spleen. It has been our experience that the ring fibers and the architectural framework of the red pulp are better demonstrated in PAS-stained sections. In addition, because of the large degree of red cell sequestration in the red pulp, the H&E stain is frequently difficult to interpret because of the prominent staining of erythrocytes by eosin. With the PAS stain, erythrocytes stain faintly, if at all, and seem to fade into the background, allowing one to observe the structure and cytology of the cords and sinuses with much greater clarity. In addition, the PAS stain demonstrates plasma cells, megakaryocytes, and granulocytes as well as the vascular framework of the red pulp better than the H&E stain.

Attention to these details of tissue handling and processing will provide pathologists with a better opportunity to appreciate both the normal morphology and pathologic changes in the spleen.

Color Plates

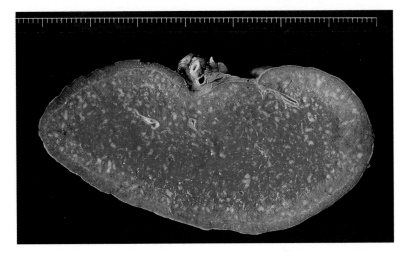

Color Plate 1. Cross section of a normal spleen placed in fixative without prior sectioning showing inadequate tissue penetration of fixative. (Courtesy of Dr. Bridget Wilkins, University of Southhampton, UK.)

Color Plate 2. Cross section of a normal spleen showing the distribution of white pulp nodules, which are easily seen in this particular specimen.

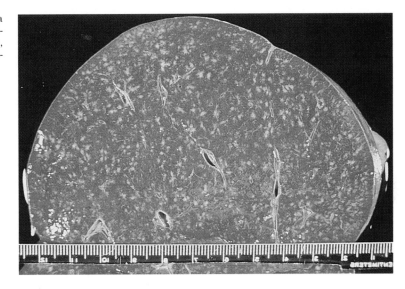

Color Plate 3. Lacerated spleen. Traumatic laceration, such as this example, frequently results in splenosis.

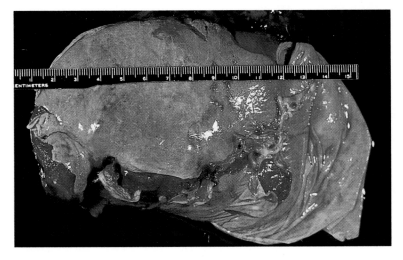

Color Plate 4. A cross section of the entire spleen from a 32-year-old patient with sickle cell disease. The organ weighed 12 grams.

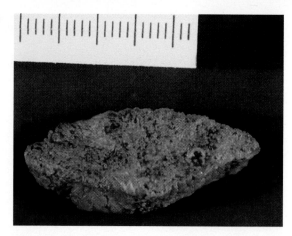

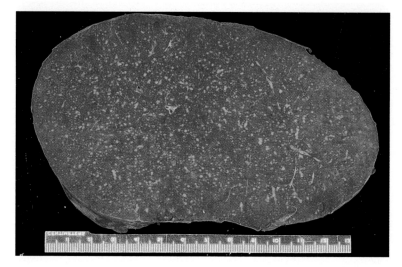

Color Plate 5. Some cases of chronic immune activation of the white pulp, such as in this spleen from a patient with rheumatoid arthritis, may produce a gross picture that mimics malignant lymphoma.

Color Plate 6. Splenic involvement by Hodgkin's disease showing multiple tumor masses of varying sizes similar to the pattern of involvement seen in malignant lymphomas of large cell type.

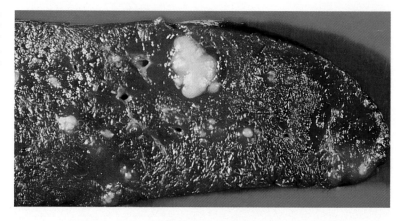

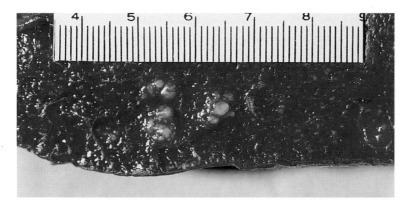

Color Plate 7. Splenic involvement in Hodgkin's disease. These three nodules, each measuring only approximately 0.5 cm in diameter and in aggregate only approximately 1.5 cm in greatest dimension, represent the only sites of involvement in this 225-gram spleen. It is clear that they would have been overlooked if the organ had not been carefully examined.

Color Plate 8. Splenic involvement in marginal zone cell lymphoma. Involvement of all of the white pulp nodules produces a miliary pattern.

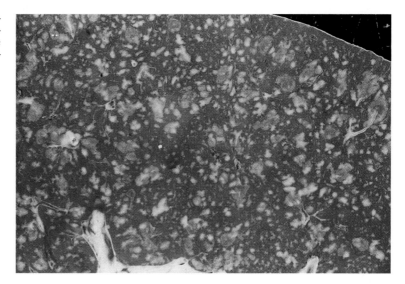

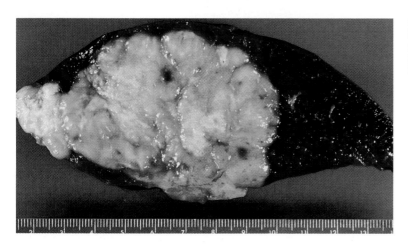

Color Plate 9. Large tumor masses in the spleen are characteristic of malignant lymphomas of large cell type and are also frequent in Hodgkin's disease.

Color Plate 10. Multifocal transformation to large cell lymphoma (large tumor nodules) in a case of follicular small cleaved cell lymphoma. Note the miliary pattern of involvement of the white pulp typical of low-grade B-cell lymphomas underlying the large tumor masses.

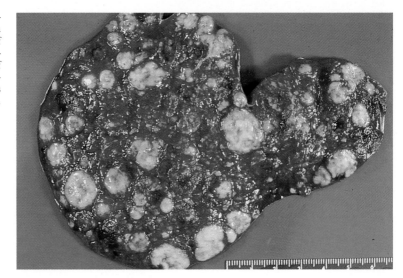

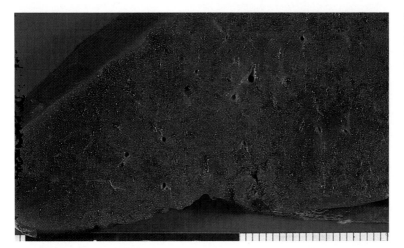

Color Plate 11. Splenic amyloidosis. Extensive deposits of amyloid in the red pulp produce a homogeneous and waxy appearance to the cut section of the organ.

Color Plate 12. Hereditary spherocytosis. Sequestration of large numbers of spherocytes in the cords of Billroth creates an intensely congested appearance.

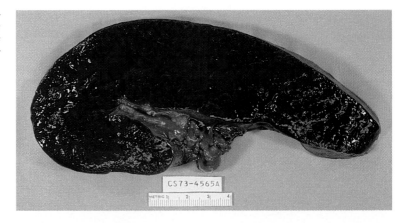

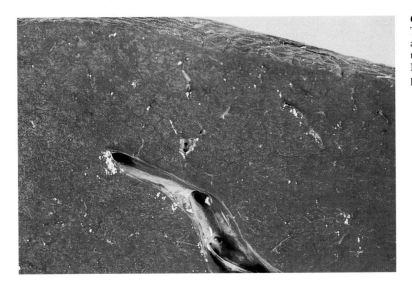

Color Plate 13. Gaucher disease. The cut surface of the spleen shows a mottled appearance because of the accumulation of Gaucher cells. Note the obliteration of the white pulp.

Color Plate 14. Langerhans cell histiocytosis. The infiltration of Langerhans cells creates a vaguely mottled appearance to the organ, with loss of the white pulp markings.

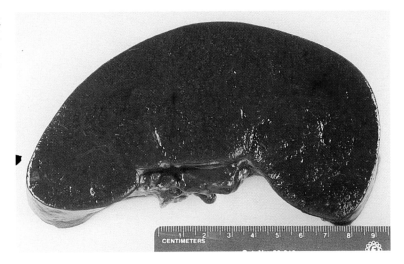

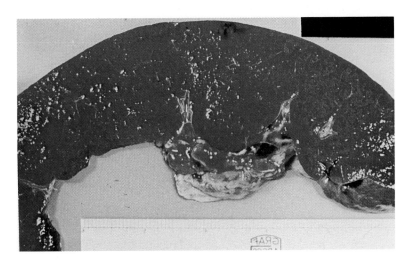

Color Plate 15. Cross section of the spleen in a typical example of acute myeloid leukemia. The cut section appears homogeneous with loss of white pulp markings. The color may vary from pale salmon to brown or purple, according to the degree of congestion and the type of cell infiltrating the red pulp.

Color Plate 16. Cross section of the spleen in chronic granulocytic leukemia. Splenomegaly is common and may reach massive proportions. The cut surface of the organ is solid and reddish without evidence of white pulp markings.

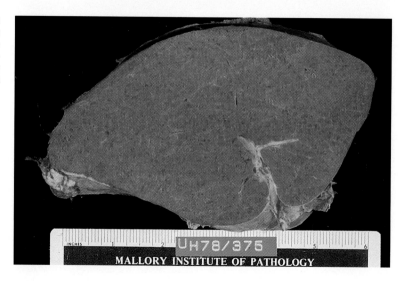

MALLORY INSTITUTE OF PATHOLOGY

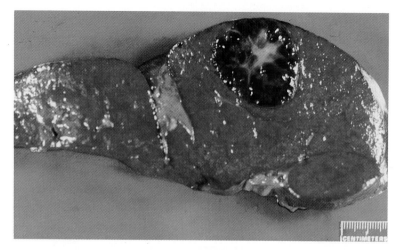

Color Plate 17. Cut section of a spleen in a case of chronic granulocytic leukemia. The large nodule or "plum" represents a focal clone of blast transformation. The vast majority of cases of blast transformation in the spleen occur as a homogeneous nontumor-forming infiltrate. It is unusual for blast transformation to occur with this tumorlike manifestation.

Color Plate 18. Chronic lymphocytic leukemia. The expansion of the white pulp and infiltration of the red pulp produce a mottled appearance.

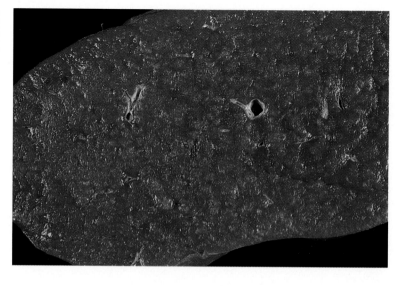

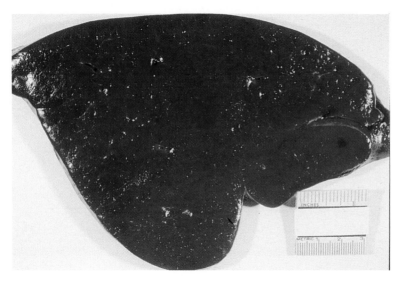

Color Plate 19. Hairy cell leukemia. The spleen in this disorder is characteristically deep purplish-red because of the presence of sequestered blood and of blood lakes.

Color Plate 20. Chronic idiopathic myelofibrosis. Splenomegaly in this condition may assume gigantic proportions. Expansion of the red pulp by hematopoietic precursors results in a homogeneous appearance indistinguishable from a leukemic infiltrate.

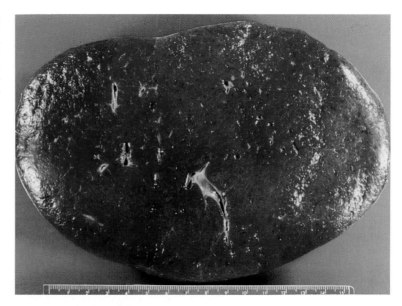

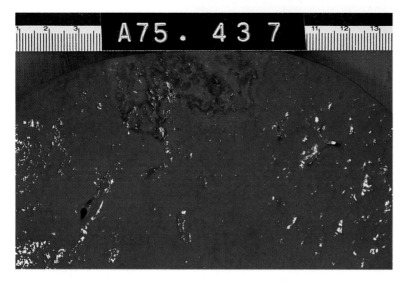

Color Plate 21. Fresh hemorrhagic infarct in a spleen involved by acute leukemia. The infarct has begun to organize, creating the lighter areas that delimit the lesion.

Color Plate 22. Organized infarct of the spleen. The yellow color is due to the presence of lipid from the degenerated red blood cells and platelets.

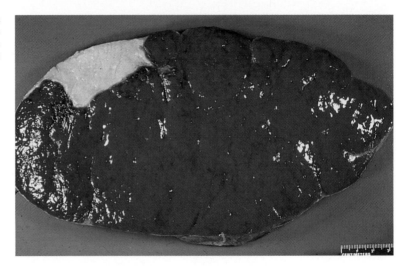

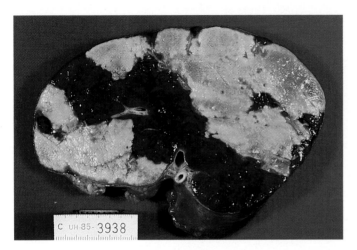

Color Plate 23. Massive organizing infarcts of the spleen. Such lesions may be mistaken for malignant lymphoma (see color plate 9). Extensive infarcts such as these may result in hyposplenism.

Color Plate 24. Peliosis of the spleen. Blood-filled cysts in all stages of organization occur scattered randomly throughout the organ.

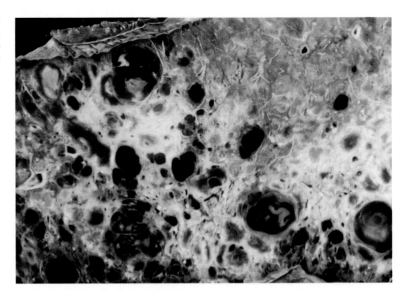

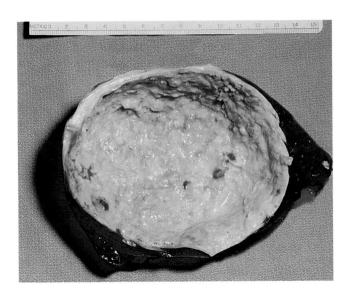

Color Plate 25. Splenic pseudocyst. The wall of the cyst is shaggy and nontrabeculated.

Color Plate 26. This splenic infarct has undergone liquefactive necrosis, causing a pseudocyst.

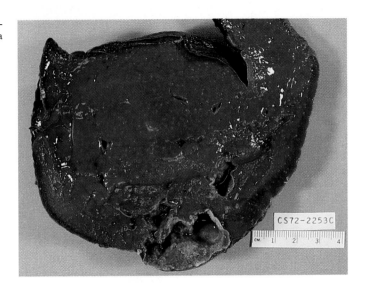

Color Plate 27. Splenic epidermoid cyst. The lesion is unilocular and has a trabeculated wall. The brown color is the result of organizing blood.

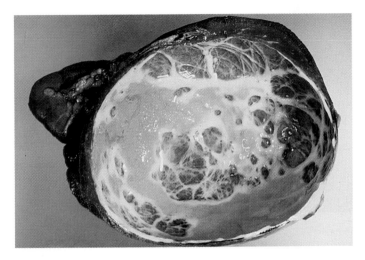

Color Plate 28. Hemangiosarcoma of the spleen. The entire organ appears involved. Cystic lesions alternate with solid areas of tumor. (Courtesy of Dr. Renato Rosso, University of Pavia, Pavia, Italy.)

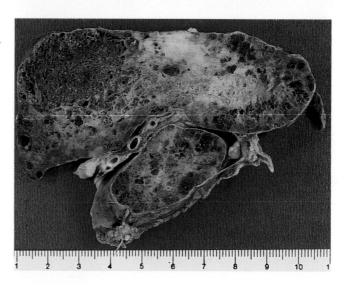

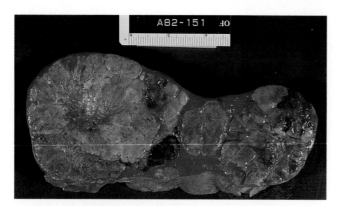

Color Plate 29. Spleen involved with metastatic melanoma. Note that several of the tumor masses display the brown color of melanotic pigment.

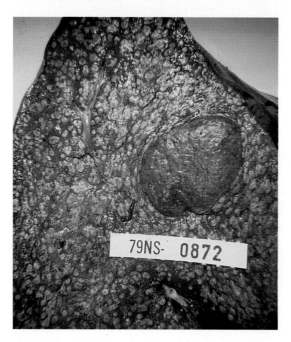

Color Plate 30. Splenic hamartoma found incidentally in a spleen removed from a patient with malignant lymphoma. Note that in addition to the single large hamartoma, there is miliary involvement by malignant lymphoma.

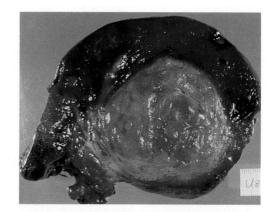

Color Plate 31. Inflammatory pseudotumor of the spleen. The lesion appears well circumscribed only on its upper border and has an infiltrative appearance elsewhere.

I

General Considerations

1

EMBRYOLOGY AND ANATOMY

EMBRYOLOGY

The spleen is first visible in human embryos during the 5th week of gestation (Fig. 1–1), which corresponds to an 8- to 10-mm embryo.[1, 2, 3] The organ arises entirely from mesodermal tissue as nodular thickenings of mesenchymal cells between layers of the left dorsal mesogastrium, the mesentery suspending the stomach from the dorsal wall of the abdominal cavity. These nodules condense and become vascularized during the 6th and 7th weeks of fetal life.[3, 4] The nodules of the splenic anlage are the origin for the development of splenic segments, or lobules.[5] The frequent presence of notches in the splenic surface in postnatal organs probably represents evidence of their incomplete fusion.[6]

The embryologic development of the human spleen has been divided into three stages.[2] The first, or preliminary developmental stage, begins at about the 6th to 7th week of fetal life and lasts until about the 14th week. Blood vessels begin to proliferate within a network of mesenchymal cells, and venous sinuses and arterioles appear. Reticular cells

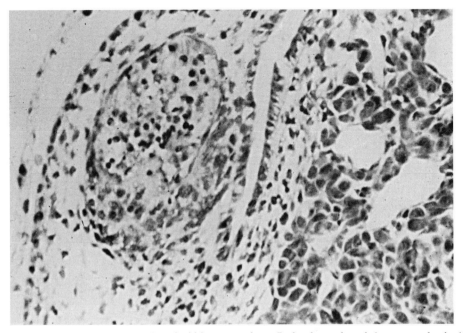

Figure 1–1. Splenic anlage from a 6-week-old human embryo. Red pulp cords and sinuses are clearly visible.

3

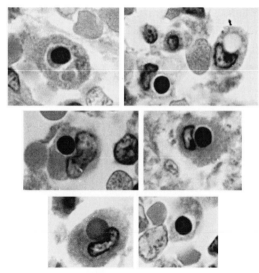

Figure 1–2. Composite photograph of six 1st-trimester fetal spleens. Phagocytosis of normoblasts and erythrocytes is clearly seen in each case.

and fibers form sheaths surrounding developing arterioles.[7] At this stage during the 1st trimester, red and white pulp cannot be distinguished.[8] Phagocytic activity by macrophages begins during the 1st trimester, and phagocytosis of nucleated red blood cells can be documented as early as the 12th week of gestation (Fig. 1–2).[9] However, full phagocytic capacity is not attained by the spleen until some time during the 1st year of postnatal life. This defi-

ciency can be documented by an elevation in red blood cell pit counts in both premature and full-term infants (see Chapter 4).[10]

During the later weeks of the preliminary developmental stage, hematopoietic cells make their appearance both in venous sinuses and within the mesenchymal tissue (Fig. 1–3). The significance of this phenomenon has been a subject of controversy. Some investigators have described extensive hematopoiesis[11, 12] and have used their observations to support the thesis that the fetal spleen is a significant hematopoietic organ. Others[2, 9, 13–15] have observed less convincing evidence of hematopoiesis and have suggested that the human fetal spleen plays no significant hematopoietic role (see Chapter 2).

The second stage of splenic embryologic development has been termed the "transformation stage"; it begins about the 15th gestational week. It is during this stage that the characteristic adult splenic organ structure becomes established. During the 15th to 17th weeks of fetal life, splenic lobules begin to form, composed of central arteries surrounded by a mass of fixed cells that will form the stromal elements of the white pulp. The lobules are not yet populated by lymphoid cells (Fig. 1–4). Between the lobules, the red pulp forms as the venous sinuses differentiate.[2, 7]

By the 18th week this stage is completed, leading to the third and last stage of splenic

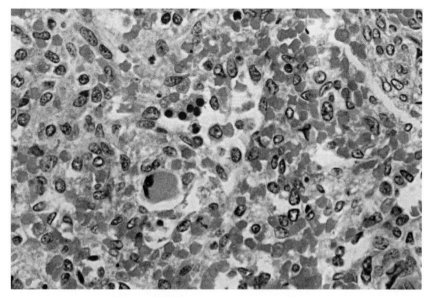

Figure 1–3. Representative section of fetal spleen in early 2nd trimester showing "hematopoiesis." There are scattered normoblasts and a mature megakaryocyte present.

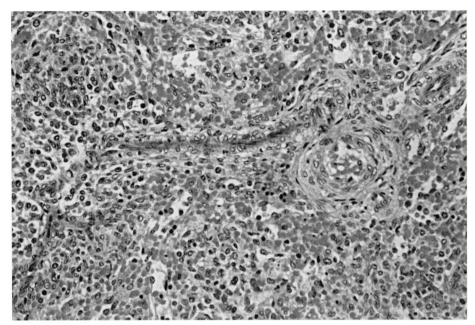

Figure 1–4. Representative spleen of 2nd-trimester fetus. Central arteries and their branches are forming. The fixed cells of the white pulp surround the vessel. Note the absence of lymphoid cells.

development, the stage of lymphoid colonization, which lasts from about the 18th to the 24th week of fetal life. Accumulation of T lymphocytes around the central arteries and their branches occurs first, beginning at about the 19th or 20th week, associated with the development of dendritic reticulum cells of the splenic lymphoid follicles. Plasma cells appear at about this time.[2, 16, 17] The development of the B-cell region of the spleen occurs later in fetal development than that of all other lymphatic organs, beginning about the 23rd gestational week. From the 20th to the 24th week the white pulp enlarges until it represents about half of the total volume of the spleen, only to decrease in percentage of volume to about 20 percent at birth. This decrease is due to the more rapid proliferation of the red pulp in the 3rd trimester.[12, 15] Splenic lymphoid tissue is both anatomically and functionally immature during fetal life and does not attain adult form and function until the 1st year after birth.[18–23] This tissue is characterized by a monomorphic population of medium-sized lymphocytes without morphologic evidence of compartmentalization. Germinal center formation does not occur. Although T cells appear similar in immunophenotypic proportions and function to those in adults,[21, 24] B cells display evidence of immunologic immaturity. Almost all express IgM and

IgD, few express IgA, and none appear to express IgG or IgE. Many B cells also coexpress CD5 at this time, but this decreases during fetal development.[18–23] At the time of birth, only inactive follicles are present, without evidence of germinal center formation (Fig. 1–5).[22] Even in cases of systemic intrauterine or neonatal infection, secondary germinal centers are not usually noted until approximately 3 weeks after birth.[18, 25] The splenic marginal zone, critical in the immune response to polysaccharide antigens, is also delayed in its full maturation until sometime after birth. Fetal marginal zone cells are few in number and display immunologic evidence of immaturity by coexpressing IgM and IgD and by not expressing CD21.[26]

Splenic Weight

The range of normal splenic weights during fetal life has been reported by several investigators[27–31] (Table 1–1). Splenic weight is insignificant until the end of the 1st trimester. By the end of the preliminary stage of splenic development, the spleen weighs between 0.1 and 0.2 gram.[27] Increase in splenic weight after this point is rapid, with normal weight approaching 1 to 2 grams by the end of the 20th week. The most rapid increase in splenic

Table 1–1. Recorded Splenic Weights for Fetuses from 20–44 Weeks

Age (WK)	Sung and Singer (GA)[29]		Gruenwald and Minh (MA)[31]	Larroche (MA)[28]	Schultz et al (GA)[30]	
	S	L			M	F
20	0.3 ± 1.0	0.7 ± 0.3			1.7 ± 1.5	1.4
21	0.4 ± 0.6	0.7 ± 0.2				
22	0.5 ± 0.4	0.8 ± 0.4				
23	0.7 ± 0.5	0.8 ± 0.4				
24	0.9 ± 0.7	0.9 ± 0.5	1.7 ± 1.1		2.5 ± 1.9	3.1 ± 1.8
25	1.2 ± 0.4	1.1 ± 1.6				
26	1.5 ± 1.1	1.3 ± 0.7	2.2 ± 1.5	1.9 ± 0.8		
27	1.9 ± 1.0	1.7 ± 1.0				
28	2.3 ± 1.1	2.1 ± 0.8	2.6 ± 1.4	2.6 ± 0.8	3.8 ± 2.3	3.9 ± 2.3
29	2.7 ± 2.0	2.6 ± 0.9				
30	3.1 ± 1.5	3.3 ± 2.0	3.4 ± 2.0	3.2 ± 1.0		
31	3.6 ± 4.0	4.0 ± 1.2				
32	4.2 ± 2.4	4.7 ± 5.4	4.1 ± 2.1	4.8 ± 1.4	5.4 ± 2.4	5.4 ± 3.1
33	4.7 ± 2.3	5.5 ± 3.5				
34	5.3 ± 2.5	6.4 ± 3.0	5.2 ± 2.1	6.5 ± 1.9		
35	5.9 ± 6.8	7.2 ± 5.2				
36	6.5 ± 2.9	8.1 ± 3.1	6.7 ± 3.0	7.3 ± 2.1	8.6 ± 4.0	8.6 ± 3.7
37	7.2 ± 6.3	8.8 ± 6.4				
38	7.8 ± 5.9	9.5 ± 3.5	8.8 ± 4.2	10.2 ± 2.4		
39	8.5 ± 4.5	10.1 ± 3.5			12.0 ± 4.0 (S)	10.0 ± 4.0 (S)
40	9.2 ± 4.1	10.4 ± 3.3	10.0 ± 3.9	10.9 ± 2.2	10.0 ± 3.0 (L)	11.0 ± 4.0 (L)
41	9.9 ± 4.5	10.5 ± 4.5				
42	10.6 ± 3.7	10.3 ± 3.6	10.2 ± 4.3			
43						
44			11.2 ± 4.1			

Results expressed as mean ± 2 standard deviation
MA = Menstrual age   GA = Gestational age   M = Male
L = Liveborn infants   S = Stillborn infants   F = Female

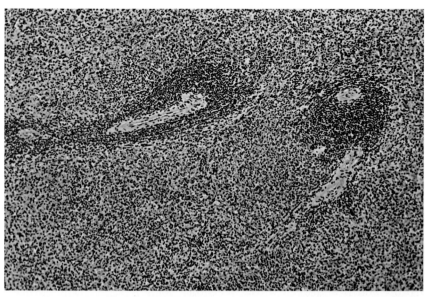

Figure 1–5. Section of spleen from 3rd-trimester fetus. Note that the red and white pulp are clearly demarcated. However, secondary germinal centers have not formed.

weight occurs during the second half of gestation, with recorded values averaging about 9 to 10 grams, plus or minus 3.5 grams at 40 weeks of gestational life.[28-31] Variation in weight appears great. However, there is little evidence documenting any significant difference in splenic weight between males and females during fetal life.[28] Variation in splenic weight appears more directly related to fetal weight and body length and to whether the study involves liveborn or stillborn infants.[32] There is a wide variation in reported splenic weight at birth, which is probably also related to fetal weight and body length but undoubtedly is also due to the underlying pathologic conditions responsible for fetal death. In only one of the studies quoted[30] was this factor addressed, and infants with certain conditions such as sepsis or congenital anomalies were eliminated from the study. During the first 12 months of life the spleen enlarges rapidly, reaching an average of about 30 grams by the end of the 1st year of life (Table 1–2). There is a further rapid increase in the size of the spleen from the first year through the years

of puberty, with weights approaching those of normal adults being reached by the end of the 1st decade of life (Table 1–3). There appears to be little statistical difference in splenic weight between males and females in this age group.[33]

There is no uniform agreement concerning the normal weight of the adult human spleen.[33-37] McCormick and Kashgarian[37] reviewed a large number of studies dealing with normal splenic weights and reported a wide range in weight from 80 to 300 grams. In our experience, the weight of the normal adult spleen may range from 50 to 250 grams. Several autopsy series of nonhospitalized populations have indicated that, other factors being equal, splenic weights tend to be greater in white persons than in black persons and greater in males than in females.[35-37] The weight of the spleen decreases with age, in association with a decrease in splenic function.[38, 39] The wide range of normal weight of the spleen can be deceptive, because a normally small spleen can enlarge to two to three times its size and still remain within the normal range.

Table 1–2. Mean Spleen Weights During First Year of Life

Age	Kayser[33] M	Kayser[33] F	Schultz et al[31] M	Schultz et al[31] F	Coppelletta and Wolbach[32]
1 Day	6.6 ± 0.7	5.8 ± 0.7			
1–3 Days					8
3–7 Days					9
2–30 Days	12.4 ± 1.4	11.5 ± 1.9			
1–3 Wk					10
31–60 Days	16.3 ± 2.1	22.9 ± 6.5			
3–5 Wk					12
1 Mo			12.0 ± 4.0	11.0 ± 4.0	
5–7 Wk					13
7–9 Wk					13
2 Mo			15.0 ± 5.0	14.0 ± 5.0	
9 Wk–3 Mo					14
61–90 Days	17.4 ± 2.6	16.3 ± 4.0			
91–120 Days	19.1 ± 4.3	14.6 ± 1.9			
121–150 Days	23.0 ± 5.0	19.9 ± 4.5			
151–180 Days	20.0 ± 3.4	18.2 ± 3.4			
3 Mo			16.0 ± 5.0	15.0 ± 5.0	
4 Mo			17.0 ± 5.0	17.0 ± 5.0	16
5 Mo			18.0 ± 7.0	19.0 ± 5.0	16
6 Mo			20.0 ± 7.0	18.0 ± 8.0	17
7 Mo			23.0 ± 10.0	22.0 ± 8.0	19
8 Mo			20.0 ± 7.0	20.0 ± 9.0	20
9 Mo			22.0 ± 5.0	18.0 ± 6.0	20
10 Mo			24.0 ± 11.0	25.0 ± 11.0	22
11 Mo			28.0 ± 10.0	23.0 ± 9.0	25
12 Mo	31.1 ± 4.7	23.5 ± 3.6	28.0 ± 7.0	27.0 ± 9.0	26

Kayser results expressed as mean ± 2 standard deviation
Schultz results expressed as mean ± 1 standard deviation
Coppelletta and Wolbach expressed as mean only

Table 1–3. Recorded Spleen Weights 1–19 Years

Age	Kayser[33]		Coppelletta and Wolbach[32]
	M	F	
1 Y	31.0 ± 4.7	23.5 ± 3.6	26
14 Mo			26
16 Mo			28
18 Mo			30
20 Mo			30
22 Mo			33
2 Y	42.6 ± 4.4	42.0 ± 7.2	33
3 Y	54.8 ± 10.1	41.8 ± 5.5	37
4 Y	58.7 ± 14.4	49.3 ± 9.2	39
5 Y	56.8 ± 9.9	50.7 ± 9.1	47
6 Y	69.3 ± 12.2	67.2 ± 10.6	58
7 Y	103.3 ± 36.8	64.2 ± 15.8	66
8 Y	73.1 ± 12.2	94.3 ± 27.3	69
9 Y	90.9 ± 29.0	80.9 ± 14.0	73
10 Y	111.3 ± 28.6	90.0 ± 29.2	85
11 Y	90.0 ± 27.9	87.5 ± 24.6	87
12 Y	114.7 ± 24.1	89.0 ± 20.3	93
13 Y	138.7 ± 55.4	129.0 ± 30.6	
14 Y	151.2 ± 40.1	162.8 ± 52.1	
15 Y	155.3 ± 36.1	129.2 ± 31.8	
16 Y	165.1 ± 29.7	219.0 ± 58.9	
17 Y	212.7 ± 48.2	158.0 ± 17.3	
18 Y	181.0 ± 25.2	146.4 ± 25.1	
19 Y	195.6 ± 29.0	156.5 ± 39.9	

Kayser results expressed as mean ± 2 standard deviation
Coppelletta and Wolbach expressed as mean only

ANATOMY

The spleen is covered by a fibrous capsule that contains the major afferent and efferent blood vessels, lymphatic vessels, and nerves.[40]

The peritoneal mesothelium covers the capsule. Although the mesothelium is seldom preserved in histologic sections, it can occasionally be visualized as a single layer of cuboidal cells that may have microvilli. The capsule of the human spleen contains little, if any, smooth muscle, in contrast to that of some animal species, and therefore has no significant contractile function.[40]

The arterial supply of the spleen is derived from the celiac axis via the splenic artery, which enters the capsule at the splenic hilum. It branches to form trabecular arteries, which are accompanied by splenic veins and efferent lymphatics[41] (Fig. 1–6). It is doubtful that the human spleen contains afferent lymphatics. The vascular structures are surrounded by collagenous tissue arranged into trabeculae or septa,[32, 34] which are invaginations of the fibrous capsule. The central arteries, the largest arteries of the white pulp, arise as branches of the trabecular arteries. The venous drainage is from the venous sinuses into the portal system via the splenic vein.

Histology

Van Krieken and te Velde[41] have commented on the confusion and misunderstanding relating to the normal histology of the human spleen. We agree with their observation and with their identification of the sources of this confusion, which include: (1) the inappropriate application of data derived from studies

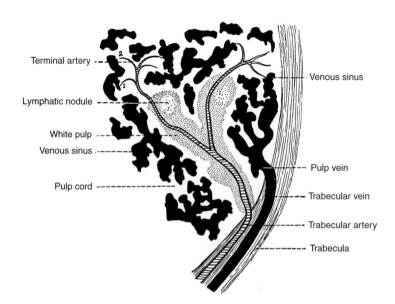

Terminal artery
Lymphatic nodule
White pulp
Venous sinus
Pulp cord
Venous sinus
Pulp vein
Trabecular vein
Trabecular artery
Trabecula

Figure 1–6. Diagram showing the arterial circulation of the spleen and its relationship to the white pulp. Illustrated are the closed (rapid) (1) and open (slow) (2) compartments of the circulation. (From Fawcett D: Bloom and Fawcett: A Textbook of Histology, 11th ed, p 474. Philadelphia, WB Saunders, 1985.)

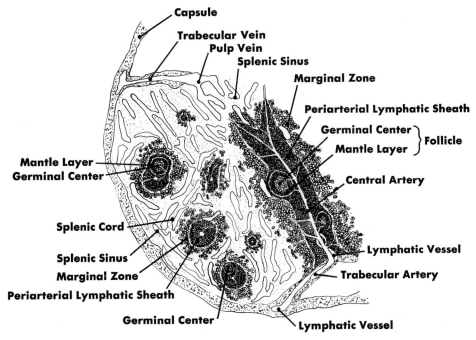

Figure 1-7. Diagram of splenic white pulp showing the association between the arterial network and the lymphoid tissue. (From Weiss L, Tavassoli M: Anatomical hazards to the passage of erythrocytes through the spleen. Semin Hematol 1974; 7:372.)

on animal spleens, which are not identical to human spleens; (2) confusion in terminology; (3) the use of postmortem specimens that are subject to autolysis; and (4) wide variations in normal histologic features with age, especially with respect to the white pulp. The following description of splenic histology is derived from our experience and from studies on human spleens only, except where specifically indicated.

The White Pulp

The white pulp of the spleen can be visualized grossly as uniformly distributed, 1- to 2-mm white nodules (Color Plate 2). Histologically the white pulp is intimately associated with the splenic arterial circulation (Fig. 1-7). A cylindrical cuff composed predominantly of T lymphocytes with some B lymphocytes, plasma cells, and macrophages—called the periarterial, or periarteriolar, lymphoid sheath (PALS)—surrounds the central arteries.[24, 42, 43] The PALS becomes gradually more attenuated as the arteries branch into smaller tributaries but may still be seen around the penicilli (penicilliary arterioles) (Fig. 1-8).[44] Periodically,

lymphoid follicles, also known as malpighian bodies or follicles, containing predominantly B lymphocytes, occur as outgrowths of the lymphatic sheath, usually at arterial branch points (Fig. 1-9).[24, 44] These follicles appear as bipolar spheroids resembling grapes or a gas flame as they project from the PALS (Fig. 1-10), their shape in histologic sections depending on the angle at which they are cut. A meshwork of CD21-positive dendritic reticulum cells with long cytoplasmic processes, and extracellular reticulin fibers, which can be demonstrated using silver impregnation stains, forms a scaffolding for all white pulp compartments.[45, 46]

The morphologic features of the splenic white pulp vary with age and with the presence of systemic antigenic stimulation.[44, 47] The white pulp, unlike other lymphoreticular organs, is not fully developed at birth and attains full function during the 1st year of postnatal life.[21] It reaches a peak of function approximately at the time of puberty and then gradually involutes. The rate of involution may vary greatly from person to person. Inactive or hypoplastic white pulp is characteristic of both infancy and senescence (Fig. 1-11).[21, 41] The white pulp of the immunologically unstimulated adult spleen may be abundant but contains no germinal centers. However, spleens

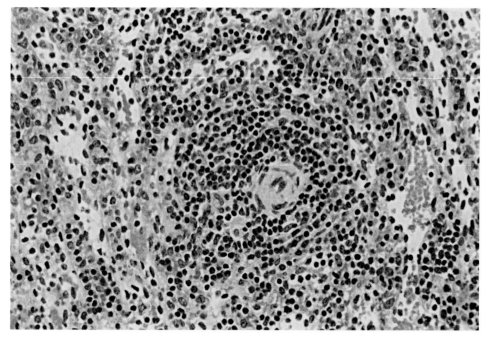

Figure 1–8. Penicilliary arteriole of red pulp with its surrounding collection of lymphoid cells. This represents the attenuated extension of the PALS.

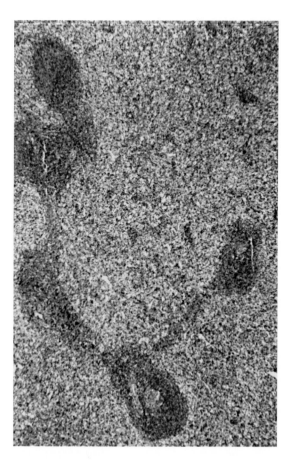

Figure 1–9. Lymphoid follicles of the white pulp appearing as budlike outgrowths of the lymphoid sheath.

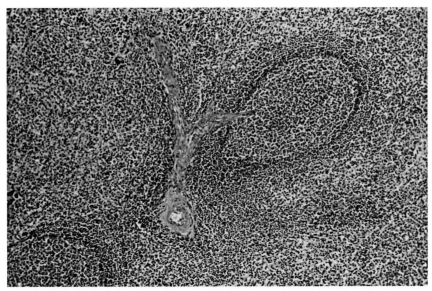

Figure 1–10. Secondary follicle arising from trabecular vessels. Note its elliptic configuration and relationship to the arterial circulation and the PALS.

of children and young adults usually contain secondary germinal centers, indicating their generally heightened immunologic state (Fig. 1–12).

In the immunologically activated state three distinct morphologic and functional zones are identifiable in the lymphoid follicles of the spleen (Fig. 1–13).[48-53] The secondary germinal center, or follicle, is similar in structure to germinal centers in other lymphoid organs, such as lymph nodes. It is composed predominantly of a variety of follicular B lymphocytes

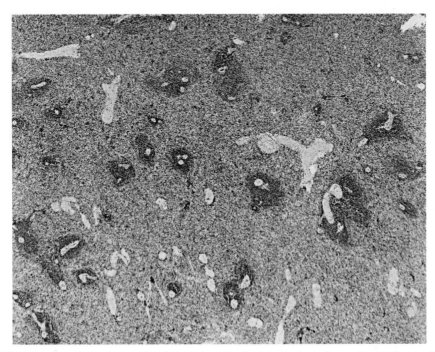

Figure 1–11. Low-power photomicrograph of the spleen in the immunologically unstimulated state. No secondary follicles are noted.

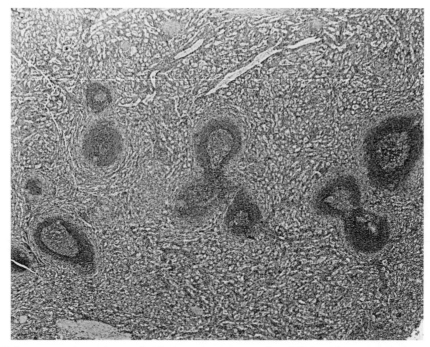

Figure 1–12. Low-power photomicrograph of spleen showing secondary follicles. This morphologic picture is typical in children and young adults and indicates a heightened immunologic state.

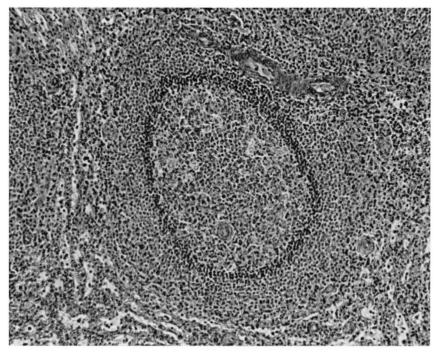

Figure 1–13. Activated (secondary) lymphoid follicle showing an outer marginal zone; a well-defined dark zone, the mantle zone; and the central germinal center.

containing either surface, cytoplasmic, or no immunoglobulin in a meshwork of dendritic reticulum cells.[46, 52] However, there are a variable but usually small number of CD3-positive T cells and NK cells present in the germinal centers as well.[52] Millikin[49] described a division of the germinal centers of the spleen into light- and dark-staining zones. The light zone reportedly contains predominantly pale reticular cells with admixed small lymphocytes and tingible-body macrophages, and the darker zone contains larger basophilic cells. Most of the lymphocytes in the light zone contain cytoplasmic IgM and IgG, whereas most of the lymphocytes in the dark zone contain surface IgM and IgD.[52] These zones are best recognized in large germinal centers; in smaller germinal centers the two types of cells may be mixed homogeneously instead of forming distinct zones. In lymph nodes the light zones are polarized toward the capsule and in mucous membranes toward the epithelial surfaces, presumably the regions in which antigens are first encountered.[53] In contrast to the orderly arrangement in other lymphoid organs, the arrangement of the lymphoid follicles in the spleen is at varying angles owing to the eccentric location of the follicles as they project from the PALS. As a result, in a given histologic preparation of the spleen, secondary follicles are usually seen in multiple different planes of section.

The germinal center is surrounded by a darker rim of small lymphocytes: the mantle zone, also composed of B lymphocytes that express surface IgD and IgM.[52, 53] The mantle zone is then encased by the outer marginal zone at the interface between the white and the red pulp. Lymphoid cells with the same morphologic and immunologic characteristics as marginal zone cells occur in the periphery of the follicular mantle zone of lymph node[54] and in the gastrointestinal tract.[55] However, only in the spleen do they form a distinct anatomic zone.[54] The marginal zone is an extension of the PALS and thus contains T lymphocytes.[52] However, the predominant cell is a B lymphocyte.[52-55] Marginal zone B cells are medium-sized lymphocytes with round to oval or occasionally slightly irregular nuclei with finely dispersed chromatin and small nucleoli. They are CD20-positive, CD21-positive, CD22-positive, and CD24-positive and CD3-negative, CD5-negative, CD9-negative, CD10-negative, CD11b-negative, CD11c-negative, CD23-negative, KiB3-negative, and IgD-

negative.[54] These cells are also alkaline phosphatase–positive.[56]

The central arteries branch within their lymphoid sheaths, some tributaries ending with the PALS and others within the marginal zones (Fig. 1–14).[40-42] Some branches go to the periphery of the lymphoid sheaths, curve around, and follow the perimeter of the marginal zones, forming the marginal sinus at the interface of the red and white pulp. Still others leave the white pulp and enter the red pulp as penicilli. Some of these small vessels may still be surrounded by a small collection of lymphocytes, representing the attenuated PALS. Before terminating, some of these vessels may be surrounded by a sheath of phagocytic cells. These sheathed arteries end in the red pulp or in the marginal zones. The marginal zone of the white pulp receives the termination of many arterial vessels.[34, 45] As will be further discussed in Chapter 2, this region is considered to be the functional site of initial antigen trapping and processing.[26, 57, 58] In most animal studies, the marginal zone is surrounded by a marginal sinus.[59] The existence of a marginal sinus in human spleens has been a subject of controversy. There is no evidence of this sinus in conventionally processed light-microscopy sections, and van Krieken et al[60] found no evidence of a marginal sinus in their study of plastic embedded spleens. However, Schmidt et al,[61] using scanning electron microscopy, described a marginal sinus composed of a flattened system of anastomosing channels (as did Burke and Simon[62] by using transmission electron microscopy). Branches of the central artery leave the white pulp and enter the red pulp as penicilliary arteries or arterioles, or penicilli. These vessels are usually still surrounded by a small collection of T lymphocytes, representing the attenuated PALS. The penicilli, in turn, branch, giving rise to several capillaries. Some of these are termed "sheathed capillaries" because they are surrounded by a sheath of fixed reticular cells and macrophages (the Schweigger-Seidel sheath or ellipsoid).[63] These and other unsheathed branches of the penicilli end in the red pulp or in the marginal zones.

The Red Pulp

The red pulp of the spleen is composed of venous sinuses, the pulp cords (of Billroth), and the terminal branches of the arterial sys-

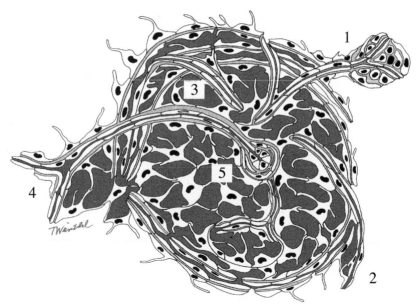

Figure 1–14. The white-pulp reticular framework showing the arterial network. This figure demonstrates a cross section of the entire PALS with the central artery at the center. The dendritic reticulum cells are illustrated with their black nuclei. The lymphocytes are omitted. Numerous branches ramify from the central artery. The sheathed artery (1) has a sheath of phagocytic cells around it and ends in either the marginal zone or the red pulp. Another branch, which is nonsheathed (2), ends in the marginal zone. A third branch (3) has access to a circumferential condensation of reticulum separating the PALS from the marginal zone. A fourth branch (4) penetrates the red pulp, where it terminates in a pulp cord. Other branches (5) are circumferential and provide blood to the germinal center. (Copyright to this illustration is the sole property of Indiana University School of Medicine.)

tem, the penicilliary arterioles (Fig. 1–15). The organization of the three provides an ideal mechanism for blood filtration. The cords of Billroth represent a meshwork of macrophages with interconnected cytoplasmic processes. These cells display the functional and immunologic features of actively phagocytic cells.[46] The structure of the splenic sinuses is unique in the human vascular system.[64] They are lined by spindle-shaped endothelial cells aligned along the longitudinal axis of the sinus.[65] The endothelial cells have long cytoplasmic processes. The basement membrane, which encircles the sinus, is composed of a grid of transversely oriented reticular "ring fibers" anchored by their attachment to the dendritic processes of the cordal macrophages.[66] The ring fibers can be visualized in histologic sections stained with periodic acid–Schiff or argyrophilic stains (Fig. 1–16). There is little, if any, mature collagen in the sinus wall. The structure of the sinus has been likened to a barrel, with the ring fibers resembling the hoops and the sinus lining cells the staves (Fig. 1–17).[66] In histologic sections there appear to be pores or apertures in the sinus wall. However, this is artifactual, resulting from shrinkage of the lin-

ing cell cytoplasm during fixation. The ring fibers are also closely opposed but shrink during fixation. Electron microscopic studies have shown that there are no true spaces between the endothelial cells.[44, 67, 68] The long cytoplasmic processes of these cells are closely opposed. However, there are only minimal interdigitations and no junctional complexes between cells.[67] This organization results in the potential for apertures between these cells.[44] Erythrocytes, granulocytes, and platelets may be observed by electron microscopy squeezing through these spaces (Fig. 1–18) and occasionally may be seen in histologic sections as well.

Some authors have postulated that the sinus lining cells in lymphoid tissues, including those of the spleen, are actually histiocytes rather than true vascular endothelial cells.[69] It is not unusual, in our experience, to see phagocytosis by these cells in pathologic specimens, and ultrastructural studies may occasionally show phagocytized material in them. In addition, several studies have documented erythrophagocytosis by sinus lining cells in hereditary spherocytosis and autoimmune hemolytic anemia.[70–72] However, sinus lining cells of the spleen also have ultrastructural features of endothelial cells, including pinocytotic vesicles

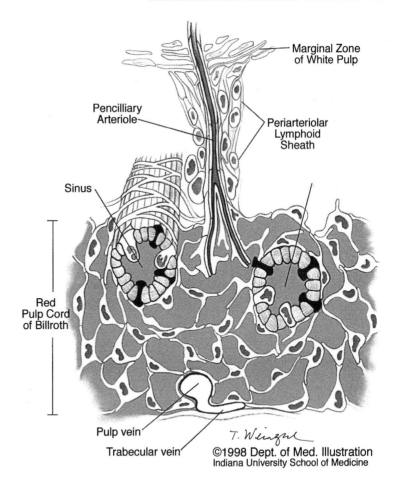

Figure 1–15. Diagram illustrating the circulation of the red pulp and demonstrating open (left) and closed (right) phases of venous circulation. (Copyright to this illustration is the sole property of Indiana University School of Medicine.)

©1998 Dept. of Med. Illustration
Indiana University School of Medicine

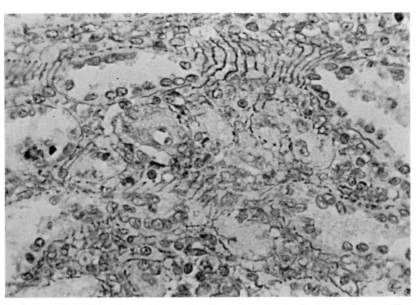

Figure 1–16. Periodic acid–Schiff—stained thin section of splenic red pulp illustrating the ring fibers that compose part of the walls of the red-pulp sinuses.

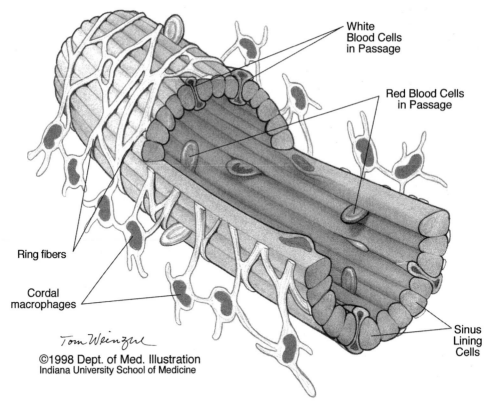

White
Blood Cells
in Passage

Red Blood Cells
in Passage

Ring fibers

Cordal
macrophages

Sinus
Lining
Cells

Tom Weinzurl

©1998 Dept. of Med. Illustration
Indiana University School of Medicine

Figure 1–17. Schematic representation of splenic sinus wall. Sinus lining cells with long cytoplasmic processes are parallel to one another and from the wall of the sinus. They have no desmosomes or tight junctions. The basement membrane is discontinuous and fenestrated in a fashion similar to that of screening or fish netting. Cordal macrophages anchor themselves to the ring fibers by their long cytoplasmic processes. The result is an imperfect barrier through which only cells with the ability to deform can pass. (Copyright to this illustration is the sole property of Indiana University School of Medicine.)

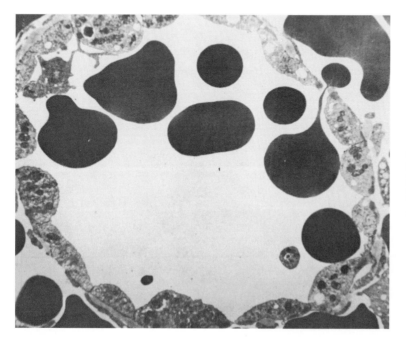

Figure 1–18. In this scanning electron micrograph of a splenic sinus, an erythrocyte is seen in the process of passing from the cord of Billroth into the sinus lumen. The degree of deformability required is graphically illustrated.

and intracytoplasmic filaments, which are not found in histiocytes. The pinocytotic vesicles are located primarily beneath the plasma membrane on the luminal and lateral surfaces. Chen and Weiss[73] described two types of cytoplasmic filaments in splenic sinus lining cells: larger filaments oriented along the long axis of the cell and finer filaments localized basally in organized bands approximately 0.3 μm in diameter. These authors postulated that the larger filaments are contractile, whereas the smaller filaments have a cytoskeletal function and may also control the passage of cells through potential apertures in the vascular walls. Dorfman[74] provided cytochemical evidence for the vascular nature of the sinus lining cells. The lining cells failed to stain with nonspecific esterase, acid phosphatase, and alkaline phosphatase, but the histiocytes of the cords of Billroth contained both nonspecific esterase and acid phosphatase. The lining cells were not identical to the capillary endothelial cells, however, because the latter possessed strong alkaline phosphatase activity. Giorno[75] demonstrated that the sinus lining cells contain factor VIII and stain for HLA-DR antigens, which are found in vascular endothelium. However, in contrast to the vascular endothelium, the lining cells failed to stain with CD14 (Leu-M3). Immunostaining with antibodies to vimentin, a marker of mesenchymal cells, and CD8, a marker for suppressor/cytotoxic T lymphocytes, revealed unusual rodlike and banded structures not found in vascular endothelial cells. Buckley et al[76, 77] have shown that splenic sinus lining cells not only express endothelial markers but also markers of monocyte-macrophage origin as well as those of T cells. In addition we have noted (unpublished observations) that although splenic vascular endothelium of arterioles and venules stains strongly with CD34, sinus lining cells stain only weakly and, in some cases, not at all. Therefore, the bulk of the evidence indicates that the sinus lining cells are special cells with a unique combination of vascular and macrophage characteristics.

The adventitial surface of the sinus wall is covered by processes of the reticular cells of the pulp cords—fixed cells of the monocyte/macrophage series—suspending the sinuses in a reticular meshwork.[60, 68] The cordal reticular fibers appear to attach to and may be continuous with reticular fibers of the sinus wall. Ultrastructurally, the cordal macrophages, some of which appear stellate, have irregular broad processes that appear as ruffled surfaces in carefully processed specimens and contain numerous lysosomes.[68] These cells appear to anchor to the adventitia of the sinuses. The reticular network of the pulp cords circumferentially surrounds the PALS and the marginal zones of the follicles. Reticular fibers do not enter the germinal centers but appear compressed at the periphery.[68]

Historically, there has been controversy as to whether the nature of the red pulp circulation is "closed" (i.e., lined by endothelium) or "open."[43, 78, 79] Ultrastructural studies are conflicting and have not resolved the debate. In animal studies, Chen and Weiss[73] reported that the termini of all arterial capillaries open into the pulp cords; and Weiss[80] reported that arterial vessels project into cordal lumens, forming a channel between the two, but do not appear to connect with the sinuses. In human studies, Burke and Simon[62] were unable to identify any arterial terminations ultrastructurally. However, Chen,[79] using injection of plastic microspheres to trace the splenic circulation, found that some arterial capillaries opened directly into the pulp cords, whereas others connected to venous sinuses. Bishop and Lansing[44] reported similar findings.

The bulk of evidence indicates that both an open and a closed circulatory system exists in the human spleen.[45, 64, 73, 81] The closed system, which accounts for most of the splenic blood flow and corresponds to the functionally rapid component of the circulation, consists of arterial branches that end in close opposition to walls of the venous sinuses. The open system, corresponding to the functionally slow component, is composed of arterial branches that end directly in the cords of Billroth. The cordal macrophages, anchored to the venous sinuses, have long dendritic cytoplasmic processes, creating a passage through which blood percolates slowly before entering the sinuses. Stagnation in the pulp cords results in an acidotic, hypoxic environment in which abnormal, defective, or senescent erythrocytes or other cells are trapped and destroyed.[43, 82]

CONGENITAL ANOMALIES

Apart from the relatively common finding of accessory spleens, congenital abnormalities of the spleen are rare. Only structural anomalies are considered in this section. The congenital immunodeficiency disorders will be discussed in Chapter 4.

Accessory Spleens

Accessory spleens, or "spleniculi," are incidental findings noted in one fifth to one third of autopsies.[83] They may be single or multiple. The most common locations are the splenic hilum, gastrosplenic ligament, and the tail of the pancreas (Fig. 1–19).[83–86] They may occasionally be found in the omentum or the intestinal mesentery. They are histologically and functionally identical to the normal spleen and share the same pathologic alterations as the parent organ in any given patient.[86] Accessory spleens may be of clinical importance if overlooked in patients in whom hypersplenism necessitates splenectomy.[87] Accessory spleens have been described in children with trisomy 13.[88] A characteristic finding was the presence of ectopic splenic tissue in the pancreas, incorporating pancreatic elements within the splenic nodules.[89]

Wandering Spleen

Wandering spleen is an uncommon condition characterized by the unusual mobility and displacement of the organ because of the presence of an elongated splenic pedicle.[90–93] The condition has also been termed "aberrant," "floating," "ptotic," "displaced," "prolapsed," "drifting," "dislocated," and "dystopic spleen."[91] Wandering spleen should not be confused with an ectopic spleen, which refers to the development of splenic tissue in an abnormal location. Wandering spleen is probably due to a congenital anomaly in the development of the dorsal mesogastrium, resulting in an abnormal gastrosplenic or splenorenal ligament,[91, 94] but acquired factors may play an additional role. The condition is more frequent in women of childbearing age and in children.[90, 94] Because wandering spleen is frequently associated with splenomegaly, it has been suggested that the increased traction of an enlarged spleen on its supporting ligaments plays a role in its pathogenesis.[91] However, most of the causes of the splenomegaly seem related to vascular congestion, with few cases revealing underlying intrinsic splenic disease. Moreover, there is no evidence that there is an increased incidence of wandering spleen in populations with a high incidence of splenomegaly.[90]

Wandering spleen is frequently asymptomatic and may be detected only incidentally. In at least one half of the cases, it is associated with abdominal cramping or other nonspecific gastrointestinal symptoms. Its rarity and the relative unfamiliarity of the entity may lead to a presumptive diagnosis of a malignant process. It may also present as an acute abdomen, related to torsion of the pedicle[95] and resultant venous occlusion, which may over time cause venous thrombosis, localized peritonitis, adhesions, or splenic infarction. In several cases, torsion has been observed after blunt abdominal trauma.[96] Another uncommon complication includes thrombocytopenia, most often associated with torsion of the pedicle.[93] There are also rare reports of lymphomatous involvement in wandering spleens.[95] Therapy, if the patient does present with an acute abdomen, is surgical, with reduc-

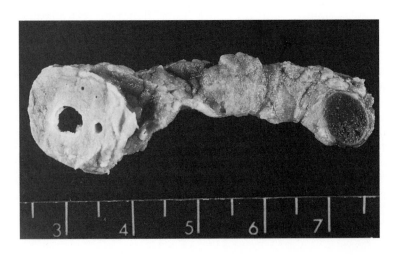

Figure 1–19. Ectopic spleen (right) in tail of pancreas found incidentally at autopsy.

tion of the torsion and splenopexy if there is no evidence of hypersplenism, infarction, or thrombosis.[97] Splenectomy should be performed in cases of splenic infarction or thrombosis or in cases where splenopexy is technically not feasible.[98]

Splenic-Gonadal Fusion

This unusual entity is fusion of the spleen with the left gonad or derivatives of the left mesonephros, which is an embryonic excretory system, the remnants of which are retained in males as the epididymis and ductus deferens.[3] In embryonic development the spleen is located near the mesonephros. Therefore, fusion of these structures could occur between the 5th week of development, when the spleen is first recognizable, and the 8th week, when the descent of the gonad and the involution of the mesonephros begins. The earliest reports of splenic-gonadal fusion were clinically unexpected postmortem findings.[99] This condition has subsequently been recognized during life.[100] Cases have been reported almost exclusively in males.[3] In a review of 97 reported cases, Walther et al[101] found only seven cases in females. In all well-documented cases, the left gonad has been involved, although one case was described as a right-sided scrotal mass. The majority of the patients are asymptomatic. The condition is often discovered when males present with cryptorchidism or during repair of a congenital hernia. Occasionally, however, patients present with a painful scrotal or inguinal mass[101] or, in rare cases, seminoma[102] or bowel obstruction.[103] Two of the three reported females had incompletely descended ovaries.[3] Two authors have described an enlarging painful mass during an attack of malaria.[104, 105]

Putschar and Manion[3] described two forms of splenic-gonadal fusion. The continuous variant, constituting 60 percent of the cases, consists of a cordlike structure connecting the spleen and the gonadal-mesonephric remnant. In the discontinuous form, the connection with the main spleen is lost, and splenic tissue is found as an encapsulated mass attached to the testis or epididymis. We have seen a case in which normal splenic tissue was embedded entirely within the parenchyma of a normally descended testicle, with no apparent relation to the main spleen (Fig. 1–20). The discontinuous form should probably be considered a variant of an accessory spleen.

Putschar and Manion[3] also described a syndrome consisting of splenic-gonadal fusion and severe malformation of the extremities. Three of the five reported patients, four males and one female, also had micrognathia. An even rarer condition, fusion of the spleen and liver, was reported as an incidental autopsy finding by Cotelingham and Saito.[106]

Asplenia

Congenital absence of the spleen associated with malformations of the cardiovascular system is a well-documented syndrome.[107–109] More than 130 cases have been reported.[107] The cardiovascular abnormalities include (1) transposition of the great vessels, (2) pulmonary stenosis or atresia,[110] (3) abnormalities of the pulmonary and/or systemic venous connections, (4) atrial and ventricular septal defects, and (5) a single atrioventricular valve. The majority of the patients die in infancy, with few living longer than 1 year. These cases may also have abnormalities of body symmetry, with a tendency toward symmetry of the lungs and abdominal viscera. Both lungs may have three lobes, the liver may be symmetrical, and there may be malposition of the stomach and intestines. This has been termed bilateral "rightsidedness" by Moller and coworkers.[111] Pulmonary lymphangiectasis may also be associated with this syndrome.[112]

Congenital hypoplasia of the spleen is more common than complete absence of the organ. Patients with anatomic or functional asplenia show characteristic peripheral blood findings in erythrocytes, including Howell-Jolly bodies, target cells, and siderotic granules (Pappenheimer bodies), reflecting absence of the spleen's filtration function.[107] Bisno and Freeman[113] reported a case of a 29-year-old female who developed fatal pneumococcal sepsis with disseminated intravascular coagulation and bilateral adrenal hemorrhages (Waterhouse-Friderichsen syndrome). The patient was found to have an atrophic spleen, and the authors postulated that the sepsis was due to the absence of the ability of the spleen to produce opsonizing antibodies as well as to perform its filtration function.

Polysplenia

Polysplenia refers to the congenital division of the bulk of the splenic tissue into two or

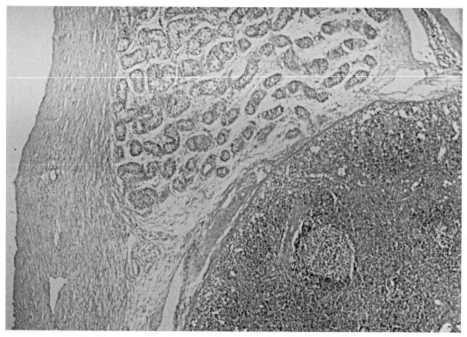

Figure 1–20. Splenic-gonadal fusion, discontinuous form. Normal splenic tissue (lower right) is found within the parenchyma of a normal testicle.

more roughly equal-sized masses (Fig. 1–21). Moller and associates[111] reported 12 cases in which the number of spleens ranged from 2 to 9. As in the asplenia syndrome, there were also cardiovascular abnormalities and a tendency toward abnormal body symmetry. The cardiovascular abnormalities included (1) dextrocardia, (2) bilateral superior venae cavae, (3) atrial and ventricular septal defects, and (4) anomalous pulmonary venous connections. The tendency toward body symmetry included two lobes to each lung, symmetry of the liver, and malrotation of the bowel. These authors termed these findings bilateral "left-sidedness." Eight of the 12 patients died before 1 year of age. Polysplenia has also been associated with polycystic disease of the kidneys.[114–116]

Splenosis

The term splenosis was introduced by Buchbinder and Lipkoff[117] and refers to the regrowth of splenic tissue following splenectomy or, more commonly, after traumatic rupture (Color Plate 3). The phenomenon has been attributed to the seeding or "autotransplantation"[118] of splenic tissue from the lacerated organ; it has been estimated to occur in as

many as two thirds of all cases of rupture.[117–121] Splenotic implants usually occur within the peritoneal cavity.[117] However, they have occasionally been noted in the thorax,[122–129] usually in patients who have had trauma to both abdomen and diaphragm. Within the thorax, they have been noted on pleural surfaces[122–124] and rarely on the pericardial sac.[130, 131] Rare cases have been reported in the skin[132] and in skin scars.[133] One unusual case was reported within the brain 15 years after post-traumatic splenectomy.[134] Hematogenous spread of splenic tissue was proposed as the cause of this lesion. Splenotic implants are usually numerous and may number up to several hundred.[120] The ectopic nodules of splenic tissue are usually small and measure less than several centimeters in most cases. However, nodules as large as 12 cm in greatest diameter have been reported.[135] Splenotic implants are usually encapsulated and may be either sessile or pedunculated.[136] Microscopically, some appear to display normal splenic architecture, but they may lack trabecular structures. Lymphoid follicles may or may not be present.[136]

It may be difficult or impossible in a given case to distinguish splenosis from accessory spleens, which are frequent incidental findings. Accessory spleens are typically few in number, occur in the left upper quadrant, usu-

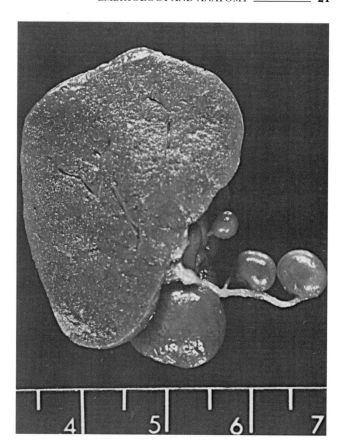

Figure 1–21. Polysplenia. The specimen is from a patient with no history of trauma or prior surgery. Note the multiple nodules of splenic tissue along the splenic artery and the division of the bulk of the spleen into two lobes.

ally contain all the components of the normal organ, and derive their arterial blood supply from the splenic artery or its branches. Splenotic implants, however, are more widely distributed, are usually more numerous, may vary greatly in size and shape, may or may not contain all the components of the normal spleen, and derive their blood supply from the surrounding tissue.[136]

The vast majority of cases of splenosis are incidental findings found at autopsy or surgery with no clinical significance.[137] However, there are numerous case reports of splenosis mimicking both benign and malignant tumors.[135, 137–141] They have been reported causing symptoms relating to intestinal obstruction[142–144] and have been associated with gastrointestinal or intra-abdominal hemorrhage[145, 146] and hemoptysis.[127] There is one exceptional case report of sudden enlargement of splenotic implants during an attack of malaria.[136]

The functional capacity of splenic autoimplants is a subject of controversy. Several lines of evidence suggest that splenic autoimplants are in fact functional. There are occasional well-documented cases of recurrence of con-

genital hemolytic anemia,[146] idiopathic thrombocytopenic purpura,[147, 148] and Felty syndrome,[117] which have been attributed to the development of functioning splenotic nodules. In addition, the frequency of postsplenectomy sepsis appears higher after elective splenectomy then after splenectomy following splenic rupture, implying a protective rate of splenotic implants.[149] Further evidence that splenosis retains some normal splenic function was provided by Pearson et al,[150] who assessed splenic activity by studying the percentage of pitted red blood cells in three groups of children: a normal eusplenic group, children subjected to splenectomy for hematologic conditions, and those who had emergency splenectomy following injury. The latter group had demonstrable splenic activity in the majority of cases, which the authors attributed to splenosis and which they documented in some cases by ^{99m}Tc sulfur colloid scans. Zoli et al[151] found similar results in their study and showed that residual splenic function correlated with serum tuftsin activity. In an attempt to test the hypothesis that splenosis could provide retention of splenic function, Ludtke et al[121] autotransplanted splenic tissue in a group of patients undergoing surgery following traumatic rupture of the spleen and compared them with a splenectomized group with no splenosis and no autotransplantation. They demonstrated successful reimplantation by scintigraphy in all cases and preservation of filtration; however, they could not demonstrate preservation of immunologic function. Traub et al[152] documented that splenic reticuloendothelial function was better preserved after autotransplantation than after total splenectomy but that it was less effective than after partial splenectomy with spleen repair. It is clear that the presence of splenosis per se is not a reliable indication that splenic function is preserved.[120, 152-154] However, the degree of function probably relates to the total bulk of splenic tissue present; radioisotopic scans have demonstrated uptake by larger nodules in many cases.[155] The quantity of splenic tissue necessary to prevent the findings of hyposplenism or to cause recurrent hypersplenism in such cases is unknown. It has been suggested that a total of 20 to 30 cm^3 is needed[156] but that bacterial clearance by implanted splenic tissue may be deficient if there is no main arterial supply.[121, 157]

REFERENCES

1. Barzanji J, Emery JL: Changes in the spleen related to birth. J Anat 1979; 129:819.
2. Vellguth S, von Gaudecker B, Muller-Hermelink H-K: The development of the human spleen: Ultrastructural studies in fetuses from 14th to 24th week of gestation. Cell Tissue Res 1985; 242:579.
3. Putschar WGJ, Manion WC: Splenic-gonadal fusion. Am J Pathol 1956; 32:15.
4. Dawson H, Eggleton MG: Principles of Human Physiology, 14th ed, p 227. London, J and A Churchill, 1968.
5. Voboril Z: On the question of segmentation of the human spleen. Folia Morphol 1982; 30:295.
6. Voboril Z: Relationship of the notches and fissures of the human spleen to the splenic segments. Folia Morphol 1983; 31:163.
7. Weiss L: The development of the primary vascular reticulum in the spleen of human fetuses (38 to 57 mm crown–rump length). Am J Anat 1973; 136:315.
8. Weiss L, Chen DT: The differentiation of white pulp and red pulp in the spleen of human fetuses (72–145 mm crown–rump length). Am J Anat 1974; 141:393.
9. Wolf BC, Luevano E, Neiman RS: Evidence to suggest that the human fetal spleen is not a hematopoietic organ. Am J Clin Pathol 1983; 80:140.
10. Holroyde CP, Oski FA, Gardner FH: The "pocked" erythrocyte: Red-cell surface alterations in reticuloendothelial immaturity of the neonate. N Engl J Med 1969; 10:516.
11. Knoll W: Die embryonale Blutbildung beim Menschen. Berichte über die Tatigkeit der St Gallischen Ges 1950; 73:1.
12. Ono K: Untersuchungen über die entwicklung der menschlichen milz z.f. Zellforschung. Mikr Anatomie 1930; 10:573.
13. Zamboni L, Westin B: The ultrastructure of the human fetal spleen. I. One type of mesenchymal cell in the early stages of development of the spleen. Ultra Res 1964; 11:469.
14. Djaldetti M: Hemopoietic events in human embryonic spleens at early gestational stages. Biol Neonate 1979; 36:133.
15. Calhoun DA, Li Y, Braylan RC, et al: Assessment of the contribution of the spleen to granulocytopoiesis and erythropoiesis of the mid-gestation human fetus. Early Hum Dev 1996; 46:217.
16. Silverstein AM, Lukes RJ: Fetal response to antigenic stimulus: 1-plasmo-cellular and lymphoid reactions in the human fetus to intrauterine infection. Lab Invest 1962; 11:918.
17. Jones JF: Development of the spleen. Lymphology 1983; 16:83.
18. van Furth R, Schuit HRE, Hijmans W: The immunological development of the human fetus. J Exp Med 1965; 122:1173.
19. Hayward AR, Ezer G: Development of lymphocyte populations in the human fetal thymus and spleen. Clin Exp Immunol 1974; 17:169.
20. Owen JJT, Jenkinson EJ: Embryology of the lymphoid system. Prog Allerg 1980; 29:1.
21. Timens W, Rozenboom T, Poppema S: Fetal and neonatal development of human spleen: An immunohistological study. Immunology 1987; 60:603.
22. Barzanji AJ, Emery JL: Germinal centers in the spleens of neonates and stillbirths. Early Hum Dev 1978; 1:363.
23. Timens W, Boes A, Rozeboom-Uiterwijk T, et al: Immuno-architecture of human fetal lymphoid tissues. Virchows Arch 1988; 413:563.
24. Weissman IL: T cell maturation and the ontogeny of splenic lymphoid architecture, in Battisto JR, Streilen JW, (eds): Immune Aspects of the Spleen, p 77. Amsterdam, North Holland Press, 1976.
25. Barzanji J, Penny SR, Emery JL: Development of germinal centers in the spleen in infants related to birth and unexpected death. J Clin Pathol 1977; 29:675.
26. Timens W, Boes A, Rozeboom-Uiterwijk T, et al: Immaturity of the human splenic marginal zone in infancy: Possible contribution to deficient infant immune response. J Immunol 1989; 143:3200.
27. Potter EL, Craig JM: Pathology of the Fetus and Infant, 3rd ed. Chicago, Year Book Medical Publishers 10, 1975.
28. Larroche J-C: Developmental pathology of the neonate. Amsterdam, Elsevier North-Holland, 1977.
29. Sung CJ, Singer DB: Liveborn infants by gestational age. 1975–1984 data from Women and Infant's Hospital, Providence, RI, 1, 1988, quoted in Stocker JT, Dehner LP: Pediatric Pathology. Philadelphia, Lippincott, 1992.
30. Schultz DM, Giordano DA, Schulz DH: Weights of organs of fetuses and infants. Arch Pathol 1962; 74:244.
31. Gruenwald P, Minh HN: Evaluation of body and organ weights in perinatal pathology. I. Normal standards derived from autopsies. Am J Clin Pathol 1960; 34:247.

32. Coppelletta JM, Wolbach SB: Body length and organ weights of infants and children. Am J Pathol 1933; 9:55.

33. Kayser K: Height and weight in human beings: Autopsy report. Munich, R. Oldenbourg, 1987.

34. Myers J, Segal RJ: Weight of the spleen. I. Range of normal in a non-hospital population. Arch Pathol 1974; 98:33.

35. Boyd E: Normal variability in weight of the adult liver and spleen. Arch Pathol 1933; 16:350.

36. DeLand FH: Normal spleen size. Radiology 1970; 97:589.

37. McCormick WF, Kashgarian M: The weight of the adult human spleen. Am J Clin Pathol 1965; 43:332.

38. Zago MA, Figueiredo MS, Covas DT, et al: Aspects of splenic hypofunction in old age. Klin Wochenschr 1985; 63:590.

39. Markus HS, Toghill PJ: Impaired splenic function in elderly people. Aging 1991; 20:287.

40. Raviola E: Spleen, in Fawcett DW (ed): A Textbook of Histology, 12th ed, p 460. New York, Chapman and Hall, 1994.

41. van Krieken JH, te Velde J: Normal histology of the human spleen. Am J Surg Pathol 1988; 12:777.

42. Christensen BE, Jonsson V, Matre R, et al: Traffic of T and B lymphocytes in the normal spleen. Scand J Haematol 1978; 20:246.

43. Weiss L, Tavassoli M: Anatomical hazards to the passage of erythrocytes through the spleen. Semin Hematol 1970; 7:372.

44. Bishop MB, Lansing LS: The spleen: A correlative overview of normal and pathologic anatomy. Hum Pathol 1982; 13:334.

45. Eikelenboom P, Dijkstra CD, Boorsma DM, et al: Characterization of lymphoid and non-lymphoid cells in the white pulp of the spleen using immunohistoperoxidase techniques and enzyme histochemistry. Experientia 1985; 41:209.

46. Buckley PJ, Smith MR, Braverman MF, et al: Human spleen contains phenotypic subsets of macrophages and dendritic cells that occupy discrete microanatomic locations. Am J Pathol 1987; 128:505.

47. Lukes RJ: The pathology of the white pulp of the spleen, in Lennert K, Harms D (eds): Die Milz, p 130. Berlin, Springer-Verlag, 1970.

48. Millikin PD: Anatomy of germinal centers in human lymphoid tissue. Arch Pathol 1966; 82:499.

49. Millikin PD: The nodular white pulp of the human spleen. Arch Pathol 1969; 87:247.

50. Timens W, Poppema S: Lymphocyte compartments in human spleen: An immunohistologic study in normal spleens and non-involved spleens in Hodgkin's disease. Am J Pathol 1985; 120:443.

51. Hsu SM, Cossman J, Jaffe ES: Lymphocyte subsets in normal human lymphoid tissue. Am J Clin Pathol 1983; 80:21.

52. Hsu SM, Jaffe ES: Phenotypic expression of B lymphocytes: Immunoglobulin expression of germinal center cells. Am J Pathol 1984; 114:396.

53. Grogan TM, Rangel CS, Richter LC, et al: Further delineation of the immunoarchitecture of the human spleen. Lymphol 1984; 17:61.

54. van Krieken JH, von Schilling C, Kluin M, et al: Splenic marginal zone lymphocytes and related cells in the lymph node: A morphologic and immunohistochemical study. Hum Pathol 1989; 20:320.

55. Spencer J, Finn T, Pulford KAF, et al: The human gut contains a novel population of B-lymphocytes which resemble marginal zone cells. Clin Exp Immunol 1985; 62:607.

56. Hsu SM: Phenotypic expression of B lymphocytes. III. Marginal zone B cells in the spleen are characterized by the expression of Tac and alkaline phosphatase. J Immunol 1985; 135:123.

57. Weissman IL, Warnke R, Butcher EC, et al: The lymphoid system, its normal architecture and the potential for understanding the system through the study of lymphoproliferative diseases. Hum Pathol 1978; 9:25.

58. Nossal GJV, Abbot A, Mitchell J, et al: Antigens in immunity. XV. Ultrastructural features of antigen capture in primary and secondary lymphoid follicles. J Exp Med 1968; 127:277.

59. Kraal G: Cells in the marginal zone of the spleen. Int Rev Cytol 1992; 132:31.

60. van Krieken JH, te Velde J, Kleiverda K, et al: Cells in the marginal zone of the spleen. Histopathology 1985; 9:571.

61. Schmidt EE, MacDonald IC, Groom AC: Cells in the marginal zone of the spleen. Am J Anat 1988; 181:252.

62. Burke JS, Simon GT: Electron microscopy of the spleen. I. Anatomy and microcirculation. Am J Pathol 1970; 58:127.

63. Buyssens N, Paulus G, Bourgeois N: Ellipsoids in the human spleen. Virchows Arch 1984; 403:27.

64. Rappaport H: The pathologic anatomy of the splenic red pulp, in Lennert K, Harms D (eds): Die Milz, p 25. Berlin, Springer-Verlag, 1970.

65. Hirasawa Y, Tokuhiro H: Electron microscopic studies on the normal human spleen: Especially on the red pulp and the reticulo-endothelial cells. Blood 1970; 35:201.

66. King JT, Puchtler H, Sweat F: Ring fibers in human spleens. Arch Pathol 1968; 85:237.

67. Wennberg E, Weiss L: The structure of the spleen and hemolysis. Ann Rev Med 1969; 20:29.

68. Weiss L: A scanning electron microscopic study of the spleen. Blood 1974; 43:665.

69. Braunstein H, Freiman DG, Gall EA: A histochemical study of the enzymatic activity of lymph nodes. Cancer 1958; 11:829.

70. Ishihara T, Matsumoto N, Adachi H, et al: Erythrophagocytosis by the sinus endothelial cell of the spleen in haemolytic anaemias. Virchows Arch 1979; 382:261.

71. Schiffman FJ, Weiss L, Cadman EC: Erythrophagocytosis by venous sinus endothelial cells of the spleen in autoimmune hemolytic anemia. Hematol Rev 1988; 2:327.

72. Ferreira JA, Feliu E, Rozman C, et al: Morphologic and morphometric light and electron microscopic studies of the spleen in patients with hereditary spherocytosis and autoimmune haemolytic anaemia. Br J Haematol 1989; 72:146.

73. Chen LT, Weiss L: Electron microscopy of the red pulp of the human spleen. Am J Anat 1972; 134:425.

74. Dorfman RF: Nature of the sinus lining cells of the spleen. Nature 1961; 190:1021.

75. Giorno R: Unusual structure of human splenic sinusoids revealed by monoclonal antibodies. Histochem 1984; 81:505.

76. Buckley PJ, Dickson SA: Monoclonal antibodies to T-helper/inducer and T-suppressor/cytotoxic lymphocyte subsets recognize antigens on splenic sinusoidal lining cells. Am J Clin Pathol 1984; 8:167.

77. Buckley PJ, Dickson SA, Walker WS: Human splenic sinusoidal lining cells express antigens associated with monocytes, macrophages, endothelial cells, and T lymphocytes. J Immunol 1984; 134:2310.

78. Knisley MH: Spleen studies: Microscopic observations on the circulatory systems of living unstimulated mammalian spleens. Anat Rec 1936; 65:23.

79. Chen LT: Microcirculation of the spleen: An open or closed circulation? Science 1968; 201:157.

80. Weiss L: The structure of the normal spleen. Semin Hematol 1965; 2:205.

81. Koyama S, Aoki A, Deguchi K: Electron microscopic observations of the splenic red pulp with special reference to the pitting function. Mie Med J 1964; 14:143.

82. Crosby WH: Splenic remodeling of red cell surfaces. Blood 1977; 50:643.

83. Wadheim BM, Adams PB, Johnson MA: Incidence and location of accessory spleens. N Engl J Med 1981; 304:111.

84. Eraklis AJ, Filler RM: Splenectomy in childhood: A review of 1413 cases. J Pediatr Surg 1977; 7:382.

85. Halpert B, Gyorkey F: Accessory spleen in the tail of the pancreas. Arch Pathol 1957; 64:266.

86. Halpert B, Gyorkey F: Lesions observed in accessory spleens of 311 patients. Am J Pathol 1959; 32:165.

87. Robertson RF: The clinical importance of accessory spleens (with report of a case). Can Med Assoc J 1938; 39:222.

88. Mottet NK, Jensen H: The anomalous embryonic development associated with trisomy 13–15. Am J Clin Pathol 1965; 43:334.

89. Hashida Y, Jaffe R, Yunis EJ: Pancreatic pathology in trisomy 13: Specificity of the morphologic lesion. Pediatr Pathol 1983; 1:169.

90. Buehner M, Baker MS: The wandering spleen. Surg Gynecol Obstet 1992; 175:273.

91. Robinson A: Wandering spleen: Case report and review. Mt Sinai J Med 1988; 55:428.

92. Abell I: Wandering spleen with torsion of pedicle. Ann Surg 1933; 98:722.

93. Moll S, Igelhart JD, Ortel T: Thrombocytopenia in association with a wandering spleen. Am J Hematol 1996; 53:259.

94. Thompson J, Ross R, Pizzaro S: The wandering spleen in infancy and childhood. Clin Pediatr 1980; 19:221.

95. McClain G, Lebherz T: Radiographic evidence of splenic torsion. Obstet Gynecol 1967; 29:475.

96. Walcher F, Schneider G, Marzi I, et al: Torsion of a wandering spleen after blunt abdominal trauma. J Trauma 1997; 43:983.

97. Seashore J, McIntosh S: Elective splenopexy for wandering spleen. J Pediatr Surg 1990; 25:270.

98. Stringel G, Soucy P, Mercer S: Torsion of the wandering spleen: Splenectomy or splenopexy. J Pediatr Surg 1982; 17:373.

99. Emmett JM, Dreyfus ML: Accessory spleen in the scrotum: Review of literature on ectopic spleens and their associated surgical significance. Ann Surg 1943; 117:754.

100. Bennett-Jones MJ, St. Hill CA: Accessory spleen in the scrotum. Br J Surg 1952; 40:259.

101. Walther MM, Trulock TS, Finnerty DP, et al: Splenic gonadal fusion. Pediatr Urol 1988; 32:521.

102. Falowski W, Carter M: Spleno-gonadal fusion associated with an anaplastic seminoma. J Urol 1980; 124:562.

103. Hines JR, Eggum PR: Splenic-gonadal fusion causing bowel obstruction. Arch Surg 1961; 83:889.

104. Talmann IM: Nebenmilzen im Nebenhoden und Samenstrang. Virchows Arch 1926; 259:237.

105. Settle EB: The surgical importance of accessory spleens with report of two cases. Am J Surg 1940; 50:22.

106. Cotelingham JD, Saito R: Hepatolineal fusion: Case report of an unusual lesion. Hum Pathol 1980; 9:234.

107. Bush JA, Ainger LE: Congenital absence of the spleen with congenital heart disease: Report of a case with antemortem diagnosis on the basis of hematologic morphology. Pediatrics 1955; 15:93.

108. Elliott LP, Anderson RC, Edwards JE: The common cardiac ventricle with transposition of the great vessels. Br Heart J 1964; 26:289.

109. Mauck HP Jr, Segatol-Islami Z, Lester RG: Splenic agenesis associated with severe congenital heart disease: Long survival unassociated with pulmonary stenosis. Dis Chest 1966; 49:436.

110. Campbell M, Reynolds G, Trounce JR: Six cases of single ventricle with pulmonary stenosis. Guy's Hosp Rep 1953; 102:97.

111. Moller JH, Nakib A, Anderson RC, et al: Congenital cardiac disease associated with polysplenia: A development complex of bilateral "left-sidedness." Circulation 1967; 36:789.

112. Esterly JR, Oppenheimer EH: Lymphangiectasis and other pulmonary lesions in the asplenia syndrome. Arch Pathol 1970; 90:553.

113. Bisno AL, Freeman JC: The syndrome of asplenia, pneumococcal sepsis, and disseminated intravascular coagulation. Ann Intern Med 1970; 72:389.

114. Vito F, Federico A: Association of splenic syndromes with renal cystic disease. Hum Pathol 1989; 20:496.

115. Haratake J, Horie A, Okada T: An adult autopsy case of polysplenic syndrome. Rynsho Byori 1985; 3:1269.

116. Hiraoka K, Haratake J, Horie A, et al: Bilateral renal dysplasia, pancreatic fibrosis, intrahepatic biliary dysgenesis, and situs inversus totalis in a boy. Hum Pathol 1988; 19:871.

117. Buchbinder JH, Lipkoff CJ: Splenosis; multiple peritoneal splenic implants following abdominal injury: A report of a case and review of the literature. Surgery 1939; 6:927.

118. Fleming CR, Dickson ER, Harrison EG Jr: Splenosis: Autotransplantation of splenic tissue. Am J Med 1976; 61:414.

119. Brewster DC: Splenosis: Report of two cases and review of the literature. Am J Surg 1973; 126:14.

120. Livingston CD, Levine BA, Lecklitner ML, et al: Incidence and function of residual splenic tissue following splenectomy for trauma in adults. Arch Surg 1983; 118:617.

121. Ludtke FE, Mack SC, Schuff-Werner P, et al: Splenic function after splenectomy for trauma: Role of autotransplantation and splenosis. Acta Chir Scand 1989; 155:533.

122. Kwan AJ, Drum DE, Ahn CS, et al: Intrathoracic splenosis mimicking metastatic lung cancer. Clin Nucl Med 1994; 19:93.

123. Yousem SA: Thoracic splenosis. Ann Thorac Surg 1987; 44:411.

124. Hietala EM, Hermunen H, Kostiainen S: Intrathoracic splenosis: Report of a case simulating esophageal leiomyoma. Scand J Thorac Cardiovasc Surg 1993; 27:61.

125. Cordier JF, Gamondes JP, Marx P, et al: Thoracic

splenosis presenting with hemoptysis. Chest 1992; 102:626.

126. Ahmadi A, Faker LP, Milloy F: Intrathoracic splenosis. J Thorac Cardiovasc Surg 1964; 55:677.

127. Dalton ML Jr, Strange WH, Downs EA: Intrathoracic splenosis: Case report and review of the literature. Am Rev Respir Dis 1971; 103:827.

128. Skinner EF, Hurteau WW: Autotransplantation of splenic tissue into the thorax. J Thorac Surg 1957; 33:807.

129. Garamella JJ, Hay LJ: Autotransplantation of the spleen: Splenosis: Case report and preliminary report of an experimental study in revascularization of the heart. Ann Surg 1954; 140:104.

130. Ovnatanian KT: Splenosis of the pericardium. Vestn Khir 1966; 97:59.

131. Baack BR, Varsa EW, Burgdorf WH, et al: Splenosis: A report of subcutaneous involvement. Am J Dermatopathol 1990; 12:585.

132. Cohen EA: Splenosis: Review and report of subcutaneous splenic implant. Arch Surg 1954; 69:777.

133. Raper AB: Splenosis: A sequel of rupture of the spleen. East Afr Med J 1951; 28:265.

134. Rickert CH, Maasjosthusmann U, Probst-Cousin S, et al: A unique case of cerebral spleen. Am J Surg Pathol 1998; 22:894.

135. Bock DB, King BF, Hezmall HP, et al: Splenosis presenting as a left renal mass indistinguishable from renal cell carcinoma. 1991; 146:152.

136. Carr NJ, Turk EP: The histological features of splenosis. Histopathology 1992; 21:549.

137. Widmann WD, Laubscher FA: Splenosis: A disease or a beneficial condition? Arch Surg 1971; 102:152.

138. Forino M, David GL, Zins JH: Renal splenic heterotopia, a rare mimic of renal neoplasia: Case report of imaging and fine-needle aspiration biopsy. Diagn Cytopathol 1993; 9:565.

139. Mathurin J, Lallemand D: Splenosis simulating an abdominal lymphoma. Pediatr Radiol 1990; 21:69.

140. Agha FP: Regenerated splenosis masquerading as gastric fundic mass. Am J Gastroenterol 1984; 79:576.

141. Yoshimitsu K, Aibe H, Nobe T, et al: Intrahepatic splenosis mimicking a liver tumor. Abdom Imaging 1993; 18:156.

142. Prasad C, Beck AR: Splenosis and intestinal obstruction. J Mt Sinai Hosp 1968; 35:534.

143. Trimble C, Easan FJ: A complication of splenosis. J Trauma 1972; 12:358.

144. Sirinek KR, Livingston CD, Bova JG, et al: Bowel obstruction due to infarcted splenosis. South Med J 1984; 77:764.

145. Basile RM, Morales JM, Zupanec R: Splenosis: A cause of massive gastrointestinal hemorrhage. Arch Surg 1989; 124:1087.

146. Feferman I, Cramer J: Splenosis: An unusual cause of intraabdominal hemorrhage. J Emerg Med 1991; 9:239.

147. Hassan NMR, Neiman RS: The pathology of the spleen in steroid-treated immune thrombocytopenic purpura. Am J Clin Pathol 1985; 84:433.

148. Mazur EM, Field WW, Cahow CE, et al: Idiopathic thrombocytopenic purpura occurring in a subject previously splenectomized for traumatic splenic rupture: Role of splenosis in the pathogenesis of thrombocytopenia. Am J Med 1978; 65:843.

149. Balfanz, JR, Nesbit ME, Jarvis C, et al: Overwhelming sepsis following splenectomy for trauma. J Ped 1996; 88:458.

150. Pearson HA, Johnston D, Smith KA, et al: The born-again spleen: Return of splenic function after splenectomy for trauma. New Engl J Med 1978; 298:1389.

151. Zoli G, Corazza GR, D'Amato G, et al: Splenic autotransplantation after splenectomy: Tuftsin activity correlates with residual splenic function. Br J Surg 1994; 81:716.

152. Traub A, Giebink GS, Smith C, et al: Splenic reticuloendothelial function after splenectomy, spleen repair, and spleen autotransplantation. New Engl J Med 1987; 317:1559.

153. Sab W, Bergholz M, Kehl A, et al: Overwhelming infection after splenectomy in spite of some spleen remaining and splenosis. Klin Wochenschr 1983; 61:1075.

154. Schwartz AD, Goldthorn JF, Winkelstien JA, et al: Lack of protective effect of autotransplanted splenic tissue to pneumococcal challenge. Blood 1978; 51:475.

155. Nielsen JL, Ellegaard J, Marqversen J, et al: Detection of splenosis and ectopic spleens with ^{99m}Tc-labelled heat-damaged autologous erythrocytes in 90 splenectomized patients. Scand J Haematol 1981; 27:51.

156. Corazza GR, Tarozzi C, Vaira D, et al: Return of splenic function after splenectomy: How much tissue is needed? BMJ 1984; 289:861.

157. Horton J, Ogden ME, Williams S: The importance of splenic blood flow in clearing pneumococcal organisms. Ann Surg 1982; 195:172.

FUNCTIONS OF THE SPLEEN

2

The mammalian spleen is regarded as having four physiologic functions (Table 2–1). They are: (1) filtration, (2) immunologic, (3) reservoir (storage), and (4) hematopoietic. Many diseases of the spleen can best be understood in light of these functions.[1] Which functions apply to the human spleen remain controversial. In this chapter, we have restricted our attention to a discussion of human spleens exclusively. It is generally accepted that in humans, the reservoir function is of less impor-

tance. Although controversial, an increasing quantity of data suggests that the human spleen does not have an intrinsically hematopoietic function.

FILTRATION FUNCTION

The primary function of the spleen is as a filter of the peripheral blood. In the adult, approximately 2 L of blood pass through the spleen each minute.[2] Splenic filtration is predominantly a function of the marginal zone of the white pulp and the macrophages of the cords of Billroth.[3] Studies of splenic phagocytosis using electron microscopy have shown that when rabbits were injected intravenously with colloidal carbon particles, the particles were seen within 20 to 30 seconds in the sinuses, the marginal zone of the white pulp, and the red pulp. The particles were never distributed throughout the white pulp, but only at its periphery (the marginal zone). The particles were phagocytized almost entirely by cordal macrophages that extended cytoplasmic processes into the lumina of the sinuses. Only minimal phagocytosis by endothelial cells was seen.[4] The authors also described some phagocytosis of carbon particles by platelets and postulated that platelets might play an initial role in phagocytosis. Other investigators[5–8] have also shown that platelets are capable of phagocytosing particulate material.

Splenic filtration of red blood cells involves three processes: culling, pitting, and erythroclasis. Through these processes the spleen exerts a type of quality control over bone-marrow production by removing defective erythrocytes or other circulating blood cells. Culling refers to the destruction of erythro-

Table 2–1. Splenic Functions

I. Filtration
  A. Culling: erythrocyte (or other blood cell) destruction
    1. Physiologic (as red blood cells age)
    2. Pathologic
      a. Associated with blood cell abnormalities
      b. Associated with primary splenic changes
  B. Pitting ("facelifting" of erythrocytes)
    1. Removal of cytoplasmic inclusions
    2. Remodeling of cell membranes
  C. Erythroclasis: destruction of abnormal red blood cells with liberation into circulation of erythrocyte fragments
  D. Removal of other particulate material (e.g., bacteria, colloidal particles)
II. Immunologic
  A. Trapping and processing of antigen
  B. "Homing" of lymphocytes
  C. Lymphocyte transformation and proliferation
  D. Antibody and lymphokine production
  E. Macrophage activation
III. Reservoir
  A. Storage or normal sequestration of platelets, granulocytes
  B. Recycling of iron
  C. Red blood cell storage (minor in humans)
IV. Hematopoietic
  A. Erythropoiesis, granulopoiesis, megakaryopoiesis (not abnormal function in fetal or adult spleens)
  B. Lymphocyte and macrophage production

cytes, either physiologically as they age or in pathologic conditions involving increased red blood cell destruction.[9, 10] Such conditions include those in which a normally functioning spleen destroys abnormal erythrocytes (e.g., hereditary spherocytosis) and those in which normal erythrocytes are sequestered and destroyed by a pathologically altered spleen.[1, 11] The term "culling" also refers to the removal of other circulating cells, such as immature granulocytes or antibody-coated platelets, or to the removal of particulate material, such as bacteria, from the blood. The removal of such particulate material has been demonstrated experimentally using injected colloidal carbon particles.[4, 12]

The term "pitting" is used to describe the removal of inclusions from erythrocytes with return of the viable cells to the circulation.[10, 13] These inclusions may include remnants of nuclear material (Howell-Jolly bodies), denatured hemoglobin (Heinz bodies), siderotic granules (Pappenheimer bodies), and intracellular parasites such as malarial organisms.[14–21] Such inclusions appear in erythrocytes in the peripheral blood in splenectomized patients, indicating the absence of splenic function.

Erythroclasis involves the destruction of erythrocytes by fragmentation.[10] In contrast to culling, the cellular fragments are returned to the peripheral blood and are removed on subsequent passage through the spleen. This phenomenon occurs in such diseases as autoimmune hemolytic anemia, thalassemia, and the hemoglobinopathies, including hemoglobin C disease, hemoglobin H disease, and sickle cell disease.[22–25]

The structure of the splenic red pulp facilitates filtration, providing anatomic hazards to the passage of erythrocytes.[2] The marginal zone receives many arterial terminations, and many macrophages are concentrated in this region.[26] In addition, Weiss and Tavassoli[2] described high arterial endothelial cells in the marginal zone, which may act as a mechanical hazard. The cords of Billroth provide barriers to the passage of erythrocytes.[27] To enter the splenic sinuses, erythrocytes must pass around the cytoplasmic processes of the cordal macrophages, through the fenestrated basement membrane of the sinus, and squeeze through the potential spaces between the endothelial cells.[28] The ability of a red blood cell, or any cell, to traverse the sinus wall depends on its deformability, which in turn may be a function of the nature of the cell membrane or the

cell's age.[3, 4, 13, 29, 30] Cells without the ability to deform are not able to enter the sinuses. A number of factors may affect the plasticity of an erythrocyte. For example, the erythrocytes in hereditary spherocytosis are rigid because of membrane alterations.[31–33] Cytoplasmic inclusions such as Heinz bodies may also render the cells in which they occur less deformable and unable to traverse the sinus wall. Cells coated with antibody also lack the ability to deform, resulting in their increased exposure to phagocytes in the cords of Billroth. This may account for the cellular destruction in idiopathic thrombocytopenic purpura and autoimmune hemolytic anemias. Several studies have indicated that cells coated with small quantities of isoantibodies are destroyed slowly by the spleen, whereas more heavily sensitized cells are destroyed more rapidly by the liver.[34–36]

The cords of Billroth constitute a hostile environment for senescent erythrocytes.[1, 3, 37] The blood in the pulp cords has a higher hematocrit level than peripheral or splenic venous blood and is more viscous.[2] This is probably due to skimming off of plasma. Stagnation of erythrocytes causes lowering of the oxygen tension and increasing lactic acidosis, resulting in an acidotic, hypoxic environment.[38] The cords contain numerous macrophages that are rich in lysosomal acid hydrolytic enzymes that may be released into the cords if these cells are disrupted.[2, 39] Reticulocytes are not destroyed during their temporary sequestration in the spleen, possibly because they may still contain some mitochondria and are capable of oxidative phosphorylation and are therefore less vulnerable to glucose deprivation. More mature erythrocytes lack mitochondria and depend on glycolysis, rendering them vulnerable to a lack of substrate in the splenic cords. Moreover, as erythrocytes age, they gradually decay, becoming thinner and more fragile and therefore more susceptible to destruction.[40–43]

In addition to the physiologic removal of senescent red blood cells, the spleen may play an additional role in normal erythrocyte maturation through its ability to remodel red blood cell membranes.[13, 44, 45] Mature erythrocytes have a negative surface charge and therefore repel each other.[9, 46] Reticulocytes have a less negative surface charge and are, as a result, somewhat "sticky," with less tendency to repel each other.[9, 13] In addition, reticulocytes have excess membrane and are larger than mature erythrocytes. Lux and John[47] postulated that reticulocytes have a high molecular weight membrane-protein complex that is removed by the spleen, resulting in a change in cell surface and decrease in surface area. The orientation of fatty acids at the surface affects the surface charge.[13] As the cell matures, the membrane lipid content decreases in proportion to the surface area loss but with a relative increase in the concentration of essential fatty acids and cholesterol.[9] The changes in the reticulocyte surface charge appear to result from the temporary sequestration in the spleen.

IMMUNOLOGIC FUNCTION

The immunologic function of the human spleen involves the interaction of splenic lymphoid tissue with the macrophages of the cords of Billroth. The white pulp is the single largest lymphoid organ of the body. Similar to other lymphoid organs, the spleen is capable of trapping and processing antigens, with the resultant production of lymphokines and antibodies and activation of the complement system. However, in contrast to lymph nodes and mucosal-associated lymphoid tissue, which respond to localized antigenic stimulation, the spleen reacts to disseminated blood-borne antigens such as circulating bacteria in septicemia.[48, 49]

The advent of monoclonal antibody and immunohistologic techniques has allowed pathologists to study the immunoarchitecture of the spleen and to map its immunotopography.[50–55] The white pulp of the spleen is compartmentalized into B- and T-cell zones, although there is some overlap.[50, 56–58] The periarterial lymphoid sheath (PALS) is composed predominantly of T lymphocytes. The marginal zone contains both B and T lymphocytes.[51, 52] A few T cells are scattered in germinal centers and in the mantle zones.[55] T helper cells predominate in these areas, with a ratio of T helper to T suppressor cells of 3:1 to 4:1. There is some spillover of T cells into the red pulp. Red-pulp T cells are mainly suppressor/cytotoxic cells.[53] Only occasional suppressor cells are found in the PALS, and they are virtually absent from the germinal centers. Interestingly, sinus endothelial cells have also been shown to have strong positivity with the CD4 antibody, which identifies suppressor/cytotoxic T cells, in contrast to normal vascular endothelial cells, which are CD4-negative.[52, 53, 59, 60]

The majority of B cells are located in the germinal centers and mantle zones,[51, 52] although B cells also account for a large proportion of the marginal zone lymphocytes.[53] CD20, which is a marker of B cells at all stages up to but not including plasma cells, shows intense staining of cytoplasmic membranes in these areas.[54] Rare B cells are found in the PALS. CD21, which stains activated B lymphocytes and may identify the receptor for the complement fragment C3d,[61] shows a more reticular pattern within the germinal centers and reacts with most mantle zone lymphocytes but less intensely than does CD20. The reticular pattern of CD21-positivity in the germinal centers appears to be associated primarily with cell processes, probably those of dendritic reticulum cells.

The distribution of immunoglobulin-containing B cells follows a pattern similar to that in reactive lymph nodes. The majority of the lymphocytes of the dark zone of the germinal center (which are predominantly centroblasts or noncleaved cells) express surface IgM and IgD. The lymphocytes of the light zone of the germinal center (centrocytes or cleaved cells) express a cytoplasmic IgM and IgG. However, many germinal-center cells express no immunoglobulin.[53] Surface immunoglobulin-bearing B lymphocytes are found in the mantle and marginal zones with some spillover into the adjacent red pulp.[52] The B cells in the marginal and mantle zones show staining of their cytoplasmic membranes with IgM but lack IgG. IgG expression is limited to scattered cells in the red pulp. IgD is expressed predominantly in the mantle zones. Only rare IgA-containing cells are found at the periphery of the follicles. Lymphocytes bearing surface κ and λ light chains are found predominantly in the marginal and mantle zones, with a few in the PALS and red pulp.[53] κ Light chain–containing cells predominate over λ light chain–containing cells in a ratio of 2:1 or 3:1.[52] There may also be interstitial or dendritic staining for IgG, IgM, κ, and λ in the germinal centers. Plasma cells are scattered throughout the B-cell zones but are most dense at the edge of the germinal centers. They may also be scattered throughout the red pulp. Although the red pulp contains numerous cells of macrophage/monocyte lineage,[51] only a few of these cells are found in the white pulp. Natural killer (NK) cells are scattered throughout the red pulp. In the white pulp, NK cells are restricted to germinal centers. The red pulp contains a far greater number of lymphocytes and macrophages than NK cells.

The lymphocytes in the splenic white pulp are not a static population but are constantly in transit. The normal spleen contains about 15 percent of the exchangeable B-cell pool and as much as one quarter of the total exchangeable T-cell pool.[50, 62] The marginal zone and marginal sinus receive many arterial terminations. Circulating lymphocytes enter the spleen and selectively "home" into the white pulp.[63] T and B cells traverse the walls of vessels of the marginal zone and are admixed there. T cells then migrate to the PALS, and B cells migrate to the lymphoid follicles.[64–67] If antigen is present, the lymphocytes undergo activation and proliferation, with resultant germinal center formation and antibody and lymphokine production. If no antigen is present, lymphocytes return to the circulation, either via efferent lymphatics or by passing through the gaps between the endothelial cells of the venous sinuses. Studies using laboratory animals have indicated that the mean time of passage for T lymphocytes through the spleen is 3 to 4 hours, whereas that for B lymphocytes is considerably longer.[66] Grogan and coworkers[51] observed mitoses in the lymphocytes of the PALS but not in the marginal zones and suggested that T-cell proliferation may occur in the former region, whereas the marginal zones may contain mature T cells involved in antigen processing in addition to an IgM-positive B-cell population.

The marginal zone appears to play a key role in the initial trapping and processing of antigens.[63] This may be due to its numerous arterial terminations and high concentration of macrophages, which are important in the initial processing of antigens. Experimental studies using isotope-labeled particulate antigens have shown that they appear initially in the red pulp and then concentrate in the marginal zone.[48, 69, 70] Several studies have suggested that marginal zone lymphocytes have a unique immunologic phenotype and that they may be of central importance in the immune response to carbohydrate antigens.[54, 71]

Following initial localization in the marginal zones, antigens then penetrate the germinal center. Full B-cell response to antigens requires T helper cells, and the presence of these scattered T helper cells in the germinal centers facilitates their interaction with B cells. The antigens disappear from the splenic zones in the same order in which they appear. In an experimental system, following exposure to a given antigen, the first morphologic change occurs within 24 hours with the appearance of plasmablasts and plasma cells in the PALS and later in the red pulp.[72] The primary follicles enlarge and develop germinal centers within 3 to 4 days.[73] The germinal centers diminish in size approximately 10 days after the removal of the antigenic stimulation and return to the inactive state in approximately 4 weeks. Once the host has been sensitized, further exposure to a given antigen will result in the same sequence of morphologic changes in the spleen, but these changes occur much more rapidly.

The spleen appears to play a key role in the body's defense against polysaccharide-encapsulated bacteria as well as in the removal of other circulating particulate antigens.[69, 74, 75] More specifically, the spleen is most important in the rapid antibody production following challenge with previously unencountered antigen.[76] Rowley[77] demonstrated that splenectomized patients showed no significant rise in antibody titers following the injection of sheep red blood cells. In contrast, nonsplenectomized control subjects showed a significant rise in antibody titer within 9 to 14 days. Experimental studies have shown that the spleen is more efficient in the clearance of particulate matter than is the liver, especially when the level of specific antibody is low or absent, as may be the case in the early stages of bacteremia or in the case of initial exposure to a particular antigenic strain of organism.[49, 76, 78] In the spleen, antigens have a prolonged exposure to antigen-processing cells in the marginal zone and to the cordal macrophages, facilitating their phagocytosis. In contrast, the circulation through the liver is more rapid, and there is a far lower concentration of macrophages. When the level of specific antibody is high and antigens bear a higher concentration of antibody, the liver becomes more efficient in clearing antigen-antibody complexes. Some investigators have reported that splenectomized animals produce antibody as efficiently as control animals if particulate antigen is injected subcutaneously or intraperitoneally.[77, 79, 80] The spleen, however, appears to be the primary organ responsible for the production of early-appearing antibody in response to an intravenous challenge by particulate antigens.[78, 81–83]

The precise role of the spleen in the development and maintenance of specific immunity has been a subject of debate. Some investigators have stated that normal adults are not more susceptible to infection following traumatic splenectomy, although it is recognized that young children and adults with underlying hematologic disorders are at an increased risk.[76, 79, 84–86] However, as will be discussed in Chapter 4, there are reports of normal individuals who develop overwhelming postsplenectomy infections, sometimes many years after splenectomy.[69, 87, 88] The most common organisms responsible for these infections are the polysaccharide-encapsulated bacteria, predominantly *Streptococcus pneumoniae* and less often *Haemophilus influenzae*.[80]

The particular susceptibility of splenectomized individuals to bacteria appears related to the protective antiphagocytic properties of the organisms' polysaccharide coat.[75, 89] The impaired ability to clear such bacteria appears to be due to inefficient production of initial opsonizing antibody as well as to the absence of the splenic phagocytic activity. In asplenic patients, the liver assumes the bulk of the antigen-clearing function once performed by the spleen, but it cannot produce the opsonizing antibody of the spleen. Because the liver is inefficient in clearing circulating antigen to which little or no antibody has previously been made, it can protect the asplenic patient only from organisms against which high titers of antibody are already present.[49] It is significant that many postsplenectomy infections have been caused by strains of bacteria that are not usually encountered and to which an individual is less likely to have a significant titer of type-specific antibody.[79]

The exact mechanism of the deficiency in antibody response following splenectomy is not clear. The majority of studies report an impaired production of antigen-specific IgM, which normally appears before the IgG response to antigenic stimulation.[49, 83, 84, 90] There have been reports of a decreased serum level of IgM in splenectomized children and in uremic patients with hypersplenism who are splenectomized.[91–93] It has also been demonstrated that splenectomized animals may show a deficient and delayed production of opsonizing 19S antibody (IgM) during the initial challenge with a given antigen.[91, 94] However, other investigators have reported that splenectomized individuals have a deficiency in mounting an IgG response to circulating antigens, suggesting that IgG is the type-specific antibody most important in the opsonization of particulate antigens.[73, 95] Offered in support of this theory is the observation that phagocytic cells have surface receptors for the Fc portion of IgG but not of IgM, suggesting that IgG is

therefore a more important bridge between antigen and phagocyte than IgM.[96] Sullivan and colleagues[79] did not find a decreased serum level of IgM following splenectomy, although they did report a deficient primary response to intravenously injected antigens. They found a quantitatively normal response to secondary immunization. However, the class of antibody produced failed to change from IgM to IgG as normally occurs in an evolving immune response.

The complement system is also involved in the opsonization of particulate antigens. The C3b fragment of complement, which is released following activation of the third portion of complement by either the classic or alternate pathway, binds to bacteria and other antigens as well as to antigen-antibody complexes.[75] Neutrophils and macrophages have surface receptors for C3b, which act as a bridge between antigens and the phagocytes.[97–100] Although some investigators have reported a deficiency in properdin following splenectomy,[101] most evidence indicates that the complement system remains intact.[75, 102]

The spleen is thought to be the site of production of the immunoregulatory protein tuftsin.[103] Tuftsin is a tetrapeptide that is an integral part of a circulating gamma globulin called leukokinin.[104–107] Both animal and human studies have indicated that this peptide is synthesized in the spleen.[108–110] There have also been reports of a deficiency of tuftsin in splenectomized patients[69, 103] which has been reversed by splenic autotransplantation after splenectomy for abdominal trauma.[111] It is believed that tuftsin plays a role in phagocytosis by binding to receptor sites on polymorphonuclear leukocytes, monocytes, macrophages, and NK cells, stimulating phagocytosis.[112] A deficiency in tuftsin could, therefore, enhance susceptibility to severe infection.

In summary, although the exact mechanism of the impaired immune response following splenectomy is controversial, the spleen appears to play a major role in the early antibody response to circulating antigens to which the host has not been previously exposed. The bulk of the evidence indicates a deficiency in the production of antigen-specific IgM, although there is also some evidence to suggest a deficient IgG response as well.

RESERVOIR FUNCTION

Blood cells of all hematopoietic lines are stored in the spleen, but the numbers stored vary among animal species and with the hematopoietic cell line. The normal human spleen does not act as a significant storage site for erythrocytes[113] because the average adult spleen holds only 20 to 40 mL of blood.[114, 115] The capsule contains little or no smooth muscle and is, therefore, not capable of contraction.[27] This is in contrast to some animal species, such as the dog, in which the spleen functions as an expansible organ capable of holding a large volume of blood. In the dog, the spleen pools a significant volume of blood during sleep and contracts to return the blood to the circulation when the animal awakens. Thus, red-cell pooling is reversible and physiologic in these animals but pathologic in humans. The human spleen is capable of concentrating platelets, however, and approximately one third of the body platelet mass is normally held in the red pulp, as are large numbers of granulocytes.[116, 117] Platelets reside in both the reticular meshwork of the lymphoid follicles and in the red pulp cords and adhere to venous endothelial cells.[28] As in dogs, vigorous exercise in humans results in an increase in the platelet count, but the count is transient and quickly returns to the baseline number at rest.[118] As a transient increase in platelet count also occurs during exercise in splenectomized patients,[119] the spleen cannot be the sole site of platelet pooling. There is little evidence to suggest that the spleen has a special role in the storage of granulocytes, apart from its participation in the general total body marginating pool.

In contrast to the normal state in humans, blood is sequestered in the spleen in splenomegalic conditions, regardless of the cause of the splenomegaly.[37] Hypersplenism often results from the destruction of blood cells by the enlarged spleen (see Chapter 3).[120–122] Widening of the pulp cords results in prolonged exposure of circulating cells to the hostile conditions of the red pulp and results in increased opportunity for their phagocytosis by cordal macrophages. If the bone marrow cannot compensate with sufficiently increased production to offset the splenic pooling, cytopenias may result. Such hypersplenic conditions represent an exaggeration of the splenic reservoir function.

The ability of the spleen to store formed elements of the blood in splenomegalic conditions has important implications if splenectomy is performed. In normal individuals, leukocyte and platelet counts may show a postsplenectomy surge, which is usually transient (see Chapter 4).[123] However, if a large volume of platelets is sequestered in an enlarged spleen, removal of that organ may result in a dangerous postsplenectomy thrombocytosis. This is particularly true in polycythemia vera and essential thrombocythemia, in which increased sequestration of platelets by an enlarged spleen partially compensates for the increased production of hematopoietic cells by the bone marrow.[124, 125] Removal of the spleen in these conditions may result in fatal thrombotic complications.

As a result of its destruction of senescent red cells, the spleen plays an important role in iron metabolism.[9] Hemoglobin is degraded in the spleen, and the breakdown products are normally transferred to the plasma and returned to the bone marrow for reutilization in erythropoiesis. In the normal steady state, the spleen contains little storage iron: the senescent red cells are broken down, the iron is released, and most of the iron is bound to plasma transferrin within minutes.[126] However, in conditions in which macrophage iron stores increase, such as aplastic anemia, hemolytic anemias, and post–blood transfusion, significant iron in the form of hemosiderin may be noted. In some hemolytic diseases, including autoimmune hemolytic anemias, the splenic macrophages may become engorged with iron, outstripping their ability to return the iron to the marrow.[9] Extensive iron deposition in the spleen in these cases may result in an apparent systemic iron deficiency.[127]

HEMATOPOIETIC FUNCTION

The human spleen has commonly been regarded as a hematopoietic organ. This belief has been based on two lines of evidence: the presence of hematopoietic precursor cells in fetal spleens and the development of what has been termed "extramedullary hematopoiesis," or "myeloid metaplasia," in the spleens of patients with a variety of diseases. Careful analysis of the data presented in the literature however, leads us to conclude that there is no reliable evidence to support the concept that the normal human spleen is a hematopoietic organ, either during fetal or adult life. Several widely quoted studies used to support the belief in human fetal splenic hematopoiesis were actually performed on such animals as fetal pigs and marsupials.[128–130] Extrapolation from these studies to conditions in the human fetal spleen is unwarranted and misleading. Numerous authors have described hematopoietic cells in the human fetal spleen, and there is no doubt that these cells do, in fact, make their appearance in that organ. Controversy exists, however, over the extent of the hematopoiesis, the origin of the cells in question, and the physiologic implications.

A number of light microscopic studies have described hematopoiesis in human spleens in the later portion of the 1st trimester and early 2nd trimester.[131–133] Other studies of human fetal spleens, employing light microscopic, ultrastructural, immunohistologic, or molecular techniques, have reported different observations and have reached different conclusions. Gilmour[134] reported what he termed "slight haemopoiesis" scattered in the splenic pulp and in sinuses, and that it was composed primarily of erythroid precursors. He concluded that the erythroblasts present were probably not formed in the spleen from precursors but were carried into the spleen via the blood from the yolk sac or liver. Weiss[135] noted "no evidence of significant hematopoiesis" in a study of spleens in 8- to 11-week-old human fetuses. Djaldetti,[136] using electron microscopy, also reported that hematopoietic cells observed in his study were virtually all of the erythroid series, with no granulocytic precursors identified. He postulated that the finding of many early erythroid precursors in splenic sinuses and capillaries supported the thesis that these cells were produced elsewhere and that they colonized the spleen from the blood stream. Vellguth et al,[137] in their ultrastructural study of human splenic development, were not able to confirm the existence of significant hematopoietic activity. They commented on the presence of scattered normoblasts and myelocytes in the red pulp but pointedly stated that they saw no erythropoietic islands or evidence of multiple stages of erythroid precursors. Keleman et al[138] also described nucleated red cells in splenic vascular sinuses, which they termed "seeding" from extraembryonic mesenchyme. They noted erythroblastic islands and occasional megakaryocytes occurring in the 8th to 14th weeks of gestation. Although they referred to the presence of active erythropoiesis and granulopoiesis, they concluded that the spleen makes only a small contribution to blood formation in human fetal development.

Wolf and colleagues,[139] in an immunohisto-logic study using antibodies to hemoglobin, lysozyme, and platelet factor VIII, found no convincing evidence of splenic blood cell production in 48 fetuses ranging in age from 12 to 40 gestational weeks. We could discern no erythropoietic islands, no immature members of the dividing cell pool, and no evidence of progressive hematopoietic cell development. We also noted microscopic evidence of phagocytosis of erythroid precursor cells by splenic macrophages, also described by Gilmour,[134] which provided further insight into what we believe occurs. Citing both morphologic and functional studies describing the presence of hematopoietic precursor cells in fetal blood throughout the 2nd and 3rd trimesters of intrauterine life,[140–142] we postulated that the hematopoietic precursor cells in the fetal spleen resulted from filtration or trapping of these elements from fetal blood and not from intrinsic splenic hematopoiesis, which cannot occur in an effective manner in the splenic microenvironment. More recently, using an antibody to CD34 (QUBEND10), a marker for hematopoietic stem cells, we immunostained 13 fetal spleens ranging from 12 to 18 weeks of gestational age. We were unable to demonstrate the presence of CD34-positive hematopoietic stem cells in any of the cases studied using this technique (unpublished observations).

Several subsequent studies have confirmed our findings and have supported our thesis. Using both morphologic and immunofluorescent monoclonal antibody techniques, Rosenthal et al[143] studied cell suspensions of spleens from 2nd trimester human fetuses. They found no evidence of immature myeloid cells by either method. Ishikawa[144] conducted a light microscopic and ultrastructural study of spleens from 62 embryos and fetuses ranging from 30 days to 20 weeks postovulation. As in the previous studies cited, he noted that the hematopoietic precursors were preponderantly of erythroid lineage. He found no hematopoietic stem cells nor immature hematopoietic cells of the dividing marrow cell pool, such as proerythroblasts, myeloblasts, or megakaryoblasts. He concluded that the hematopoietic precursor cells present in fetal spleens resulted from filtration from the fetal blood by the spleen. Using immunohistologic techniques, Wilkins et al[145] studied fetal spleens, adult normal spleens, and spleens with extramedullary hematopoiesis associated with chronic myeloproliferative disorders. They found hematopoiesis only in the latter group.

They concluded that the fetal spleen is not a hematopoietic organ and that the presence of hematopoietic cells in both fetal and adult spleens results from splenic trapping.

Further support that the human fetal spleen is not a significant hematopoietic organ is derived from functional studies such as those by Hann et al[146] studying pluripotent hematopoietic progenitor cells (CFU-GEMM), myeloid progenitor cells (CFU-GM), and erythroid progenitor cells (BFU-E). In a series of fetuses from 12 to 23 weeks of gestational age, they were unable to document significant functional activity in 6 of 9 spleens studied. In a seventh case, splenic CFU-GM, BFU-E, and CFU-GEMM activity in the spleen was no greater than that in the fetal circulating blood. The same results were obtained by Freedman and Saunders[147] using similar colony culture techniques in seven surgically removed pediatric spleens, which demonstrated no extramedullary hematopoiesis by morphologic examination. They concluded that spleens in postnatal life have no blood-forming function.

Calhoun et al[148] studied a number of human spleens obtained from fetuses of 13 to 22 weeks' gestational age. They attempted to demonstrate that the human fetal spleen functions either as a site for clonal generation of hematopoietic progenitor cells or for production of specific hematopoietic growth factors such as granulocyte-colony-stimulating factor (G-CSF) or erythropoietin. They also performed clonogenic assays to assess concentrations of multipotent hematopoietic progenitors (CFU-MIX), erythroid progenitors (BFU-E), and granulocyte-macrophage progenitors (CFU-GM) in 14 spleens and compared them with the results in the livers and the bone marrows of the same fetuses. They also used both Northern analysis and reverse transcriptase-polymerase chain reaction (RT-PCR) to access G-CSF and erythropoietin messenger RNA in six cases. Examination of cell suspensions in 10 of their cases revealed only occasional normoblasts and rare myelocytes. They found significantly fewer progenitor cell colonies in the spleens than in the livers and the bone marrows of the same cases, and they found no transcripts of either G-CFS or erythropoietin. They concluded that the spleen of the midgestational human does not function as a significant granulopoietic or erythropoietic organ.

We believe that this experimental evidence indicates that in humans, both the fetal and adult spleen are incapable of normal hematopoiesis. The filtration function of the organ results in the trapping of circulating hematopoietic precursor cells that occurs normally in the fetus and in a range of pathologic states in adults. Any hematopoietic activity noted is transient in the fetus; such activity is ineffective and not intrinsic to the spleen in the pathologic states in which it occurs.

Because the normal human spleen has no innate hematopoietic capability, the hematopoietic precursor cells found in that organ in a wide variety of pathologic states must be derived from another source. We believe they originate from the bone marrow and that they enter the spleen via the peripheral blood, from which they are filtered by the spleen as part of its normal function. Filtration of circulating immature hematopoietic cells by the spleen is probably a constant phenomenon in all normal humans. The number of circulating precursor cells and the extent of infiltration must be too small to be noticed by conventional methods. It is only under certain conditions that increased numbers of marrow hematopoietic precursor cells gain access to the circulating blood, where they are filtered out in the spleen and, under appropriate circumstances, may initiate splenic hematopoiesis. There are at least two mechanisms by which this may occur. The first mechanism is characterized by alterations in the bone marrow stroma. Diseases in which this occurs include chronic idiopathic myelofibrosis,[149] metastatic carcinoma,[150] and osteopetrosis (marble bone disease)[147] as well as therapeutically administered granulocyte marcophage-colony stimulating factor (GM-CSF)[151-153] and interleukin-3.[151] The second mechanism is characterized by the liberation of bone marrow stem cells into the peripheral blood resulting from pathologic states such as chronic hemolytic anemias, from the activity of cytokines such as GM-CSF and G-CSF[154-159] that mobilize increased numbers of CD34-positive stem cells, or from direct infusion of CD34-positive stem cells into the blood as in bone marrow transplantation.[159, 160] It has been shown that splenic extramedullary hematopoiesis is a frequent phenomenon in patients who have undergone bone marrow transplantation.[160, 161] Reports of splenic extramedullary hematopoiesis subsequent to cytokine administration[159-167] and bone marrow transplantation [159, 160] are accumulating, and we have seen several examples in both conditions. We predict that with the more widespread use of these modalities, increasing numbers of such cases of splenic "hematopoiesis" will be reported in the future.

In light of this newer understanding of the pathogenetic mechanisms responsible for the presence of hematopoietic precursor cells in the spleen, it is necessary to review the appropriateness of the terms historically used to refer to this phenomenon. The terms "myeloid metaplasia" and "extramedullary hematopoiesis" are used interchangeably to refer to the presence of hematopoietic precursor cells in organs other than the bone marrow, and in particular in the spleen. Neither of the terms accurately defines the pathophysiologic process occurring in that condition. "Myeloid metaplasia" is inappropriate because it does not define what occurs. Metaplasia is the transformation of one mature cellular form into another, such as occurs in squamous metaplasia.[168] There is no evidence to suggest that the presence of hematopoietic precursor cells in the spleen results from the transformation of another intrinsic splenic cell type into blood cells; we therefore believe this term should be discarded. "Extramedullary hematopoiesis" is somewhat better. It denotes blood cell production in a site other than the bone marrow; in some conditions, such as chronic idiopathic myelofibrosis, it is accurate. However, in many disease states there is little, if any, evidence that a true dividing cell component is present that is actually producing blood. Moreover, in many disease processes in which these terms are used, there is no evidence of the presence of all three primary hematopoietic cell lines. In particular, in severe hemolytic processes such as thalassemia or autoimmune hemolytic anemia, erythroid cells proliferate with little or no evidence of granulocytic or megakaryocytic precursors. In these conditions, the term "erythropoiesis" is more appropriate than "hematopoiesis."

Accumulations of hematopoietic precursor cells in the spleen may be broadly divided into two types: those that are non-neoplastic and result from the passive infiltration of circulating hematopoietic precursor cells from the spleen; and those that are neoplastic (clonal) and that have spread into the spleen in a manner similar to that of leukemic infiltrates or as an unusual form of metastasis.

Some investigators have suggested that the normal adult spleen may exert a mild inhibitory effect on the bone marrow. Dameshek[169] postulated an endocrine role for the spleen. He believed that the organ produced a humoral factor, resembling a type of hormone, which he termed "splenin," and postulated that the effect of this inhibitory factor becomes pathologically increased in hypersplenic conditions. Because the bone marrow is usually hyperplastic in hypersplenic conditions, Dameshek felt that splenin might inhibit the release of hematopoietic precursors into the peripheral blood. However, little supporting documentation of the existence of a humoral factor of splenic origin exists.[170, 171]

REFERENCES

1. Neiman RS, Orazi A: Diseases of the Spleen, in Damjanov I, Linder J (eds): Anderson's Pathology, 10th ed, p 1201. St. Louis, Mosby Year–Book, 1996.
2. Weiss L, Tavassoli M: Anatomical hazards to the passage of erythrocytes through the spleen. Semin Hematol 1970; 7:372.
3. van Krieken, te Velde J: Normal histology of the human spleen. Am J Surg Pathol 1988; 12:777.
4. Burke JS, Simon GT: Electron microscopy of the spleen. II. Phagocytosis of colloidal carbon. Am J Pathol 1970; 58:157.
5. Movat HZ, Mustard JF, Taichman NS, et al: Platelet aggregation and release of ADP, serotonin, and histamine associated with phagocytosis of antigen-antibody complexes. Proc Soc Exp Biol Med 1965; 120:232.
6. Movat HZ, Weiser WJ, Glynn MF, et al: Platelet phagocytosis and aggregation. J Cell Biol 1965; 27:531.
7. Mustard JF, Packham MA: Platelet phagocytosis. Ser Hematol 1968; 1:168.
8. Vegge T, Monn E, Hjoft PF: Evidence that platelets may continue to circulate after phagocytosis of particles. Thromb Diath Haemorrh 1968; 20:354.
9. Crosby WH: Normal functions of the spleen relative to red blood cells: A review. Blood 1959; 14:399.
10. Rappaport H: The pathologic anatomy of the splenic red pulp, in Lennert K, Harms D (eds): Die Milz, p 25. Berlin, Springer-Verlag, 1970.
11. Enriquez P, Neiman RS: The Pathology of the Spleen: A Functional Approach. Chicago, American Society of Clinical Pathologists, 1976.
12. Klausner MA, Hirsch LJ, Leblond PF, et al: Contrasting splenic mechanisms in the blood clearance of red blood cells and colloidal particles. Blood 1975; 26:965.
13. Crosby WH: Splenic remodeling of red cell surfaces. Blood 1977; 50:643.
14. Koyama S, Aoki S, Deguchi K: Electron microscopic observations of the splenic red pulp with special reference to the pitting function. Mie Med J 1964; 14:143.
15. Chen LT, Weiss L: The role of the sinus wall in the passage of erythrocytes through the spleen. Blood 1973; 41:529.
16. Crosby WH: Siderocytes and the spleen. Blood 1957; 12:165.
17. Kniseley MH: Spleen studies. I. Microscopic observa-

tions of the circulatory system of living unstimulated mammalian spleens. Anat Rec 1936; 65:23.

18. Lawson NS, Schnitzer B, Smith EB: Splenic ultrastructure in drug-induced Heinz body hemolysis. Arch Pathol 1969; 87:491.

19. Rifkind RA: Heinz body anemia: An ultrastructural study. II. Red cell sequestration and destruction. Blood 1965; 26:433.

20. Schnitzer B, Sodeman TS, Mead ML, et al: An ultrastructural study of the red pulp of the spleen in malaria. Blood 1973; 41:207.

21. Schnitzer B, Sodeman TS, Mead ML, et al: Pitting function of the spleen in malaria: Ultrastructural observations. Science 1972; 177:175.

22. Weed RI, Weiss L: The relationship of red cell fragmentation occurring within the spleen to cell destruction. Trans Assoc Am Physicians 1966; 79:426.

23. Slater LM, Muir WA, Weed RI: Influence of splenectomy on insoluble hemoglobin inclusion bodies in B-thalassemic erythrocytes. Blood 1968; 31:766.

24. Charache S, Conley CL, Waugh DF, et al: Pathogenesis of hemolytic anemia in homozygous hemoglobin C disease. J Clin Invest 1967; 46:1795.

25. Wennberg E, Weiss L: Splenic erythroclasia: An electron microscopy study of hemoglobin H disease. Blood 1968; 31:778.

26. Weiss L: The structure of the normal spleen. Semin Hematol 1965; 2:205.

27. Burke JS, Simon GT: Electron microscopy of the spleen. I. Anatomy and microcirculation. Am J Pathol 1970; 58:127.

28. Weiss L: A scanning electron microscopic study of the spleen. Blood 1974; 43:665.

29. Jacob HS: The defective red blood cell in hereditary spherocytosis. Ann Rev Med 1969; 20:41.

30. Bishop MB, Lansing LS: The spleen: A correlative overview of normal and pathologic anatomy. Hum Pathol 1982; 13:334.

31. Emerson CP, Shen SC, Ham TH, et al: Studies on destruction of red blood cells. Arch Intern Med 1956; 97:1.

32. Jandl JH, Simmons RL, Castle WB: Red cell filtration and the pathogenesis of certain hemolytic anemias. Blood 1961; 18:133.

33. Weiss L: The structure of fine splenic arterial vessels in relation to hemoconcentration and red cell destruction. Am J Anat 1962; 111:175.

34. Aster RH, Jandl JH: Platelet sequestration in man. II. Immunological and clinical studies. J Clin Invest 1964; 43:856.

35. Crome P, Mollison PL: Splenic destruction of Rh-sensitized and of heated red cells. Br J Haematol 1964; 10:137.

36. Jandl JH, Kaplan ME: The destruction of red cells by antibodies in man. III. Quantitative factors influencing the pattern of hemolysis in vivo. J Clin Invest 1960; 39:1145.

37. Jandl JH, Aster RH: Increased splenic pooling and the pathogenesis of hypersplenism. Am J Med Sci 1967; 253:383.

38. Crowell JW, Ford RG, Lewis VM: Oxygen transport in hemorrhagic shock as a function of the hematocrit ratio. Am J Physiol 1959; 196:1033.

39. Sutton JS, Weiss L: Transformation of monocytes in tissue culture into macrophages, epithelioid cells, and multinucleated giant cells: An electron microscopic study. J Cell Biol 1966; 28:303.

40. Allison AC, Burn GP: Enzymatic activity as a function

of age in the human erythrocyte. Br J Haematol 1955; 1:291.

41. Finch CA, Hegsted M, Kinney TD, et al: Iron metabolism: The pathophysiology of iron storage. Blood 1950; 5:983.

42. Singer K, Weiss L: The life cycle of the erythrocyte after splenectomy and the problems of splenic hemolysis and target cell formation. Am J Med Sci 1945; 210:301.

43. Stewart WB, Stewart JM, Izzo MJ, et al: Age as affecting the osmotic and mechanical fragility of dog erythrocytes tagged with radioactive iron. J Exp Med 1950; 91:147.

44. Come SE, Shohet SB, Robinson SH: Surface remodelling of reticulocytes produced in response to erythroid stress. Nat New Biol 1972; 236:157.

45. Crosby WH: The pathogenesis of spherocytes and leptocytes (target cells). Blood 1952; 7:261.

46. Ponder E, Ponder RU: Electrophoretic mobility of red cells and their ghosts as observed with improved apparatus. J Exp Biol 1955; 32:175.

47. Lux SE, John KM: Isolation and partial characterization of a high molecular weight red cell membrane protein complex which is normally removed by the spleen. Blood 1977; 50:625.

48. Nossal GJV, Austin CM, Pye J, et al: Antigens in immunity. XII. Antigen trapping. Int Arch Allerg Appl Immunol 1966; 29:368.

49. Schulkind ML, Ellis EF, Smith RT: Effect of antibody upon clearance of I^{125}-labeled pneumococci by the spleen and liver. Pediatr Res 1967; 1:178.

50. Christensen BE, Jonsson V, Matre R, et al: Traffic of T and B lymphocytes in the normal spleen. Scand J Haematol 1978; 20:246.

51. Grogan TM, Jolley CS, Rangel CS: Immunoarchitecture of the human spleen. Lymphology 1983; 16:72.

52. Grogan TM, Rangel CS, Richter LC, et al: Further delineation of the immunoarchitecture of the human spleen. Lymphology 1984; 17:61.

53. Hsu SM, Cossman J, Jaffe ES: Lymphocyte subsets in normal human lymphoid tissue. Am J Clin Pathol 1983; 80:21.

54. Timens W, Poppema S: Lymphocyte compartments in human spleen: An immunohistologic study in normal spleens and non-involved spleens in Hodgkin's disease. Am J Pathol 1985; 120:443.

55. Van Ewijk W, Nieuwenhuis P: Compartments, domains and migration pathways of lymphoid cells in the splenic pulp. Experientia 1985; 41:199.

56. Gutman GA, Weissman IL: Lymphoid tissue architecture: Experimental analysis of the origin and distribution of T-cells and B-cells. Immunology 1972; 23:645.

57. Stein H, Bonk A, Tolksdorf G, et al: Immunohistologic analysis of the organization of normal lymphoid tissue in non-Hodgkin's lymphomas. J Histochem Cytochem 1980; 26:746.

58. Toder P, Morse PA, Humphrey LJ: Similarities of Fc receptors in human malignant tissue and normal lymphoid tissue. J Immunol 1974; 113:1162.

59. Buckley PJ, Sickson SA: Monoclonal antibodies to T-helper/inducer and T suppressor/cytotoxic lymphocyte subsets recognize antigens on splenic sinusoidal lining cells. Am J Clin Pathol 1984; 167:172.

60. Buckley PJ, Dickson SA, Walker WS: Human splenic sinusoidal lining cells express antigens associated with monocytes, macrophages, endothelial cells, and T lymphocytes. J Immunol 1984; 134:2310.

61. Ilda K, Nadler LM, Nussenzweig V: Identification of the membrane receptor for the complement fragment C3d by means of a monoclonal antibody. J Exp Med 1983; 158:1021.

62. Ford WL: Lymphocyte migration and immune responses. Prog Allergy 1975; 19:1.

63. Weissman IL, Warnke R, Butcher EC, et al: The lymphoid system, its normal architecture and the potential for understanding the system through the study of lymphoproliferative diseases. Hum Pathol 1978; 9:25.

64. Goldschneider I, McGregor DD: Migration of lymphocytes and thymocytes in the rat. I. The route of migration from blood to spleen and lymph nodes. J Exp Med 1968; 127:155.

65. Gutman G, Weissman I: Homing properties of thymus-independent follicular lymphocytes. Transplantation 1973; 16:621.

66. Howard JC, Hunt SV, Gowans JL: Identification of marrow-derived and thymus-derived small lymphocytes in the lymphoid tissue and thoracic duct lymph of normal rats. J Exp Med 1972; 175:200.

67. Sprent J: Circulating T and B lymphocytes of the mouse. I. Migratory properties. Cell Immunol 1973; 7:10.

68. Nieuwenhuis P, Ford WL: Comparative migration of B and T lymphocytes in the rat spleen and lymph nodes. Cell Immunol 1976; 23:254.

69. Eichner ER: Splenic function: Normal, too much, and too little. Am J Med 1979; 66:311.

70. Stuart AE, Davidson AE: Effect of simple lipids on antibody formation after injection of foreign red cells. J Pathol Bacteriol 1964; 87:305.

71. MacLennan ICM, Gray D, Kumaratane DS, et al: The lymphocytes of splenic marginal zones: A distinct B-cell lineage. Immunol Today 1982; 3:305.

72. Langevoort HL: The histopathology of the antibody response. I. Histogenesis of the plasma cell reaction in rabbit spleen. Lab Invest 1963; 12:106.

73. Stuart AE, Cooper GN: Susceptibility of mice to bacterial endotoxin after modification of reticulo-endothelial function by simple lipids. J Pathol Bacteriol 1962; 83:245.

74. Shinefield HR, Steinberg CR, Kaye E: Effect of splenectomy on susceptibility of mice inoculated with *D. pneumoniae*. J Exp Med 1966; 123:777.

75. Whitaker AN: The effect of previous splenectomy on the course of pneumococcal bacteraemia in mice. J Pathol Bacteriol 1968; 95:357.

76. Kitchens CS: The syndrome of post-splenectomy fulminant sepsis: Case report and review of the literature. Am J Med Sci 1977; 274:303.

77. Rowley DA: The formation of circulating antibody in the splenectomized human being following intravenous injection of heterologous erythrocytes. J Immunol 1950; 65:515.

78. Ellis EF, Smith RT: The role of the spleen in immunity with special reference to the post-splenectomy problem in infants. Pediatrics 1966; 37:111.

79. Sullivan JL, Schiffman G, Miser J, et al: Immune response after splenectomy. Lancet 1978; 1:178.

80. Rowley DA: The effect of splenectomy on the formation of circulating antibody in the adult male albino rat. J Immunol 1950; 64:289.

81. Biggar WD, Ramirez RA, Rose V: Congenital asplenia: Immunologic assessment and a clinical review of eight surviving patients. Pediatrics 1981; 67:548.

82. Corrigan JJ Jr, Van Wyck DB, Crosby WH: Clinical disorders of splenic function: The spectrum from asplenism to hypersplenism. Lymphology 1983; 16:101.

83. Taliaferro W: Functions of the spleen in immunity. Am J Trop Med Hyg 1956; 5:391.

84. Bisno AL, Freeman JC: The syndrome of asplenia, pneumococcal sepsis, and disseminated intravascular coagulation. Ann Intern Med 1970; 72:389.

85. Hosea SW: Role of the spleen in pneumococcal infection. Lymphology 1983; 16:115.

86. Winkelstein JA: Splenectomy and infection. Arch Intern Med 1977; 137:1516.

87. Gopal V, Bisno AL: Fulminant pneumococcal infection in "normal" asplenic hosts. Arch Intern Med 1977; 137:1526.

88. Van Wyck DB: Overwhelming postsplenectomy infection (OPSI): The clinical syndrome. Lymphology 1983; 16:107.

89. Knecht JC, Schiffman G, Austrian R: Some biological properties of the pneumococcus type 37 and the chemistry of its capsular polysaccharide. J Exp Med 1970; 132:475.

90. Likhite VV: Immunological impairment and susceptibility to infection after splenectomy. JAMA 1976; 236:1376.

91. Schumacher MJ: Serum immunoglobulin and transferrin levels after childhood splenectomy. Arch Dis Child 1970; 45:114.

92. Claret I, Morales L, Montaner A: Immunological studies in the post-splenectomy syndrome. J Pediatr Surg 1975; 10:59.

93. Neiman RS, Bischel MD, Lukes RJ: Hypersplenism in the uremic hemodialyzed patient: Pathology and proposed pathophysiologic mechanisms. Am J Clin Pathol 1973; 60:502.

94. Lozzio BB, Wargon LB: Immune competence of hereditarily asplenic mice. Immunology 1974; 27:167.

95. Hosea S, Burch C, Brown EJ, et al: Impaired immune response of splenectomized patients to polyvalent pneumococcal vaccine. Lancet 1981; 1:804.

96. LoBuglio AF, Cotran RS, Jandl JH: Red cells coated with immunoglobulin G: Binding and sphering by mononuclear cells in man. Science 1967; 158:1582.

97. Mantovani B: Different roles of IgG and complement receptors in phagocytosis by polymorphonuclear leukocytes. J Immunol 1975; 115:15.

98. Scribner DJ, Fahrney D: Neutrophil receptors for IgG and complement: Their roles in the attachment and ingestion phases of phagocytosis. J Immunol 1976; 116:892.

99. Ehlenberger AG, Nussenzweigh V: The role of membrane receptors for C3b and C3d in phagocytosis. J Exp Med 1977; 145:357.

100. Newmann SL, Johnston RB Jr: Role of binding through C3b and IgG in polymorphonuclear neutrophil function: Studies with trypsin-generated C3b. J Immunol 1979; 132:1839.

101. Winkelstein JA, Lambert GH: Pneumococcal serum opsonizing activity in splenectomized children. J Pediatr 1975; 87:430.

102. Erickson WD, Burgert EO Jr, Lynn HB: The hazard of infection following splenectomy in children. Am J Dis Child 1968; 116:1.

103. Constantopoulos A, Najjar VA, Wish JB, et al: Defective phagocytosis due to tuftsin deficiency in splenectomized subjects. Am J Dis Child 1973; 125:663.

104. Fidalgo BV, Najjar VA: The physiological role of the lymphoid system. III. Leucophilic gamma-globulin

and the phagocytic activity of the polymorphonuclear leucocyte. Proc Nat Acad Sci 1967; 57:957.

105. Fidalgo BV, Najjar VA: The physiological role of the lymphoid system. VI. The stimulatory effect of leucophilic gamma-globulin (leucokinin) on the phagocytic activity of human polymorphonuclear leucocytes. Biochemistry 1967; 6:3386.

106. Florentin I, Martinez J, Maral J, et al: Immunopharmacological properties of tuftsin and of some analogues. Ann N Y Acad Sci 1983; 419:177.

107. Najjar VA, Nishioka K: Tuftsin: A natural phagocytosis stimulating peptide. Nature 1970; 228:672.

108. Najjar VA, Fidalgo BV, Stitt E: The physiological role of the lymphoid system. VII. The disappearance of leucokinin activity following splenectomy. Biochemistry 1968; 7:2367.

109. Najjar VA, Constantopoulos A: A new phagocytosis-stimulating tetrapeptide hormone, tuftsin, and its role in disease. J Reticuloendothel Soc 1972; 12:197.

110. Zoli G, Corazza GR, D'Amato G, et al: Splenic autotransplantation after splenectomy: Tuftsin activity correlates with residual splenic function. Br J Surg 1994; 81:716.

111. Szendroi T, Miko I, Hajdu Z, et al: Splenic autotransplantation after abdominal trauma in childhood: Clinical and experimental data. Acta Chir Hung 1997; 36:349.

112. Bar-Shavit Z, Stabinsky Y, Fridkin M, et al: Tuftsin-macrophage interaction: Specific binding and augmentation of phagocytosis. J Cell Physiol 1979; 100:55.

113. Ebert RV, Stead EA: Demonstration that in normal man no reserves of blood are mobilized. Am J Med Sci 1941; 201:655.

114. Bowdler AJ: The spleen and haemolytic disorders. Clin Haematol 1975; 4:231.

115. Prankerd TAJ. The spleen and anaemia. Br Med J 1963; 253:517.

116. Aster RH: Pooling of platelets in the spleen: Role in the pathogenesis of "hypersplenic" thrombocytopenia. J Clin Invest 1966; 45:645.

117. Penny R, Rozenberg MC, Firkin BG: The splenic platelet pool. Blood 1966; 27:1.

118. Sarajas HSS, Konttinen A, Frick MH: Thrombocytosis evoked by exercise. Nature 1961; 192:721.

119. Freedman M, Altszuler, Karpatkin S: Presence of a non-splenic platelet pool. Blood 1977; 50:419.

120. Amorosi EL: Hypersplenism. Semin Hematol 1965; 2:249.

121. Christensen BE: Pathophysiology of the "hypersplenism syndrome": Remarks about definition and estimation of the splenic erythrocyte pool. Scand J Haematol 1973; 11:5.

122. Doan CA: Hypersplenism. Bull N Y Acad Med 1949; 25:625.

123. Lipson RL, Bayrd ED, Watkins CH: The post-splenectomy blood picture. Am J Clin Pathol 1959; 32:526.

124. Hardisty RM, Wolff HH: Haemorrhagic thrombocythaemia: A clinical and laboratory study. Br J Haematol 1955; 1:390.

125. Kutti J, Weinfeld A, Westin J: The relationship between splenic platelet pool and splenic size. Scand J Haematol 1972; 9:351.

126. Fillet G, Beguin Y, Baldelli L: Model of reticuloendothelial iron metabolism in humans: Abnormal behavior in idiopathic hemochromatosis and in inflammation. Blood 1989; 74:844–851.

127. Rappaport H, Crosby WH: Auto-immune hemolytic anemia. II. Morphologic observations and clinicopathologic correlations. Am J Pathol 1957; 33:429.

128. Theil GA, Downey H: The development of the mammalian spleen with special reference to its hematopoietic activity. Am J Anat 1921; 28:279.

129. Block M: Studies on the blood and blood-forming tissues of newborn opossum. I. Normal development. Ergebnisse der Anatomie und Entwicklungsgeschichte 1974; 34:237.

130. Ono K: Untersuchungen über die entwicklung der menschlichen milz z.f. Zellforschung. Mikr Anatomie 1930; 10:308.

131. Knoll W: Die embryonale Blutbildung beim Menschen. Berichte über die Tatigkeit der St Gallischen Ges 1950; 73:1.

132. Herrath E von: Bau und Funktion der Milz. Z Zellforsch 1935; 23:375.

133. Tischendorf F: Die Milz, in Handbuch der mikroskopischen Anatomie des Menschen, begr Mollendorf Wv, fortgeb Bargmann W, Bd VI, Blutgefarb- und Lymphgefassapparat, inner sekretorische Drusen. Springer, Berlin, Heidelberg, New York.

134. Gilmour JR: Normal haemopoiesis in intra-uterine and neonatal life. J Pathol Bacteriol 1941; 52:25.

135. Weiss L: The development of the primary vascular reticulum in the spleen of human fetus. Am J Anat 1973; 136:315.

136. Djaldetti M: Hemopoietic events in human embryonic spleens at early gestational stages. Biol Neonate 1979; 36:133.

137. Vellguth S, von Gaudecker B, Muller-Hermelink H-K: The development of the human spleen: Ultrastructural studies in fetuses from the 14th to 24th week of gestation. Cell Tissue Res 1985; 242:579.

138. Keleman E, Calvo W, Fliedner TM: Atlas of Human Haematopoietic Development, p 156. New York, Springer-Verlag, 1979.

139. Wolf BC, Luevano E, Neiman RS: Evidence to suggest that the human fetal spleen is not a hematopoietic organ. Am J Clin Pathol 1983; 80:140.

140. Linch DC, Knott RJ, Rodeck CH, et al: Studies of circulating hematopoietic progenitor cells in human fetal blood. Blood 1982; 59:976.

141. Playfair JHL, Wolfendale MR, Kay HEM: The leucocytes of the peripheral blood in the human foetus. Br J Haematol 1963; 9:336.

142. Thomas DB, Yoffey JM: Human foetal haemopoiesis. I. The cellular composition of foetal blood. Br J Haematol 1962; 8:290.

143. Rosenthal P, Rimm IJ, Umiel T, et al: Ontogeny of human hematopoietic cells: Analysis utilizing monoclonal antibodies. J Immunol 1983; 113:232.

144. Ishikawa H: Differentiation of red pulp and evaluation of hemopoietic role of human prenatal spleen. Arch Histol Jpn 1985; 48:183.

145. Wilkins BS, Green A, Wild AE, et al: Extramedullary haemopoiesis in fetal and adult human spleen: A quantitative immunohistology study. Histopathology 1994; 24:24.

146. Hann IM, Bodger MP, Hoffbrand AV: Development of pluripotent hematopoietic progenitor cells in the human fetus. Blood 1983; 62:188.

147. Freedman MH, Saunders EF: Hematopoiesis in the human spleen. Am J Hematol 1981; 11:271.

148. Calhoun DA, Li Y, Braylan RC, et al: Assessment of the contribution of the spleen to granulocytopoiesis and erythropoiesis of the mid-gestation human fetus. Early Hum Dev 1996; 46:217.

149. Wolf BC, Neiman RS: Myelofibrosis with myeloid metaplasia: Pathophysiologic implication between bone marrow changes and progression of splenomegaly. Blood 1985; 65:803.

150. O'Keane JC, Wolf BC, Neiman RS: The pathogenesis of splenic extramedullary hematopoiesis in metastatic carcinoma. Cancer 1989; 63:1539.

151. Orazi A, Cattoretti G, Schiro R, et al: Recombinant human interleukin-3 and recombinant human granulocyte-macrophage colony-stimulating factor administered in vivo after high-dose cyclophosphamide cancer chemotherapy: Effect on hematopoiesis and microenvironment in human bone marrow. Blood 1992; 79:2610.

152. Dedhar F, Gabori L, Galloway T, et al: Human granulocyte-macrophage colony-stimulating factor is a growth factor acting on a variety of cell types of nonhematopoietic origin. Proc Natl Acad Sci U S A 1988; 85:9253.

153. Falk S, Seipelt G, Ganser A, et al: Bone marrow findings after treatment with recombinant human interleukin-3. Am J Clin Pathol 1991; 95:355.

154. Gianni AM, Siena S, Bregni M, et al: Granulocyte-macrophage colony-stimulating factor to harvest circulating haemopoietic stem cell for autotransplantation. Lancet 1989; 2:580.

155. Orazi A, Gordon MS, John K, et al: In vivo effects of recombinant human stem cell factor treatment: A morphologic and immunohistochemical study of bone marrow biopsies. Am J Clin Pathol 1995; 103:177.

156. Anderlini P, Przepiorka D, Champlin R: Biologic and clinical effects of granulocyte colony-stimulating factor in normal individuals. J Am Soc Hematol 1996; 88:2819.

157. Korbling M, Huh YO, Durett A, et al: Allogeneic blood stem cell transplantation: Peripheralization and yield of donor-derived primitive hematopoietic progenitor cells (CD34+ Thy-1^{dim}) and lymphoid subsets, and possible predictors of engraftment and graft-versus-host disease. Blood 1995; 86:2842.

158. Rackoff WR, Orazi A, Robinson CA, et al: Prolonged administration of granulocyte colony-stimulating factor (filgrastim) to patients with Fanconi anemia: A pilot study. Blood 1996; 88:1588.

159. Siena S, Bregni M, Brando M, et al: Circulation of CD34+ hematopoietic stem cells in the peripheral blood of high-dose cyclophosphamide-treated patients: Enhancement by intravenous recombinant human granulocyte-macrophage colony-stimulating factor. Blood 1989; 74:1905.

160. Arnold R, Calvo W, Heymer B, et al: Extramedullary haemopoiesis after bone marrow transplantation. Scand J Haematol 1985; 34:9.

161. Antin JH, Weinberg DS, Rappeport JM: Evidence that pluripotential stem cells form splenic colonies in humans after marrow transplantation. Transplantation 1985; 39:102.

162. Redmond J III, Kantor RS, Auerbach HE, et al: Extramedullary hematopoiesis during therapy with granulocyte colony-stimulating factor. Arch Pathol Lab Med 1994; 118:1014.

163. Lieschke GJ, Burgess AW: Granulocyte colony-stimulating factor and granulocyte-macrophage colony-stimulating factor. N Engl J Med 1992; 327:28.

164. Duhrsen U, Villeval JL, Boyd J, et al: Effects of recombinant human granulocyte colony-stimulating factor on hematopoietic progenitor cells in cancer patients. Blood 1988;72:2074.

165. Glaspy JA, Golde DW: Granulocyte colony-stimulating factor (G-CSF): Preclinical and clinical studies. Semin Oncol 1992; 19:386.

166. Kazama T, Miyazawa M, Tsuchiya S, et al: Proliferation of macrophage-lineage cells in the bone marrow, severe thymic atrophy, and extramedullary hematopoiesis of possible donor origin in an autopsy case of post-transplantation graft-versus-host disease. Bone Marrow Transplant 1996; 18:437.

167. Litam PP, Friedman HD, Loughran TP: Splenic extramedullary hematopoiesis in a patient receiving intermittently administered granulocyte colony-stimulating factor. Ann Intern Med 1993; 118:954.

168. Yeldandi AV, Kaufman DG, Reddy JK: Cell injury and cellular adaptations, in Damjanov I, Linder J (eds): Anderson's Pathology, 10th ed, p 383. St. Louis, Mosby–Year Book, 1996.

169. Dameshek W: Hypersplenism. Bull N Y Acad Med 1955; 31:113.

170. Moeschlin VS: Physiopathologie des Hypersplenimus. Helv Med Acta 1956; 23:416.

171. Kunz G: Die "depressorische hypersplenie": Ein noch gerecht fertigter Begriff? Med Welt 1960; 17:913.

HYPERSPLENISM

The term "hypersplenism" refers to the excessive destruction of one or more peripheral blood cell lines by the spleen; hypersplenism is the single most common reason for elective splenectomy. Hypersplenism is not a single disease entity; it is a syndrome that may be caused by a large number of unrelated disorders. The classic definition of hypersplenism, as proposed by Dameshek,[1] includes four criteria: (1) cytopenias of one or more peripheral blood cell lines, (2) bone marrow hyperplasia commensurate with the cytopenias, (3) splenomegaly, and (4) correction of the cytopenias following splenectomy. However, there is at present no general agreement as to which disorders should be included within the category of hypersplenism, and some diseases that are usually considered forms of hypersplenism do not fulfill all four of the criteria.[2–4]

Historically, hypersplenism was divided into primary and secondary types.[3, 5, 6] The term "primary hypersplenism" was used to refer to conditions in which there is no recognizable cause for the cytopenias, either in the spleen or in the circulating blood cells. Because "primary hypersplenism" has been used in a variety of contexts, its meaning is inexact, and its existence is controversial. Doan[7, 8] defined primary hypersplenism as being an inherited condition, as opposed to secondary hypersplenism, which he believed was an acquired disorder. In his review of 270 cases of hypersplenism, he classified 65 percent as primary and only 35 percent as secondary. He believed that primary hypersplenism had an autosomal dominant inheritance in some cases and postulated a recessive mode of inheritance in others. He believed that in the latter group, hypersplenism resulted from an inherited "hyperinstability" that could be provoked by in-

fections or by other precipitating factors. However, there is no evidence in the literature to support this thesis. The introduction of other terms as synonyms for this condition has further complicated understanding of primary hypersplenism.[8, 9] Dacie and coworkers [10, 11] equated primary hypersplenism with "nontropical idiopathic splenomegaly," which these authors defined as splenomegaly of unknown origin associated with cytopenias. They distinguished this condition from the tropical splenomegaly syndrome—reported in patients in tropical countries—which has been linked by some investigators to malarial infection.[12–16] It is clear that confusing terminology and variable criteria reflect a lack of understanding of so-called primary hypersplenism. If this term is reserved for conditions in which the spleen is histologically normal and in which the splenomegaly and cytopenias have no identifiable cause, primary hypersplenism virtually disappears as an entity.

A more useful division of types of hypersplenism considers whether cytopenias are due to abnormalities in circulating blood cells, rendering them more susceptible to sequestration and destruction in a normally functioning spleen, or whether they are due to abnormalities in the spleen itself, resulting in destruction of increased numbers of normal blood cells. Some authors have argued that cytopenias associated with abnormalities in circulating blood cells should not be considered examples of hypersplenism.[1, 3] They assert that in such conditions as hereditary spherocytosis and idiopathic thrombocytopenic purpura (ITP) there is no demonstrable abnormality in the spleen, which is merely fulfilling its normal function of removing defective cells from the peripheral blood. Moreover, the spleen in such conditions as ITP and in some hemolytic anemias is often not markedly enlarged, and therefore these diseases do not meet the criteria Dameshek listed for the definition of hypersplenism. In an attempt to resolve the controversy, Crosby[17] defined hypersplenism as a detrimental increase in splenic activity. "When a person is hematologically better off without his spleen, he has hypersplenism." We agree with Crosby's pragmatic definition and consider hypersplenism to include all disorders in which destruction of circulating hematopoietic cells by the spleen results in cytopenias of one or more blood cell lines that are ameliorated or corrected by splenectomy.

PATHOGENESIS OF HYPERSPLENISM

The pathogenesis of hypersplenism has been a subject of historical controversy.[18] Dameshek[1] hypothesized that cytopenias were secondary to an inhibitory effect of the spleen on the bone marrow that resulted in either depressed hematopoiesis or in the ineffective release of hematopoietic cells from a cellular bone marrow. However, Doan[7] postulated that hypersplenism results from increased sequestration of the cellular elements of the blood in an enlarged spleen. A third proposed mechanism for the anemia associated with hypersplenism was the dilutional effect due to the increased plasma volume that was observed in some patients with splenomegaly.[19, 20]

Dameshek[1] believed that the spleen normally had an endocrine function that exercised a mild inhibitory effect on the bone marrow, and he postulated the existence of a hormonelike substance produced by the spleen, which he termed "splenin." He hypothesized that hematopoiesis was controlled by the interaction of the bone marrow, the spleen, and the adrenal cortex. He suggested that splenomegaly led to increased production of splenin, resulting in cytopenias due to an exaggeration of the inhibitory effect of the hormone on the bone marrow. There is little evidence to support the theory of the production of an inhibitory substance by the spleen.[21] In support of his thesis, Dameshek cited the fact that some cases of autoimmune hemolytic anemia are immediately cured by splenectomy. However, in many cases, antibody titers remain elevated following splenectomy.[18] It has also been reported that some cases of aplastic ane-

mia have resolved with the recovery of the bone marrow following splenectomy.[3, 22, 23] However, these cases are rare, and recovery may have been coincidental, occurring as part of the natural history of the disease. Moreover, splenectomy may be beneficial in these cases by decreasing the splenic "reservoir" of CD8+ cells that seem to be responsible for the suppressor effect on hematopoiesis in some of these patients.[24] Jacob[2] demonstrated sequestration of ^{51}Cr-labeled red cells in hypersplenic conditions coincidental with an increase in hemoglobin synthesis by the bone marrow, which is inconsistent with the theory of a substance of splenic origin inhibiting marrow hematopoiesis. Experimental studies explaining the existence and effects of a splenic hormone affecting hematopoiesis have provided variable and sometimes conflicting data.[25] Some investigators have reported that transplantation of splenic tissue to a subcutaneous location or rerouting the splenic blood flow to the systemic circulation in experimental animals leads to a depression of erythropoiesis; they have hypothesized that this results from bypassing the liver, which could degrade substances produced by the spleen.[26, 27] However, anastomosis of the splenic vein directly into the inferior vena cava, which also bypasses the portal system, has not produced similar results.[28] To date, Dameshek's theory remains unsupported.

Alternately, substantial evidence for the sequestration theory of hypersplenism has come from radioisotope studies.[2, 29–32] In these studies, radioisotope-tagged erythrocytes or platelets are injected intravenously, and radioactivity is measured by a scintillation counter placed externally over the spleen.[32–35] It can be demonstrated that experimentally injured erythrocytes, treated either with heat or sulfhydryl inhibitors, which damage the cell membrane, are trapped in the normal spleen.[31, 36] In addition, a number of studies have demonstrated that in cases of splenomegaly due to a variety of causes, there is sequestration of undamaged erythrocytes and platelets.[4] Harris and coworkers[30] showed that there was a rapid equilibration of radioactivity over the normal spleen following injection of ^{51}Cr-labeled normal erythrocytes, with no rise during subsequent days. In patients with splenomegaly, however, some cases gave two exponential curves of radioactivity over the spleen. Similarly, in some patients with normal spleens, double curves were also obtained following the injection of certain types of abnormal erythrocytes, particularly antibody-coated red cells or spherocytes obtained from patients with hereditary spherocytosis. These investigators believed that the second rise in radioactivity represented hemolysis with excess removal of labeled cells by the spleen.

Hypersplenism can be induced in experimental animals via a mechanism sometimes referred to as "reticuloendothelial blockade."[17, 37] Injection of finely divided particles of poorly metabolized polymers such as methyl cellulose or thorium dioxide (Thorotrast), which are phagocytized by macrophages, results in splenomegaly and pancytopenia.[2, 38] It is believed that these so-called blocking agents overload the hepatic Kupffer cells, resulting in increased exposure of the splenic macrophages to the particulate material and stimulating a proliferation of macrophages.

It has been postulated that hemodilution may play a role in the anemia associated with hypersplenism.[19, 20] Several investigators have demonstrated an increased plasma volume in patients with splenomegaly while the body red blood cell mass remains normal or is only slightly increased.[39–42] The increased plasma volume, measured using ^{125}I-labeled albumin associated with a normal red blood cell mass, would result in a decreased plasma hemoglobin concentration. McFadzean and colleagues[42] reported that splenectomy somewhat reduces the plasma volume, although it still remains higher than normal. Pettit[43] reported that the plasma volume returns toward normal in 30 to 60 days following splenectomy. The cause of the elevated plasma volume has been attributed to circulatory dynamics. Some authors have hypothesized that the enlarged spleen might act as an arteriovenous shunt, which is associated with an increased cardiac output and plasma volume.[44] Hess and associates,[19] however, stated that increased blood flow to the spleen induces portal hypertension, resulting in a redistribution of body water, leading to salt and water retention. They demonstrated an elevated portal venous pressure—which decreased after splenectomy—in all 12 patients with lymphoproliferative disorders. This flow-induced portal hypertension could result in a decreased effective intravascular volume, stimulating renin and aldosterone secretion and, thereby, increasing plasma volume. They also postulated that the increased plasma volume would lead to a decrease in colloid osmotic pressure, stimulating

albumin synthesis and resulting in a delay of return of the plasma volume to normal following splenectomy. They found no evidence to support the theory that the enlarged spleen acts as an arteriovenous shunt.

It is now generally accepted that the cytopenias in hypersplenism result predominantly from splenic sequestration and/or destruction of blood cells.[7, 17, 18, 29, 45–48] The spleen also plays a role in the production of autoantibodies in the autoimmune cytopenias. However, the persistence of these autoantibodies following splenectomy indicates that the spleen is not the sole site of production. In addition, there may be a dilutional effect due to an elevated plasma volume involved in the anemia associated with splenomegaly, but this appears to be of secondary importance.

The majority of diseases associated with hypersplenism involve the red pulp of the spleen (Table 3–1). Splenic sequestration and destruction of the cellular elements of the blood may be due to abnormalities in the circulating blood cells themselves, rendering them susceptible to sequestration and destruction by a normal spleen, or may be due to abnormalities in the spleen itself, resulting in accelerated destruction of normal blood cells. In both situations, the cords of Billroth are widened, and the cordal macrophages proliferate, leading to an increased transit time of circulating cells, with prolonged exposure to the acidotic, hypoxic environment of the cords and increased opportunity for phagocytosis by cordal macrophages.

The majority of diseases in which abnormal circulating cells are trapped by an intrinsically normal spleen are disorders of erythrocytes; the diseases may be either congenital or acquired. Congenital abnormalities of erythrocytes include hereditary spherocytosis and elliptocytosis as well as the hemoglobinopathies and hereditary hemolytic anemias. Acquired abnormalities of erythrocytes resulting in hypersplenism include the autoimmune hemolytic anemias and parasitic disorders.

Hereditary spherocytosis is characterized by prominent splenomegaly and anemia.[49–52] Spherocytes are less deformable than normal erythrocytes, owing to a structural abnormality of the cell membrane, rendering them incapable of transversing the splenic sinus wall.[49] A similar structural abnormality occurs in hereditary elliptocytosis, although severe anemia is unusual in this condition.[53] Interestingly, in spite of the sometimes massive splenomegaly,

Table 3–1. Disorders Associated with Hypersplenism

I. Disorders associated with sequestration of abnormal blood cells in an intrinsically normal spleen
   A. Congenital disorders of erythrocytes
      1. Hereditary spherocytosis
      2. Hereditary elliptocytosis
      3. Hemoglobinopathies, e.g., sickle cell disease, unstable hemoglobins
   B. Acquired disorders of erythrocytes
      1. Autoimmune hemolytic anemias
      2. Parasitic diseases, e.g., malaria, babesiosis
   C. Autoimmune thrombocytopenia
   D. Autoimmune neutropenia
II. Disorders of the spleen resulting in sequestration of normal blood cells
   A. Disorders of the monocyte/macrophage system
      1. Chronic congestive splenomegaly
      2. Storage diseases
      3. Parasitic diseases, e.g., kala-azar
      4. Langerhans cell histiocytosis
      5. Infection-associated and familial hemophagocytic syndromes
   B. Infiltrative disorders
      1. Leukemias
      2. Lymphomas
      3. Plasma cell dyscrasias
      4. Extramedullary hematopoiesis
         a. Severe hemolytic states
         b. Chronic idiopathic myelofibrosis
      5. Chronic infections, e.g., tuberculosis, brucellosis
      6. Metastatic carcinoma
   C. Vascular abnormalities
      1. Vascular tumors
      2. Peliosis
   D. Splenic cysts
   E. Hamartomas
III. Miscellaneous conditions
   A. Hyperthyroidism
   B. Hypogammaglobulinemia
   C. Progressive multifocal leukoencephalopathy

hematopoietic cells other than the abnormal erythrocytes are usually not sequestered, and the anemia is rarely associated with thrombocytopenia or leukopenia.

The spleen may be markedly enlarged in young children with sickle cell disease, owing to the accumulation of both normal and sickled erythrocytes.[54–57] This phenomenon may also occur in patients with other hemoglobinopathies, particularly hemoglobin S-C disease,[58] homozygous hemoglobin C disease,[59] and thalassemia major.[60–62] Later in the course of sickle cell disease the spleen becomes atrophic because of autoinfarction.

Splenic sequestration and destruction of antibody-coated cells are the causes of the anemia in autoimmune hemolytic disorders.[63, 64] The spleen plays a role both in the production

of the autoantibody and in the destruction of the abnormal cells.[64–67] Antibody-coated cells are less able to traverse the sinus walls, resulting in their accumulation in the cords.[67] The autoantibodies also act as opsonins, which may facilitate phagocytosis. In some of these disorders splenomegaly may lead to cytopenias of the other cell lines as well. Splenectomy usually results in remission of the cytopenias, although some patients may have a Coombs test with persistently positive results.

Hypersplenism has also been described in patients with chronic uremia who are undergoing hemodialysis. Bischel and coworkers[68] demonstrated sequestration of ^{51}Cr-labeled erythrocytes in the spleen of 6 of the 15 patients in their study. Splenectomy resulted in a decrease in serum level of IgM in the four patients with elevated IgM preoperatively. Histologically the spleens showed striking lymphoid hyperplasia, and these authors postulated that the spleen might be the site of production of the IgM.[69] Splenectomy in these patients would therefore decrease peripheral cell destruction by removing both a site of erythrocyte sequestration and antibody production.

Parasitic infections that affect erythrocytes, such as malaria and babesiosis, may also be associated with anemia associated with hypersplenism.[70, 71] In these conditions the parasitized erythrocytes lack the deformability necessary to enter the splenic sinuses.

Splenic sequestration and destruction of antibody-coated platelets are the causes of thrombocytopenia in ITP, an acquired disorder of platelets.[72–75] The mechanism of the hypersplenism associated with ITP, as well as with the rare cases of selective neutropenia,[76, 77] is similar to that described for autoimmune hemolytic disorders.

Intrinsic disorders of the spleen resulting in the sequestration and destruction of normal circulating hematopoietic cells include (1) disorders of the monocyte-macrophage system, (2) infiltrative disorders, (3) vascular abnormalities, and (4) primary nonhematopoietic tumors of the spleen. The majority of the disorders of cordal macrophages are systemic diseases of histiocytes. Some storage diseases, particularly lipidoses such as Gaucher disease,[78–80] Niemann-Pick disease,[81, 82] and ceroid histiocytosis,[83] result in the accumulation of histiocytes containing abnormal metabolites in the spleen and in other lymphoid organs, leading to hypersplenism that may necessitate splenectomy. Parasitic disorders that involve the reticuloendothelial system may also cause splenomegaly with hypersplenism. For example, splenomegaly in visceral leishmaniasis (kala-azar) results from parasitization and resultant proliferation of the cordal macrophages.[84] Other histiocytoses, including disseminated Langerhans cell histiocytosis[85–88] and the infection-associated and familial hemophagocytic syndromes, may also result in hypersplenism.[89, 90]

Cordal macrophages also proliferate early in the course of Banti syndrome. Banti[91, 92] noted the association of splenomegaly and cytopenias and postulated that the spleen produced a toxic substance that damaged the bone marrow and the liver, leading to cirrhosis. The term "Banti syndrome" is presently used to refer to fibrocongestive splenomegaly secondary to liver disease with portal hypertension. Later in the course of the disease, fibrosis of the red pulp occurs, resulting in rigid splenic cords and apparently dilated sinuses. In this late stage, the spleen also often contains nodules of fibrous tissue.[93, 94]

Infiltrative disorders that result in hypersplenism include lymphoreticular malignancies, particularly the leukemias and lymphomas, and, although rarely, plasma cell dyscrasias. In particular, hairy cell leukemia,[95–97] prolymphocytic leukemia,[98, 99] and mantle cell and marginal zone cell lymphomas may be associated with hypersplenism, and cytopenias may be the presenting features of these disorders.[100–102] Splenic myeloid metaplasia, occurring in the myeloproliferative disorders and other related conditions, may cause splenomegaly with cytopenias.[103–106] Splenectomy in these infiltrative conditions may ameliorate the cytopenias, although the course of the disease is rarely affected.[107, 108] Certain chronic infections such as miliary tuberculosis[109] and brucellosis[110] are occasionally associated with hypersplenism. Metastatic carcinoma is an uncommon cause of hypersplenism.[111, 112]

Vascular lesions, including peliosis and benign and malignant vascular tumors, may cause cytopenias due to splenomegaly.[113–117] In addition, these lesions may cause a microangiopathic hemolytic anemia owing to the irregularity of the neoplastic endothelial cells. Hypersplenism may also occur occasionally with other primary nonhematopoietic tumors of the spleen, such as splenic cysts[118] and hamartomas.[119]

There are occasional reports of hypersplenism associated with disorders in which the cause of the splenomegaly is unclear. Such conditions include hyperthyroidism,[120] hypogammaglobulinemia,[121] and progressive multifocal leukoencephalopathy.[122]

REFERENCES

1. Dameshek W: Hypersplenism. Bull N Y Acad Med 1955; 31:113.
2. Jacob HS: Hypersplenism: Mechanisms and management. Br J Haematol 1974; 27:1.
3. Amorosi EL: Hypersplenism. Semin Hematol 1965; 2:249.
4. Jandl JH, Aster RH: Increased splenic pooling and the pathogenesis of hypersplenism. Am J Med Sci 1967; 253:383.
5. Dameshek W: The spleen: Facts and fancies. Bull N Engl Med Center 1941; 3:304.
6. Singer K, Miller EB, Dameshek W: Hematologic changes following splenectomy in man. Am J Med Sci 1941; 202:171.
7. Doan CA: Hypersplenism. Bull N Y Acad Med 1949; 25:625.
8. Doan CA, Wright CS: Primary congenital and secondary acquired splenic panhematopenia. Blood 1946; 1:10.
9. Evans WH: The blood changes after splenectomy in splenic anemia, purpura hemorrhagica and acholuric jaundice, with special reference to platelets and coagulation. J Pathol Bacteriol 1928; 31:815.
10. Dacie JV, Brain MC, Harrison CV, et al: "Nontropical idiopathic splenomegaly" ("primary hypersplenism"): A review of ten cases and their relationship to malignant lymphomas. Br J Haematol 1969; 17:317.
11. Dacie JV, Galton DAG, Gordon-Smith EC, et al: Nontropical "idiopathic splenomegaly": A follow-up study of ten patients described in 1969. Br J Haematol 1978; 38:185.
12. Gebbie DAM, Hamilton PJS, Hutt MSR, et al: Malarial antibodies in idiopathic splenomegaly in Uganda. Lancet 1964; 2:392.
13. Hamilton PJ, Hutt MSR, Wilks NE, et al: Idiopathic splenomegaly in Uganda. I. Pathological aspects. East Afr Med J 1965; 42:191.
14. Marsden PD, Hutt MSR, Wilks NE, et al: An investigation of tropical splenomegaly at Mulago Hospital, Kampala, Uganda. Br Med J 1965; 1:89.
15. Pryor DS: Splenectomy in tropical splenomegaly. Br Med J 1967; 3:825.
16. Richmond J, Donaldson GWK, Williams R, et al: Haematological effects of idiopathic splenomegaly seen in Uganda. Br J Haematol 1967; 13:348.
17. Crosby WH: Hypersplenism. Ann Rev Med 1962; 13:127.
18. Crosby WH: Is hypersplenism a dead issue? Blood 1962; 20:94.
19. Hess CE, Ayers CR, Sandusky WR, et al: Mechanism of dilutional anemia in massive splenomegaly. Blood 1976; 47:629.
20. Huber H, Lewis SM, Szur L: The influence of anaemia, polycythaemia and splenomegaly on the relationship between venous haematocrit and red-cell volume. Br J Haematol 1964; 10:567.
21. Ruhenstroth-Bauer G: The role of humoral splenic

factors in the formation and release of blood cells. Semin Hematol 1965; 2:229.

22. Ferrata A, Fieschi A: Risultati e insegnamenti della splenectomia nelle mielosi aplastiche. Haematologica 1941; 23:979.

23. McFarland W, Granville N, Schwartz R, et al: Therapy of hypoplastic anemia with bone marrow transplantation. Arch Intern Med 1961; 108:23.

24. Roman S, Grigoriu G, Puscariu T, et al: The role of spleen in the pathogeny of aplastic anemia related to increased number of CD3+, CD8+, and FcR+ cells. Rom J Intern Med 1994; 32:275.

25. Jacob HS, MacDonald RA, Jandl JH: Regulation of spleen growth and sequestering function. J Clin Invest 1963; 42:1476.

26. Altman KI, Watman RN, Salomon K: Surgically induced splenogenic anaemia in the rabbit. Nature 1951; 168:827.

27. Schneiberg K, Watras J: Erythropoiesis in mice C$_{57}$-black investigated with radio-iron after exclusion of the spleen from the portal circulation. Folia Biol 1960; 8:339.

28. Lorber M: Peripheral blood and bone marrow in dogs subsequent to the routing of splenic blood into the systemic circulation. Acta Haematol 1959; 21:232.

29. Christensen BE: Pathophysiology of the "hypersplenism syndrome:" Remarks about definition and estimation of the splenic erythrocyte pool. Scand J Haematol 1973; 11:5.

30. Harris IM, McAlister J, Prankerd TAJ: Splenomegaly and the circulating red cell. Br J Haematol 1958; 4:97.

31. Harris IM, McAlister JM, Prankerd TAJ: The relationship of the abnormal red cell to the normal spleen. Clin Sci 1957; 16:223.

32. Jandl JH, Greenberg MS, Yonemoto RH, et al: Clinical determination of the sites of red cell sequestration in hemolytic anemias. J Clin Invest 1956; 35:842.

33. Aster RH, Jandl JH: Platelet sequestration in man. II. Immunologic and clinical studies. J Clin Invest 1964; 46:856.

34. Baldini M: Banti's view of splenic anemia ("hypersplenism" and the humoral factor). Proceedings of the VIth International Congress of the International Society of Hematology, p 422. New York, Grune & Stratton, 1958.

35. Prez-Tamayo R, Mejia S, Montfort I: Influence of spleen on thrombocytopenia induced by humoral factor(s) of experimental hypersplenism. Blood 1961; 18:364.

36. Jacob HS, Jandl JH: Effects of sulfhydryl inhibition of red cells. II. Studies in vivo. J Clin Invest 1962; 41:1514.

37. Fisher S, Riley WB, Shorey CD: Studies on the mechanism of increased splenic particle uptake in mice after the injection of some finely divided agents. J Pathol Bacteriol 1968; 96:463.

38. Motulsky AG, Giblett E, Cassard F, et al: Studies on the pathophysiology of splenic anemia. Proceedings of the VIth International Congress of the International Society of Hematology, p 419. New York, Grune & Stratton, 1958.

39. Blendis LM, Clark MB, Williams R: Effects of splenectomy on the haemodilutional anaemia of splenomegaly. Lancet 1969; 1:795.

40. Blendis LM, Ramboer C, Williams R: Studies on the haemodilution anaemia of splenomegaly. Eur J Clin Invest 1970; 1:54.

41. Bowdler AJ: Blood volume studies in patients with splenomegaly. Transfusion 1970; 10:171.

42. McFadzean AJS, Todd D, Tsang KC: Observations on the anemia of cryptogenic splenomegaly. II. Expansion of the plasma volume. Blood 1958; 13:524.

43. Pettit JE: Spleen function. Clin Haematol 1977; 6:639.

44. Garnett ES, Goddard BA, Markby D, et al: The spleen as an arteriovenous shunt. Lancet 1969; 1:386.

45. Christensen BE: Quantitative determination of splenic red blood cell destruction in patients with splenomegaly. Scand J Haematol 1975; 14:295.

46. Kunz G: Die "depressorische Hypersplenie:" Ein noch gerechtfertiger Begriff? Med Welt 1960; 17:913.

47. Moeschlin VS: Pathophysiologie des hypersplenimus. Helv Med Acta 1956; 23:416.

48. Motulsky AG, Cassard F, Giblett ER, et al: Anemia and the spleen. N Engl J Med 1958; 259:1164.

49. Palek J, Jarolim P: Red cell membrane disorders, in Hoffman R, et al (eds): Hematology Basic Principles and Practice, 2nd ed, p 667. New York, Churchill Livingstone, 1995.

50. Molnar Z, Rappaport H: Fine structure of the spleen in hereditary spherocytosis. Blood 1972; 1:81.

51. Chang C, Li C, Liang Y, et al: Clinical features and splenic pathologic changes in patients with autoimmune hemolytic anemia and congenital hemolytic anemia. Mayo Clin Proc 1993; 68:757.

52. LaCelle PL: Alteration of membrane deformabilities in hemolytic anemias. Semin Hematol 1970; 7:355.

53. Weiss HJ: Hereditary elliptocytosis with hemolytic anemia: Report of six cases. Am J Med 1963; 35:455.

54. Finch CA: Pathophysiologic aspects of sickle cell anemia. Am J Med 1972; 53:1.

55. Hathorn M: Patterns of red cell destruction in sickle-cell anemia. Br J Haematol 1967; 13:746.

56. Rossi E, Westing DW, Santos AS, et al: Hypersplenism in sickle cell anemia. Arch Intern Med 1964; 114:408.

57. Watson RJ, Lichtman HC, Shapiro HD: Splenomegaly in sickle cell anemia. Am J Med 1956; 20:196.

58. River GL, Robbins AB, Schwartz SO: S-C hemoglobin: A clinical study. Blood 1961; 18:385.

59. Wheby MS, Thorup OA, Leavell BS: Homozygous hemoglobin-C disease in siblings: Further comment on intraerythrocytic crystals. Blood 1956; 11:266.

60. Erlandson ME, Schulman I, Smith CH: Studies on congenital hemolytic syndromes. I. Rate of destruction and production of erythrocytes in thalassemia. Pediatrics 1958; 22:910.

61. Smith CH, Erlandson ME, Stein G, et al: The role of splenectomy in the management of thalassemia. Blood 1960; 15:197.

62. Smith CH, Schulman I, Ando RE, Stein G: Studies on Mediterranean (Cooley's) anemia. I. Clinical and hematologic aspects of splenectomy with special reference to fetal hemoglobin synthesis. Blood 1955; 10:582.

63. Sokol RJ, Booker DJ, Stamps R: The pathology of autoimmune hemolytic anemia. J Clin Pathol 1992; 45:1047.

64. Bowdler AJ: The role of the spleen and splenectomy in autoimmune hemolytic disease. Semin Hematol 1976; 13:333.

65. Evans RS, Takahashi K, Duane RT, et al: Primary thrombocytopenic purpura and acquired hemolytic anemia. Arch Intern Med 1961; 87:48.

66. Rappaport H, Crosby WH: Autoimmune hemolytic anemia. II. Morphologic observations and clinicopathologic correlations. Am J Pathol 1957; 33:429.

67. Jandl JH, Simmons RL, Castle WB: Red cell filtration and the pathogenesis of certain hemolytic anemias. Blood 1961; 18:133.

68. Bischel MD, Neiman RS, Berne TV, et al: Hypersplenism in the uremic hemodialyzed patient: The effect of splenectomy on transplantation and proposed mechanisms. Nephron 1972; 9:146.

69. Neiman RS, Bischel MD, Lukes RJ: Hypersplenism in the uremic hemodialyzed patient: Pathology and proposed pathophysiologic mechanisms. Am J Clin Pathol 1973; 60:502.

70. Looareesuwan S, Ho M, Wattanagoon Y, et al: Dynamic alteration in splenic function during acute falciparum malaria. N Engl J Med 1987; 317:675.

71. Wyler DJ: Splenic functions in malaria. Lymphology 1983; 16:121.

72. Chang C-S, Li C-Y, Cha SS: Chronic idiopathic thrombocytopenic purpura: Splenic pathologic features and their clinical correlation. Arch Pathol Lab Med 1993; 117:981.

73. Gugliotta L, Isacchi G, Guarini A, et al: Chronic idiopathic thrombocytopenic purpura (ITP): Site of platelet sequestration and results of splenectomy—a study of 197 patients. Scand J Haematol 1981; 26:407.

74. McMillan R, Longmire RL, Tavassoli M, et al: In vitro platelet phagocytosis by splenic leukocytes in idiopathic thrombocytopenic purpura. N Engl J Med 1974; 290:249.

75. Tavassoli M, McMillan R: Structure of the spleen in idiopathic thrombocytopenic purpura. Am J Clin Pathol 1975; 64:180.

76. Laszlo J, Jones R, Silberman HR: Splenectomy for Felty's syndrome: Clinicopathologic study of 27 patients. Arch Intern Med 1978; 138:597.

77. Louie JS, Pearson CM: Felty's syndrome. Semin Hematol 1971; 8:216.

78. Beutler E: Gaucher's disease. N Engl J Med 1991; 325, 1354.

79. Fleshner PR, Aufses AJ Jr, Grabowsky GA, et al: A 27-year experience with splenectomy of Gaucher's disease. Am J Surg 1991; 161:69.

80. Beutler E. Grabowski GA: Gaucher disease, in Scriver CR, Beaudet AL, Sly WS, et al (eds): The Metabolic and Molecular Bases of Inherited Disease, p 2641. New York, McGraw-Hill, 1995.

81. Wesz B, Spirer Z, Reif S: Neimann-Pick disease: Newer classification based on genetic mutations of the disease. Adv Ped 1994; 41:415.

82. Elleder M: Niemann-Pick Disease. Pathol Res Pract 1989; 185:293.

83. Silverstein MN, Ellefson RD: The syndrome of the sea-blue histiocyte. Semin Hematol 1972; 9:299.

84. Burchenal JH, Bowers RF, Haedicke TA: Visceral leishmaniasis complicated by severe anemia: Improvement following splenectomy. Am J Trop Med 1947; 27:690.

85. Nezelof C, Basset F, Rousseau MF: Histiocytosis X: Histogenetic arguments for a Langerhans cell origin. Biomedicine 1973; 18:365.

86. Nezelof C: Histiocytosis X: A histological and histogenetic study, in Rosenberg HS, Bolande RP (eds): Perspectives in Pediatric Pathology, p 153. New York, Masser, 1979.

87. Callihan TR: Langerhans cell histiocytosis (histiocytosis X), in Jaffe ES (ed): Surgical Pathology of the Lymph Nodes and Related Organs, p 534. Philadelphia, WB Saunders Co, 1995.

88. Favara BE: Langerhans cell histiocytosis: Pathology and pathogenesis. Semin Oncol 1991; 18:3.

89. Risdall RJ, McKenna RW, Nesbit ME, et al: Virus-associated hemophagocytic syndrome: A benign histiocytic proliferation distinct from malignant histiocytosis. Cancer 1979; 44:993.

90. Loy TS, Diaz-Arias AA, Perry MC: Familial erythrophagocytic lymphohistiocytosis. Semin Oncol 1991; 18:34.

91. Banti G: Dell' anemia splenica. Florence, Italy. Reprint from R. Instituto di Studi Superiori Practicie di Perfezionamento in Firenze, 1882.

92. Banti G: La splenomegalie avec cirrhose du foie. La Sem Medicale 1894; 14:318.

93. Bishop MP, Lansing LS: The spleen: A correlative overview of normal and pathologic anatomy. Hum Pathol 1982; 13:334.

94. Wolf BC, Neiman RS: Histopathologic manifestations of lymphoproliferative and myeloproliferative disorders involving the spleen, in Knowles DM (ed): Neoplastic Hematopathology, p 1517. Baltimore, Williams & Wilkins, 1992.

95. Burke JS, Byrne GE Jr, Rappaport H: Hairy cell leukemia (leukemic reticuloendotheliosis). I. A clinical pathologic study of 21 patients. Cancer 1974; 33:1399.

96. Burke JS, MacKay B, Rappaport H: Hairy cell leukemia (leukemic reticuloendotheliosis). II. Ultrastructure of the spleen. Cancer 1976; 34:2267.

97. Saven A, Piro LD: Hairy cell leukemia, in Hoffman R, Benz EJ Jr, Shattil SJ, et al (eds): Hematology, Basic Principles and Practice, 2nd ed, p 1322. New York, Churchill Livingstone, 1995.

98. Brunning RD, McKenna RW: Chronic lymphocytic leukemia/prolymphocytic leukemia, in Brunning RD, McKenna RW (eds): Atlas of Tumor Pathology, 3rd series, fascicle 9, p 276. Washington DC, Armed Forces Institute of Pathology, 1994.

99. Bearman RM, Pangalis GA, Rappaport H: Prolymphocytic leukemia: Clinical, histopathological and cytochemical observations. Cancer 1978; 42:2360.

100. Narang S, Wolf BC, Neiman RS: Malignant lymphoma presenting with prominent splenomegaly: A clinicopathologic study with special reference to intermediate cell lymphoma. Cancer 1985; 55:1948.

101. Isaacson PG, Matutes E, Burke M, et al: The histopathology of splenic lymphoma with villous lymphocytes. Blood 1994; 84:3228.

102. Neiman RS, Sullivan AL, Jaffe R: Malignant lymphoma simulating leukemic reticuloendotheliosis: A clinicopathologic study of ten cases. Cancer 1979; 43:329.

103. Ward HP, Block MH: The natural history of agnogenic myeloid metaplasia (AMM) and a critical evaluation of its relationship to the myeloproliferative syndrome. Medicine 1971; 50:357.

104. Wolf DJ, Silver RT, Coleman M: Splenectomy in chronic myeloid leukemia. Ann Intern Med 1978; 89:684.

105. Benbassat J, Penchas S, Ligumski M: Splenectomy in patients with agnogenic myeloid metaplasia: An analysis of 321 published cases. Br J Haematol 1979; 42:207.

106. Brenner B, Nagler A, Tatarsky I, et al: Splenectomy in agnogenic myeloid metaplasia and postpolycythemic myeloid metaplasia. Arch Intern Med 1988; 108:2501.

107. Baropsi G, Ambrosetti A, Buratti A, et al: Splenectomy for patients with myelofibrosis and myeloid

metaplasia: Pretreatment variables and outcome predication. Leukemia 1993; 7:200.

108. Szur L, Smith MD: Red cell production and destruction in myelosclerosis. Br J Haematol 1961; 7:417.

109. Chapman AZ, Redes PS, Baker LA: Neutropenia secondary to tuberculous splenomegaly. Ann Intern Med 1954; 41:1225.

110. Scherger A, Dearing WH, Waugh JM: Intermittent fever over a 17-year period in a patient with hypersplenism due to brucellosis. Mayo Clin Proc 1959; 34:262.

111. Carere RP, Clemes IL: An unusual case of splenomegaly and pancytopenia (secondary hypersplenism). Can Med Assoc J 1962; 86:833.

112. Dunn MA, Goldwein MI: Hypersplenism in advanced breast cancer: Report of a patient treated with splenectomy. Cancer 1975; 25:1449.

113. Lacson A, Berman LD, Neiman RS: Peliosis of the spleen. Am J Clin Pathol 1979; 71:586.

114. Taxy JB: Peliosis: A morphologic curiosity becomes an iatrogenic problem. Hum Pathol 1978; 9:311.

115. Donald D, Dawson AA: Microangiopathic haemolytic anemia associated with malignant haemangio-endothelioma. J Clin Pathol 1971; 24:456.

116. Garvin DF, King FM: Cysts and nonlymphomatous tumors of the spleen. Pathol Ann 1981; 1:61.

117. Smith VC, Eisenberg BL, McDonald EC: Primary splenic angiosarcoma: Case report and literature review. Cancer 1985; 55:1625.

118. Steidl RM, Cardy JD: Solitary cyst of the spleen associated with hypersplenism: Report of a case. Lancet 1957; 2:45.

119. Hardmeier T: Hypersplenismus bei einem Hamartom der Milz (splenom). Schweiz Med Wochenschr 1962; 92:1270.

120. Girsch LS, Myerson RM: Thyrotoxicosis associated with thrombocytopenia and hypersplenism. Am J Clin Pathol 1957; 27:328.

121. Prasad AS, Reiner ES, Watsen CJ: Syndrome of hypogammaglobulinemia, splenomegaly and hypersplenism. Blood 1957; 12:926.

122. Weinstein VF, Woolf AL, Meynell MJ: Progressive multifocal leucoencephalopathy and primary hypersplenism, with a note on the association between disease of the reticuloendothelial system and progressive multifocal leucoencephalopathy. J Clin Pathol 1963; 16:405.

4

HYPOSPLENISM

Hyposplenism refers to deficient or absent function of the spleen. The most common cause is splenectomy, but hyposplenism may also be caused by congenital absence of the organ. Defective function may occur in the presence of an intact spleen and may be congenital or, more commonly, acquired. Hyposplenism results in characteristic findings in the peripheral blood, reflecting the lack of the red pulp filtration function. There may also be an immunologic defect, the extent of which is in part related to the age of the patient when hyposplenism occurs.

ASSESSMENT OF SPLENIC FUNCTION

The adequacy of splenic function may be assessed by either radiologic imaging techniques or morphologic methods. All have some limitations, the most significant of which is that they measure only the filtration and not the immunologic function of the organ.

Imaging techniques currently used include routine x-ray, ultrasonography, computed tomography, and nuclear magnetic resonance. All provide evidence of the anatomic presence or absence of the organ and can define its size and the presence of grossly identifiable lesions. However, none quantify splenic function. Radionuclide scanning, however, can provide both anatomic and functional information regarding the spleen, and it represents the preferred radiologic method of assessing splenic function. The two most widely utilized techniques involve the infusion of technetium 99m sulfur-colloid (^{99m}Tc) or chromium^{51}-labeled (^{51}Cr) heat-damaged red blood cells, with subsequent measurement of splenic uptake of these compounds by scintillation scans. Both techniques measure splenic filtration of particulate matter and do not assess the spleen's ability to clear antigenically active material from the blood. The ^{51}Cr labeled heat-damaged technique is the more sensitive of the two methods, because the majority of these cells are sequestered in the spleen, whereas only about 10 percent of the ^{99m}Tc-labeled sulfur-colloid cells is so localized. However, the latter method is more commonly employed because it is easier to perform and to interpret and because it provides fewer false-positive results. The ability of the spleen to clear blood-borne antigens may be measured by infusing ^{51}Cr-labeled Rh(D) red blood cells sensitized with anti-D. Clearance of Rh-positive red blood cells involves Fc receptor sites on splenic macrophages, which normally remove the bulk of erythrocytes. This technique can be performed only in patients who are Rh(D)-positive; all other patients may become Rh antigen–sensitized.

Morphologic methods for assessing splenic function include examining the peripheral blood for changes associated with depressed or absent filtration function (Table 4–1) and counting pitted red blood cells.

A variety of inclusions may occur in circulating erythrocytes in the asplenic or hyposplenic state.[1] These cellular inclusions rarely occur in individuals with normal splenic function because they are removed from the red blood cells as they traverse the splenic pulp cords. The most consistent and characteristic finding is the presence of Howell-Jolly bodies.[1-3] These cytoplasmic structures are small, dense, basophilic granules composed of fragments of nuclear material and are visible in Romanovsky-stained smears (Fig. 4–1). There is usually only

Table 4–1. Postsplenectomy Blood Picture

I. Erythrocyte inclusions
   A. Howell-Jolly bodies
   B. Heinz bodies
   C. Pappenheimer bodies
II. Poikilocytosis
   A. Target cells
   B. Acanthocytes
   C. Nucleated red blood cells (rarely)
III. Thrombocytosis (usually transient)
IV. Leukocytosis
   A. Lymphocytosis (may persist)
   B. Monocytosis (may persist)
   C. Eosinophilia

one in any affected erythrocyte, but occasionally they are multiple. Howell-Jolly bodies are the only cellular inclusions occurring in patients with hyposplenism that persist for the life of the individual.[4] Their presence is a reliable indication of an anatomically or functionally absent spleen. Because they may be quite infrequent even in asplenia, careful search of the blood smear is advised.

Heinz bodies may be found in the blood smears of asplenic patients who have been given oxidative drugs.[5] They are composed of denatured hemoglobin and appear as refractile cytoplasmic inclusions that are visible only with supravital staining or with phase contrast microscopy (Fig. 4–2). Heinz bodies may also be seen in the peripheral blood smears of patients with hemoglobinopathies that are associated with unstable hemoglobins. These unstable hemoglobins have an increased sus-

ceptibility to oxidation. They precipitate and attach to the erythrocyte membrane if the patient is given an oxidative drug. The number of Heinz bodies increases following splenectomy in patients with hemoglobinopathies. The formation of Heinz bodies can be provoked by oxidative drugs in normal persons only if the spleen has been removed. They may persist in the peripheral blood for several weeks after the offending drug has been discontinued.[5]

Siderocytes, which are erythrocytes containing iron granules, may also be seen in patients with hyposplenism or asplenia.[6, 7] The iron granules stain blue with Prussian blue stain and are referred to as siderotic granules or Pappenheimer bodies. They may be seen in 1 to 2 percent of circulating erythrocytes and in even greater numbers in hemolytic states.

The peripheral blood smear also shows poikilocytosis following splenectomy.[3] Most notable is the presence of target cells or leptocytes[3, 8] (Fig. 4–3). Target cells are thinner than normal erythrocytes and have a greater surface area-to-volume ratio. Their hemoglobin cannot fill the entire cell and is deposited at the periphery and at the center of the cell, which is surrounded by a lucent halo. Target cells have decreased osmotic fragility. They increase in numbers during the weeks following splenectomy, suggesting that they are not formed from preexisting erythrocytes but are produced following splenectomy. Acanthocytes may also occur in hyposplenic states.[9] These cells are characterized by multiple irregular

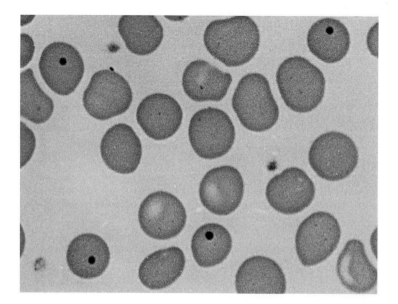

Figure 4–1. Howell-Jolly bodies in an asplenic patient. The remnants of nuclear DNA are the most characteristic findings in patients with depressed splenic function.

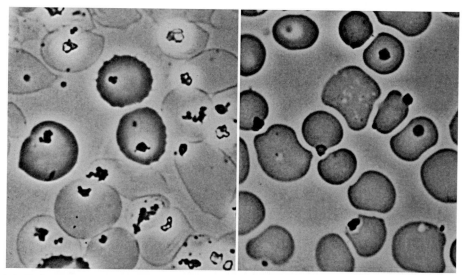

Figure 4–2. Heinz bodies seen by phase contrast microscopy (left) and supravital staining (right). (From Bessis M: Living Blood Cells and Their Ultrastructure, p 214. New York, Springer-Verlag, 1973.)

surface projections, and their presence in the peripheral blood reflects the spleen's loss of the ability to remove deformed erythrocytes (Fig. 4–4).

In contrast to some animal species, normal humans do not become anemic immediately following splenectomy because the human spleen neither stores a large volume of erythrocytes nor produces them. As the red blood cell life span is not prolonged after splenectomy, it is believed that the reticuloendothelial cells of other organs, such as the liver and lymph nodes, assume the function of the destruction of senescent erythrocytes.[10] Nucleated red blood cells are rarely seen in the peripheral blood following splenectomy, and the reticulocyte count remains normal.

Individuals with normal hematologic function do not become polycythemic following splenectomy,[10, 11] but there may be a transient leukocytosis, usually in the range of 10,000 to 15,000/mm³.[1] Approximately 60 percent of

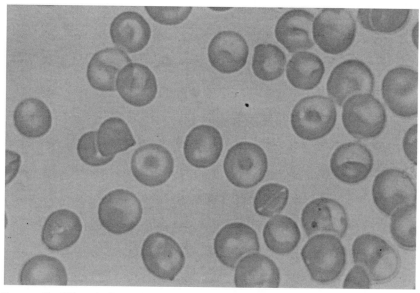

Figure 4–3. Target cells. Although these cells characteristically occur in asplenic patients, they are not unique for that condition and may be seen in a variety of disorders, including liver disease.

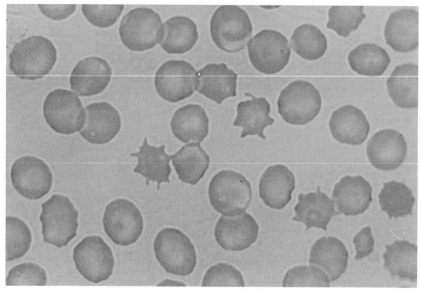

Figure 4–4. Acanthocytes. These also are not specific for splenic hypofunction, and may be seen in a variety of other disorders.

individuals develop a relative or absolute lymphocytosis, and 30 percent develop a relative or absolute monocytosis.[12] There may also be granulocytosis and a mild eosinophilia and basophilia. Although the leukocytosis is usually transient, in approximately 25 percent of patients the white blood cell count may remain mildly elevated and usually displays a lymphocytosis and monocytosis. The leukocyte count in asplenic patients may show a greater fluctuation than in persons with normal splenic function, and patients with apparently elevated or depressed counts should have repeated complete blood counts performed to confirm the persistence of these values.[1, 2] The platelet count may also show a striking elevation immediately following splenectomy, but it usually normalizes within 1 month.[13, 14]

The postsplenectomy blood picture varies in patients whose spleens are removed for underlying hematologic disorders. A postsplenectomy polycythemia (erythrocytosis) is characteristic

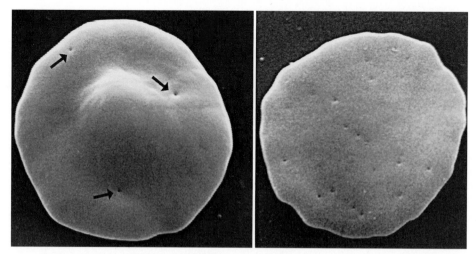

Figure 4–5. Scanning electron micrograph of red blood cells in asplenic patient, demonstrating surface pits. The cell on the left contains three pits (arrows). The cell on the right has numerous pits. An increase in the percentage of red blood cells with these pits is the most sensitive indication of decreased splenic function. (Courtesy of Michael Goheen.)

of hereditary spherocytosis.[10] Patients with myeloproliferative disorders or hemolytic conditions may develop persistent thrombocytosis after splenectomy that can be potentially dangerous. This is especially true in polycythemia vera and essential thrombocythemia.[15, 16] In these disorders the postoperative platelet count may reach dangerously high levels, resulting in thromboses.

Another morphologic expression of hyposplenism is the presence of "pits" or pock-marks in the surface membranes of erythrocytes[17–19]; these pits represent vacuolar inclusions of excess cell membrane that dispose of solid material from the red blood cell in the absence of a functional spleen.[20–22] Normally, erythrocytes lose surface area as they mature owing to the removal of protein-lipid components of the cell membrane by the spleen. The presence of a large number of these pits reflects the lack of splenic removal of cell membrane components. The pits appear as depressions in the cell membrane and are visible only with phase-contrast or scanning electron microscopy. Such pits are seen in 2 to 5 percent of erythrocytes in eusplenic persons,[23–25] but they are usually seen in more than 20 percent of erythrocytes in splenectomized patients and may approach 40 to 50 percent in some cases. The number of pits may vary greatly among red blood cells (Fig. 4–5). The number of pits appears to be inversely proportional to the relative degree of splenic function.[26] Pit counts have been shown to be increased during fetal life, averaging almost 50 percent in premature infants and about 25 percent in term infants.[18]

Because it is important to define accurately which patients, especially children, are at increased risk for infection associated with hyposplenism, there have been attempts to determine whether Howell-Jolly body counts or pitted red blood cell counts are more sensitive and specific in quantitating splenic filtration function. Howell-Jolly body counting has long been used as a screening method,[10] and some authors[27] formerly used this technique to quantitate splenic hypofunction. However, Casper et al[17] have argued that Howell-Jolly body counts are not a reliable quantitative method, with the result that pitted red blood cell counts have become the favored method of the measurement of splenic function.[23, 28, 29] It has been suggested that erythrocyte surface pits are a more reliable indication of splenic hypofunction than Howell-Jolly bodies, because the latter occur only in persons with virtually complete absence of splenic function.[24] Corazza et al[22] compared Howell-Jolly body counting with pitted red blood cell counting. They found a close correlation between the two methods overall but demonstrated that pitted cell counts had a greater degree of sensitivity in defining mild examples of splenic hypofunction. They concluded that pitted cell counting was the more sensitive method but that Howell-Jolly body counting was a simpler yet equally reliable technique for identifying and following patients with a clinically significant risk of infection associated with hyposplenism. Recently, Tham et al[30] have proposed a method of assessing splenic filtration function by counting red blood cells with argyrophilic inclusions using a silver stain. The method correlates well with pit counting, and it has the advantage of requiring no specialized equipment other than a microscope.

CAUSES OF HYPOSPLENISM

Splenectomy is by far the most common cause of hyposplenism (Table 4–2). Complete asplenia is otherwise very rare. Congenital asplenia is part of a syndrome that, in most cases, includes cardiovascular abnormalities and occasionally pulmonary malformations and situs inversus of the abdominal viscera.[31–34] Congenital hypoplasia of the spleen is somewhat less rare. It may occur in cases of Fanconi anemia in association with marrow hypoplasia. It has been postulated that this disorder may represent a generalized failure of mesenchymal organs to develop properly.[10] Normal newborn infants may have rare Howell-Jolly bodies in the peripheral blood as evidence of immaturity of the spleen, and premature infants may have a more marked deficiency in splenic function. Moreover, erythrocyte pit counts have been shown to be increased in newborns.[18] These findings are usually transient, and counts return to normal within a few months after birth.[10] However, the presence and persistence of a significant number of Howell-Jolly bodies in the peripheral blood, particularly in term infants, should be considered evidence of absent or deficient splenic function.[31]

Normal splenic function also decreases in old age in association with the decreases in splenic weight and general immune function that occur in this age.[35] That splenic filtration

Table 4–2. Disorders Associated
with Hyposplenism

I. Congenital
  A. Asplenia
  B. Hypoplasia
  C. Immunodeficiency disorders
II. Acquired
  A. Splenectomy
  B. Acquired atrophy and/or infarction
    1. Sickle cell disease
    2. Vascular disorders (vasculitides,
       thromboembolic conditions)
    3. Essential thrombocythemia
    4. Malabsorption syndromes
    5. Autoimmune diseases
    6. Irradiation
    7. Cytotoxic chemotherapy
    8. Chronic alcoholism
    9. Hypopituitarism
  C. Functional asplenia with normal-sized or enlarged
    spleen
    1. Infiltration by leukemia, lymphoma, multiple
       myeloma, mastocytosis
    2. Early (splenomegalic) sickle cell disease
    3. Amyloidosis
    4. Sarcoidosis
    5. Benign and malignant vascular tumors
    6. Malabsorption syndromes
  D. Depressed immune function
    1. AIDS
    2. Status post
      a. Irradiation
      b. Cytotoxic chemotherapy
      c. Immunosuppressive agents, including
        corticosteroids
    3. Endocrine disorders
      a. Hypothyroidism
      b. Hypopituitarism
      c. Diabetes mellitus
    4. Chronic alcoholism

function also decreases is demonstrated by studies indicating increased red blood cell pit counts and impaired clearance of heat-damaged erythrocytes in elderly people.[36] Although the decrease in splenic function in old age is real, it appears to have little clinical significance.

Hyposplenism due to acquired atrophy of the spleen is much more frequent than congenital asplenia or splenic hypoplasia and may be associated with a variety of conditions. The most common of these is sickle cell disease. In advanced stages of this disorder, the spleen becomes fibrotic and nonfunctional (Color Plate 4) owing to autoinfarction resulting from the clogging of the splenic microvasculature with sickled cells (Fig. 4–6). Splenic size and function do not correlate ideally, however, because functional hyposplenism, thought to re-

sult from the progressive atrophy of the organ, is common in children in the splenomegalic phase of sickle cell disease.[10, 37–39] There is some evidence that the progressive decrease in both the size and function of the spleen in sickle cell disease is reversible. Several studies have documented an improvement in splenic function, as measured by erythrocyte pit counts, and an increase in splenic size, as measured by palpation or spleen scans, after transfusion.[37–41] The fact that no improvement in function occurs after infusions of plasma suggests that hyposplenism is not related to decreased plasma volume or to deficiencies of opsonins or other humoral factors.[39] Correction of splenic dysfunction in sickle cell disease has also been reported following bone marrow transplantation[42] and most recently has been documented in patients receiving hydroxyurea.[43] It has been suggested that functional hyposplenism in patients with sickle cell disease is related to the high blood viscosity that causes diversion of splenic blood flow through arteriovenous shunts in the red pulp that bypass phagocytic cells.[38] Blood transfusion and marrow transplantation decrease blood viscosity by dilution or replacement of the sickle cells by normal hemoglobin-containing red blood cells. Hydroxyurea may function in a similar manner because it increases hemoglobin F levels and retards sickling.[44] There is some evidence that return of splenic function is associated with regeneration of splenic parenchyma.[43]

Splenic atrophy may also occur in the course of essential thrombocythemia, with infarction probably secondary to the stagnation of masses of platelets.[16, 45, 46] Infiltration of the spleen by leukemia or lymphoma may also occasionally produce the peripheral blood findings of functional hyposplenism. Hyposplenism in these cases may be due to defective filtration because of massive infiltration by leukemic cells or may be a result of splenic infarction. Splenic infarction in these cases probably results from compression of vessels by tumor cells, from leukostatic thrombi, or from tumor infiltration of the subendothelial zones of the trabecular vessels with subsequent thrombosis.

Splenic hypofunction has been reported in a series of patients with acute leukemias of both myeloid or lymphoid types in which spleen sizes may be either normal or increased according to clinical parameters.[47] Using erythrocyte pit counts, more than 50 percent of patients were found to have evidence of

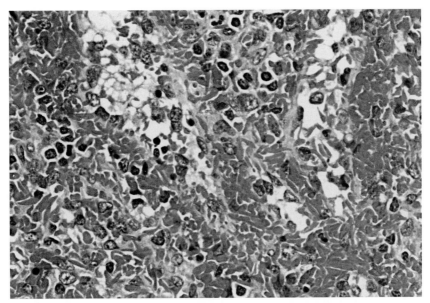

Figure 4–6. Sickle cell disease. Splenic cords and sinuses are clogged with sickled erythrocytes.

functional hyposplenism. In four of seven cases in which clearance of heat-damaged erythrocytes was also measured, similar results were found.

Partial or complete atrophy of the spleen without infarction is an uncommon complication of some of the malabsorption syndromes.[48–53] This has been reported in patients with celiac sprue, ulcerative colitis, and (rarely) Crohn disease. The degree of hyposplenism in these disorders does not correlate with splenic size; the peripheral blood findings characteristic of asplenia may occur in patients with normal-sized spleens. The degree of hyposplenism often increases and decreases with the activity of the intestinal disease.[37] The hyposplenism cannot be attributed to malnutrition because it does not occur in starvation.[10] These malabsorption syndromes are often associated with circulating autoantibodies, and it is possible that the depressed splenic function in these conditions may be an autoimmune phenomenon.[2, 54] This thesis is supported by the observation that the systemic autoimmune diseases are associated with an increased incidence of hyposplenism.[55] Wardrop and associates[54] studied 14 patients who had the peripheral blood findings of hyposplenism. Eight of these patients were found to have a malabsorption syndrome. Four others had clinically apparent autoimmune disease. However, many of the other patients in the study without clinical autoimmune diseases

had circulating autoantibodies. Antithyroglobulin antibody was seen in high titers in some cases, and antinuclear and anti–smooth muscle antibodies in low titers were also found.

Therapeutic irradiation of the spleen may result in splenic atrophy and functional hyposplenism.[56, 57] The morphologic changes are characteristic in delayed radiation injury. The spleen so treated is small, appears collapsed, and often has wrinkled, thickened capsules (Fig. 4–7). Histologically, the white pulp appears hypocellular with depletion of the lymphoid elements, leaving the relatively radioresistant nonlymphoid framework (Fig. 4–8). The red pulp shows variable fibrosis, in some instances resulting in rigid, open sinuses. In cases with severe fibrosis, the normal sinusoidal architecture may be obliterated. The vascular changes are the most reliable indication of radiation exposure. Both arteries and veins show mild intimal proliferation, often with enlarged, hyperchromatic endothelial cell nuclei and with subintimal foamy macrophages (Fig. 4–9). Arteries and arterioles may show reduplication of the elastic lamina. Some arterial intimal thickening may occur as early as 2 months after the initiation of radiotherapy, although severe damage usually does not occur before 1 year. Doses of radiation as small as 1000 to 2000 rad (centigray) may be sufficient to cause vascular damage. In cases in which radiation is given for hematologic malignancies, these changes are independent of the involvement

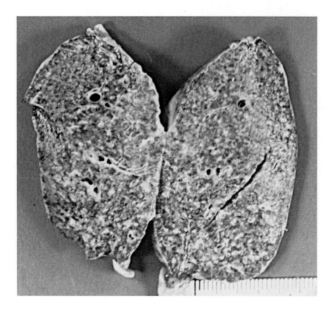

Figure 4–7. Shrunken and fibrotic spleen in patient exposed to 4500 centigrays as treatment for Hodgkin's disease. The miliary white nodules on the cut surface represent areas of fibrosis, not Hodgkin's disease.

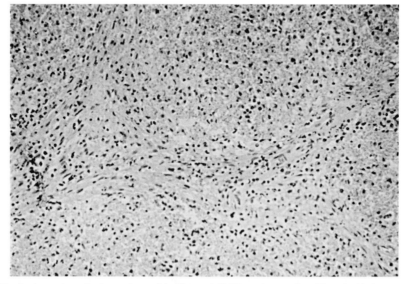

Figure 4–8. Histologic section of spleen pictured in Figure 4–7. There is atrophy of lymphoid tissue and fibrosis of the cords of Billroth.

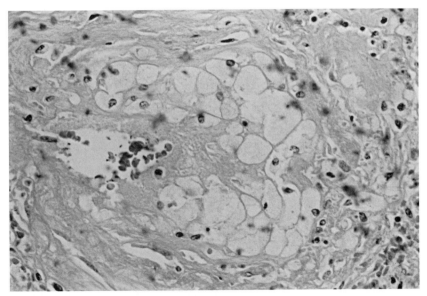

Figure 4–9. Subintimal collection of foam cells in splenic arteriole postirradiation.

of the spleen by tumor. A similar picture has been reported in the spleens of patients exposed to thorium dioxide (Thorotrast), a radioactive compound emitting alpha rays that was formerly used as an angiographic dye (Fig. 4–10).[58–60] Thorotrast is retained in the lymphoreticular system and may cause splenic atrophy and fibrosis many years after exposure. This agent has also been associated with hepatic angiosarcomas and cholangiocarcinomas, but splenic tumors have not been noted.

Splenic atrophy, particularly of the white pulp, is common following cytotoxic chemotherapy (Fig. 4–11). Splenic atrophy has also been reported in chronic alcoholism, hypopituitarism, and hyperthyroidism (Graves disease).[10] This latter condition may also be associated with the presence of autoantibodies.[61] Other, rare causes of splenic atrophy include splenic arterial embolization and splenic vein thrombosis.

Although most cases of hyposplenism are associated with splenic atrophy, evidence of functional hyposplenism may occasionally oc-

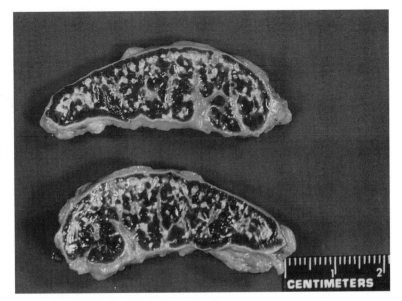

Figure 4–10. Cross section of spleen from patient exposed to Thorotrast. The organ is shrunken, and the capsule is thickened and wrinkled. The cross section of the organ is riddled with areas of fibrosis.

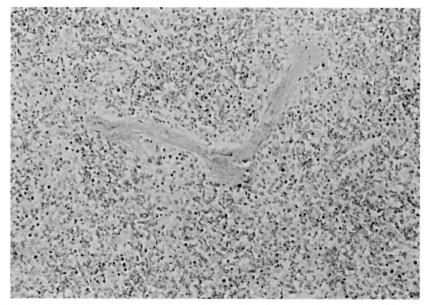

Figure 4–11. Section of spleen after several courses of multiagent chemotherapy. The white pulp is atrophic.

cur in patients whose spleens are normal or increased in size.[24, 37] This has been reported in a variety of conditions, including sarcoidosis,[62, 63] amyloidosis,[64, 65] and systemic lupus erythematosus,[55, 66] as well as in such neoplastic disorders involving the spleen as myeloma, metastatic carcinoma, angiosarcoma, systemic mastocytosis, and lymphomas and leukemias.[47, 67–70] It is also common in the early stages of sickle cell disease.[26]

Depressed Splenic Immune Function

The immunodeficiency disorders are not usually included among the causes of hyposplenism because they represent systemic diseases of the immune system and because the functions of the red pulp of the spleen are not impaired; however, they are discussed here because they represent depressed function of the splenic white pulp.

The white pulp of the spleen in the congenital immunodeficiency disorders may be severely depleted (see Fig. 4–11) or may resemble the normal immunologically unstimulated adult spleen (Fig. 4–12). The actual mass of lymphoid tissue present varies with the type and severity of the disorder. The deficiency may affect either B or T lymphocytes selectively or may involve the lymphoid stem cell.[71–74]

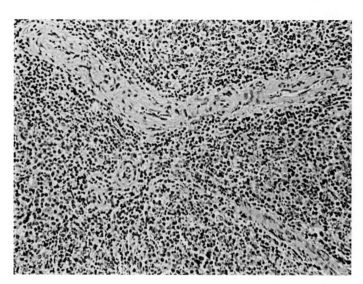

Figure 4–12. Agammaglobulinemia. The lymphoid tissue surrounding the central artery and arterioles of the follicle is depleted. There are scattered lymphocytes but no structural organization of the follicle.

Most of the primary immunodeficiency disorders are manifested by recurrent infections in infancy and childhood. The splenic morphology reflects the cell line involved. Deficiencies involving B lymphocytes show depleted or inactive white pulp without germinal center formation and without plasmacytosis. Clinically, deficiency in humoral immunity leads to recurrent infections with pyogenic bacteria. T-cell deficiencies result in depletion of the periarterial lymphoid sheaths (PALS) and are clinically reflected in deficient cell-mediated immunity as manifested by fungal infections and by impaired allograft rejection.

Each of the various congenital immunodeficiency disorders will not be discussed here in detail because the findings in the spleen are similar in many. As examples, we describe three. One of the most common and most severe is X-linked agammaglobulinemia, or agammaglobulinemia of Bruton, a B-cell deficiency. Spleens from infants with this disorder show trabeculae that are virtually devoid of lymphoid sheaths and small lymphoid follicles that lack germinal centers (see Fig. 4–12). The few lymphocytes present show no evidence of activation. In contrast, the spleen in DiGeorge syndrome of thymic hypoplasia shows depletion of the thymic-dependent T-cell zones, including the PALS (Fig. 4–13). Severe combined immunodeficiency is a heterogeneous disorder characterized by profound B- and T-lymphocyte deficiency. Spleens from children show virtual absence of lymphoid tissue (Fig. 4–14). Occasionally the PALS in the spleens of patients with severe combined immunodeficiency may appear histologically normal. However, immunohistologic stains reveal a severe depletion of T cells with only B cells remaining.[75]

In common variable immunodeficiency, 30 percent of the patients present with splenomegaly. The white pulp appears increased in size and reveals prominent germinal centers. The red pulp macrophages display diminished lysozyme and nonspecific esterase activity.[76] Sarcoidlike epithelioid cell granulomas are also frequently found.[77]

Sarcoidal-type granulomas may also be found in other congenital immunodeficiency disorders (see Chapter 6). This is particularly true for selective IgA deficiency.[77, 78] Spleens in patients with IgA deficiency may also show loosely formed clusters of epithelioid histiocytes in the cords of Billroth.

The ability of the spleen to respond to antigenic stimulation can be affected by extrinsic and intrinsic factors. Cytotoxic chemotherapy and radiotherapy may deplete lymphoid tissue. Immunosuppressive agents, including corticosteroids and antilymphocyte serum, may also diminish or abolish the ability of the white pulp to react to antigens. In addition, the patient's endocrine status may affect the splenic immune response. Patients with hypothyroidism or hypoadrenalism, or occasionally those with diabetes mellitus, may have a diminished immune response and accompanying splenic lymphoid depletion.

Patients with AIDS are susceptible to opportunistic infections and Kaposi sarcoma because of a profound derangement of their immune systems resulting from infection by the retrovirus HIV. The morphologic features of spleens

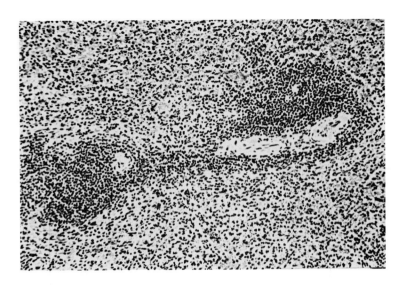

Figure 4–13. DiGeorge syndrome. Lymphoid tissue is present but is composed exclusively of B lymphocytes. The section resembles splenic white pulp in premature infants or in very old patients.

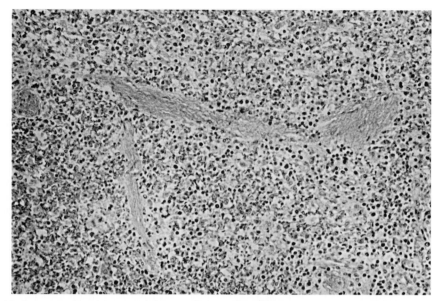

Figure 4–14. Severe combined immunodeficiency disease. The white pulp appears depleted of lymphoid elements, leaving the trabecular structures without an appreciable lymphoid sheath.

obtained at autopsy from patients with AIDS reflect the generalized lymphoid atrophy characteristic of the late stages of this disorder. The white pulp is most often markedly depleted.[79] However, in occasional cases, there may be a proliferation of immunoblasts in the red or white pulp.[80] In some cases the lymphoid follicles and PALS appear replaced by fibrillar or hyalinized material.[81] Occasionally, microabscesses may occur in the white pulp. The red pulp is congested and shows a variable degree of plasmacytosis, which is striking in some cases. The red pulp may also be fibrotic. Erythrophagocytosis can sometimes be demonstrated in touch imprints. In some cases, infectious agents such as *Pneumocystis carinii* (Fig. 4–15) can be identified.[79, 81] In addition, Kaposi sarcoma may be present, predominantly in a perivascular distribution.[81]

One of the authors of this book reviewed the morphologic features of the spleens obtained at autopsy from 14 patients with AIDS, all of whom were homosexual males. Two spleens were involved by malignant lymphoma. The remaining 12 spleens ranged in weight from 195 to 2600 g, with a mean weight of 480 g. All showed lymphoid depletion and plasmacytosis of the red pulp. Scattered foci of extramedullary hematopoiesis were common. Cryptococcosis was found in one spleen; the spleen of a patient with disseminated *Mycobacterium avium-intracellulare* (Fig. 4–16) showed

sheets of foamy histiocytes containing acid-fast bacilli. None of the spleens showed Kaposi sarcoma. Immunologic studies in two cases showed a depletion of T lymphocytes. In particular, only rare CD4-positive cells were demonstrated. These findings correlate with the depletion of CD4 cells in the peripheral blood characteristic of AIDS and with the defect in immunoregulatory T cells associated with this disease.

POSTSPLENECTOMY INFECTION

The most clinically dangerous and feared complication of the loss of splenic function occurs most frequently after splenectomy and has been termed "overwhelming postsplenectomy infection" (OPSI).[82] As early as 1919,[82] it had been suggested that splenectomy might predispose a patient to infection. However, the study of King and Shumaker,[83] reporting severe infections in five infants who had been splenectomized for hereditary spherocytosis, was the first to receive attention.

There is now no question that there is an increased risk of septicemia in patients who have had previous splenectomy.[82–90] In many cases, particularly in infants and in patients with underlying hematologic diseases, this septicemia is fulminating.[91–96] Because of the absence of the spleen, rapid unopposed pro-

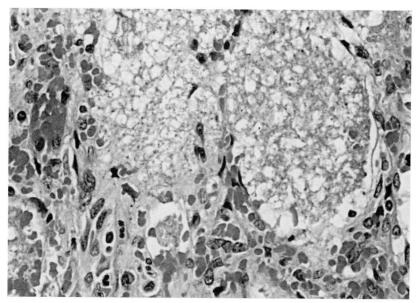

Figure 4–15. Spleen showing involvement of *Pneumocystis carinii.* The characteristic bubbly material is present in the sinuses.

liferation of bacteria may occur and may lead to shock, disseminated intravascular coagulation and, in some cases, bilateral adrenal hemorrhages (Waterhouse-Friderichsen syndrome).[97–100]

The incidence of OPSI is difficult to assess. Most reports do not indicate the number of splenectomized patients at risk at their institutions during the time interval from which their OPSI cases were obtained. In addition, most studies do not distinguish between different groups of patients with apparently varying risks. The risk of postsplenectomy infection appears highest in young children and is most frequent in the first 2 years after splenectomy.[101] However, such infections have been reported even decades after surgical removal of the spleen.[102, 103] There appears to be a correlation between the age of the splenectomized patient and the interval between splenectomy and the development of the infection: the younger the patient, the shorter the interval. The risk of infection in otherwise healthy adults, in whom the spleen is removed because of traumatic rupture or other nonhematologic disorders, has been a subject of debate. It is generally accepted that these individuals do have a slightly increased risk over age- and sex-matched control subjects, although the risk appears to be nowhere near as great as that in children, immunosuppressed individuals,[92, 93, 100, 104] and patients with

diseases involving the immune system, such as autoimmune hemolytic anemia.[105] The incidence of infection appears to be less in patients who have been splenectomized following traumatic rupture of the spleen. This is thought to be due to the protective effect of splenosis, which occurs in many such patients (see Chapter 1).

Because of these variables, the incidence of OPSI is reported to vary from 1 to 10 percent, with a mortality rate estimated to be slightly over one half of the incidence rates. The most comprehensive studies, with the longest follow-up and the inclusion of the most patients in differing risk groups, indicate that the overall incidence appears to be between 3 and 4 percent, with a mortality rate of 1.5 to 2.5 percent.[105, 106]

As discussed in Chapter 2, the spleen plays an important role in the immune response to circulating particulate antigens. In particular, the spleen is central in the host defense against polysaccharide-encapsulated bacteria. It is usually stated that the spleen functions in this regard by filtering organisms out of the peripheral blood so that they are prevented from multiplying in the circulation. The true mechanisms appear more complex. In experimental animals, the lungs and liver are the primary organs responsible for clearing pneumococci from the blood.[107] The spleen makes little further contribution. There is also little

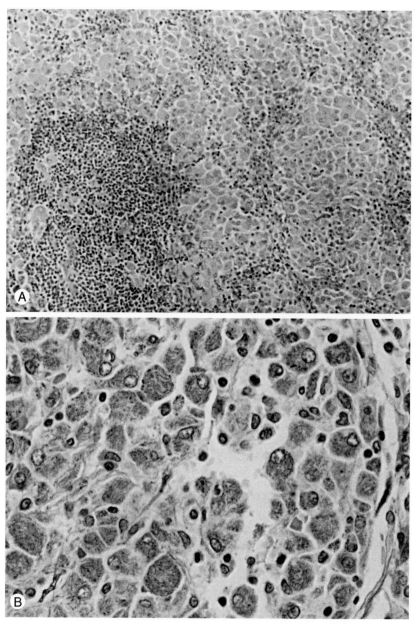

Figure 4–16. (A) *Mycobacterium avium-intracellulare* infection in the spleen in a patient with AIDS. (B) Acid-fast stain showing numerous mycobacteria in macrophages.

evidence to suggest that either total or type-specific antipneumococci antibodies decreased after splenectomy. However, there is evidence of a decrease in serum IgM levels[108, 109] and decreased IgG and IgM response to subcutaneously administered pneumococcal polysaccharide after splenectomy.[110] It appears that the spleen is important in protecting against these organisms because of its ability to rapidly produce type-specific IgM that facilitates phagocytosis and because it is the most effective site of phagocytosis and destruction of these organisms once they are antibody-coated.[111, 112]

The most common organism responsible for the OPSI syndrome in both children and adults is *Streptococcus pneumoniae*, which accounts for approximately two thirds of such infections.[113, 114] The subtypes of streptococci responsible for the postsplenectomy septicemia appear to be uncommon ones, suggesting that the prior acquisition of an infection with the more commonly occurring subtypes before the spleen is removed results in the establishment of permanent type-specific immunity.[101] The bacterial subtypes therefore most likely to cause the syndrome are those to which the individual has had least chance of presplenectomy exposure and therefore has developed no type-specific antibody. The development of polyvalent antipneumococcus vaccine (Pneumovax) had provided susceptible individuals with a means to be somewhat protected from overwhelming infection.[115]

Less commonly, postsplenectomy septicemia may be caused by other encapsulated bacteria such as *Haemophilus influenzae* as well as occasionally by *Staphylococcus aureus* and *Neisseria meningitidis*.[115] Fulminant postsplenectomy infection has been reported following a dog bite, owing to aerobic gram-negative bacilli, particularly a strain called DF-2 bacillus.[116–119] Malarial infection may also follow a more fulminant course in splenectomized patients, and *Babesia*, a malarialike parasite that usually produces self-limited infections in healthy persons, may cause fatal infection in asplenic persons.[114, 116, 120] In 10 to 15 percent of the cases, a causative organism is not identified. There does not appear to be an increased risk of viral infection in the splenectomized individual.

Because of the spleen's major role in immune function, several investigators have addressed the question of whether there is an increased cancer risk after splenectomy. Two studies[121, 122] followed groups of patients who underwent splenectomy for trauma; the studies found no long-term postsplenectomy increase in cancer incidence. There was an observed excess in some specific tumors after splenectomy in patients with certain benign and malignant disorders, but the significance of this observation was questioned in this group of patients because many received potentially carcinogenic therapeutic regimens as treatment of their underlying diseases.

REFERENCES

1. Lipson RL, Bayrd ED, Watkins CH: The post-splenectomy blood picture. Am J Clin Pathol 1959; 32:526.
2. Crosby WH: Structure and functions of the spleen, in Williams WJ, Beutler E, Erslev AJ, et al (eds): Hematology, 3rd ed, p 89. New York, McGraw-Hill, 1983.
3. Singer K, Miller EB, Dameshek W: Hematologic changes following splenectomy in man with particular reference to target cells. Am J Med Sci 1941; 202:171.
4. Pepper OHP, Austin JH: A twenty-eight year follow-up on a splenectomy for hemolytic anemia: Persistence of Howell-Jolly bodies. JAMA 1943; 122:870.
5. Selwyn JG: Heinz bodies in red cells after splenectomy and after phenacetin administration. Br J Haematol 1955; 1:173.
6. Crosby WH: Siderocytes and the spleen. Blood 1957; 12:165.
7. Douglas AS, Dacie JV: Incidence and significance of iron-containing granules in human erythrocytes and their precursors. J Clin Pathol 1953; 6:307.
8. Crosby WH: The pathogenesis of spherocytes and leptocytes (target cells). Blood 1952; 7:261.
9. Dean HM: Acanthocytes after splenectomy. N Engl J Med 1968; 279:947.
10. Crosby WH: Hyposplenism: An inquiry into normal functions of the spleen. Ann Rev Med 1963; 14:349.
11. Crosby WH: Normal functions of the spleen relative to red blood cells: A review. Blood 1959; 14:399.
12. McBride JA, Dacie JV, Shapley R: The effect of splenectomy on the leucocyte count. Br J Haematol 1968; 14:225.
13. Hirsh J, Dacie JV: Persistent post-splenectomy thrombocytosis and thromboembolism. Br J Haematol 1966; 12:44.
14. Zuricker M: Beiträge zum Einfluss der Splenectomie auf Blutbild und Knochenmarksausstrich. Folia Haematol (Leipz) 1956; 74:109.
15. Gordon DH, Schaffner D, Bennett JM, et al: Postsplenectomy thrombocytosis: Its association with mesenteric, portal, and/or renal vein thrombosis in patients with myeloproliferative disorders. Arch Surg 1978; 113:713.
16. Gunz FW: Hemorrhagic thrombocythemia: A critical review. Blood 1960; 15:706.
17. Casper TJ, Koethe SM, Rodey GE, et al: A new method for studying reticuloendothelial dysfunction in sickle cell disease patients and its clinical application: A brief report. Blood 1976; 47:183.
18. Holroyde CP, Oski FA, Gardner FH: The "pocked" erythrocyte: Red-cell surface alterations in reticuloendothelial immaturity of the neonate. N Engl J Med 1969; 281:516.
19. Koyama S, Aoki S, Deguchi K: Electron microscopic observations of the splenic red pulp with special reference to the pitting function. Mei Med J 1964; 14:143.
20. Schnitzer B, Rucknagel DL, Spencer HH, et al: Erythrocytes: Pits and vacuoles as seen with transmission and scanning electron microscopy. Science 1971; 173:251.
21. Reinhart WH, Chien S: Red cell vacuoles: Their size and distribution under normal conditions and after splenectomy. Am J Hematol 1988; 27:265.
22. Corazza GR, Ginaldi L, Zoli G, et al: Howell-Jolly body counting as a measure of splenic function: A reassessment. Clin Lab Haemat 1990; 12:269.
23. Pearson HA, Johnston D, Smith KA, et al: The born-again spleen: Return of splenic function after splenectomy for trauma. N Engl J Med 1978; 298:1389.
24. Corrigan JJ Jr, Van Wyck DB, Crosby WH: Clinical disorders of splenic function: The spectrum from asplenism to hypersplenism. Lymphology 1983; 16:101.
25. Buchanan GR, Holtkamp CA: Splenic reticuloendo-

thelial function in children with cancer. J Pediatr 1985; 106:239.

26. Pearson HA, McIntosh S, Ritchey AK, et al: Developmental aspects of splenic function in sickle cell diseases. Blood 1979; 53:358.

27. McCarthy CF, Fraser ID, Evans KT, et al: Lymphoreticular dysfunction in idiopathic steatorrhoea. Gut 1996; 7:140.

28. Corazza GR, Bullen AW, Hall R, et al: Simple method of assessing splenic function in coeliac disease. Clin Sci 1981; 60:109.

29. Pearson HA, Gallagher D, Chilcote R, et al: Developmental pattern of splenic dysfunction in sickle cell disorders. Pediatrics 1985; 76:392.

30. Tham KT, Teague MW, Howard CA, et al: A simple splenic reticuloendothelial function test. Am J Clin Pathol 1996; 105:548.

31. Bush JA, Ainger LE: Congenital absence of spleen with congenital heart disease: Report of a case with ante-mortem diagnosis on the basis of hematologic morphology. Pediatrics 1955; 15:93.

32. Esterly JR, Oppenheimer EH: Lymphangiectasis and other pulmonary lesions in the asplenia syndrome. Arch Pathol 1970; 90:553.

33. Mauck HR Jr, Segatol-Islami Z, Lester RG: Splenic agenesis associated with severe congenital heart disease: Long survival unassociated with pulmonary stenosis—report of a case. Dis Chest 1966; 49:436.

34. Putschar WGJ, Manion WC: Congenital absence of the spleen and associated anomalies. Am J Clin Pathol 1956; 26:429.

35. Markus HS, Toghill PJ: Impaired splenic function in elderly people. Age Ageing 1991; 20:287.

36. Zago MA, Figueiredo MS, Conas PT, et al: Aspects of splenic hypofunction in old age. Klin Wochenschr 1985; 63:590.

37. Eichner ER: Splenic function: Normal, too much and too little. Am J Med 1979; 66:311.

38. Pearson HA, Cornelius EA, Schwartz AD, et al: Transfusion-reversible functional asplenia in young children with sickle-cell anemia. N Engl J Med 1970; 83:334.

39. Pearson HA, Spencer RP, Cornelius EA: Functional asplenia in sickle-cell anemia. N Engl J Med 1969; 281:923.

40. Buchanan GR, McKie V, Jackson EA, et al: Splenic phagocytic function in children with sickle cell anemia receiving long-term hypertransfusion. J Pediatr 1989; 115:568.

41. Wethers DL, Grover R: Reversibility of splenic function by transfusion in two young adults with sickle cell anemia. Am J Pediatr Hematol Oncol 1987; 9:209.

42. Ferster A, Bryan W, Corazza F, et al: Bone marrow transplantation corrects the splenic reticuloendothelial dysfunction in sickle cell anemia. Blood 1993; 81:1102.

43. Claster S, Vichinsky E: First report of reversal of organ dysfunction in sickle cell anemia by the use of hydroxyurea: Splenic regeneration. Blood 1996; 88:1951.

44. Charache S, Dover GJ, Moyer MA, et al: Hydroxyurea-induced augmentation of fetal hemoglobin production in patients with sickle cell anemia. Blood 1987; 69:109.

45. Hardisty RM, Wolff HH: Haemorrhagic thrombocythaemia: A clinical and laboratory study. Br J Haematol 1955; 1:390.

46. Marsh GW, Lewis SM, Szur L: The use of ^{51}Cr-labeled heat-damaged red cells to study splenic function. I. Splenic atrophy in thrombocythaemia. Br J Haematol 1966; 12:167.

47. Simoes BP, Tone LG, Zago MA, et al: Splenic function in acute leukemia. Acta Haematologica 1955; 94:123.

48. Ferguson A, Hutton MM, Maxwell JD, et al: Adult coeliac disease in hyposplenic patients. Lancet 1970; 1:163.

49. Marsh GW, Stewart JS: Splenic function in adult coeliac disease. Br J Haematol 1970; 19:445.

50. Martin JB, Bell HE: The association of splenic atrophy and intestinal malabsorption: Report of a case and review of the literature. Can Med Assoc J 1965; 92:875.

51. McCarthy CF, Fraser ID, Evans KT, Read AE: Lymphoreticular dysfunction in idiopathic steatorrhoea. Gut 1966; 7:410.

52. Morowitz DA, Allen LW, Kirsner JB: Thrombocytosis in chronic inflammatory bowel disease. Ann Intern Med 1968; 68:1013.

53. Ryan FP, Smart RC, Holdsworth CD, et al: Hyposplenism in inflammatory bowel disease. Gut 1970; 19:50.

54. Wardrop CAJ, Dagg JH, Lee FD, et al: Immunological abnormalities in splenic atrophy. Lancet 1975; 2:4.

55. Dillon AM, Stein HB, English RA: Splenic atrophy in systemic lupus erythematosus. Ann Intern Med 1982; 96:40.

56. Dailey MO, Coleman CN, Fajardo LF: Splenic injury caused by therapeutic irradiation. Am J Surg Pathol 1981; 5:325.

57. Dailey MO, Coleman CN, Kaplan HS: Radiation-induced splenic atrophy in patients with Hodgkin's disease and non-Hodgkin's lymphomas. N Engl J Med 1980; 302:215.

58. Bensinger TA, Keller AR, Merrell LF, et al: Thorotrast-induced reticulo-endothelial blockade in man. Am J Med 1971; 51:663.

59. Langlands AO, Williamson ER: Late changes in peripheral blood after thorotrast administration. Br Med J 1967; 3:206.

60. Looney WB: An investigation of the late clinical findings following thorotrast (thorium dioxide) administration. Am J Roentgenol Rad Ther Nucl Med 1960; 83:163.

61. Brownlie BE, Hamer JW, Cook HB, et al: Thyrotoxicosis associated with splenic atrophy. Lancet 1975; 2:1046.

62. Guyton JR, Zumwalt RE: Pneumococcemia with sarcoid-infiltrated spleen. Ann Intern Med 1968; 68:1013.

63. Stone RW, McDaniel WR, Armstrong EM, et al: Acquired functional splenia in sarcoidosis. J Natl Med Assoc 1985; 77:935.

64. Gertz MA, Kyle RA, Greipp PR: Hyposplenism in primary systemic amyloidosis. Ann Intern Med 1983; 98:475.

65. Stone MJ, Frendel EP: The clinical spectrum of light chain myeloma: A study of 35 patients with special reference to the occurrence of amyloidosis. Am J Med 1975; 58:601.

66. Piliero P, Furie R: Functional asplenia in systemic lupus erythematosus. Semin Arthritis Rheum 1990; 20:185.

67. Budke, HL, Breitfeld PP, Neiman RS: Functional hyposplenism due to a primary epithelioid hemangi-

oendothelioma of the spleen. Arch Pathol Lab Med 1995; 119:755.

68. Yucel AE, Durak H, Bernay I, et al: Functional asplenia and portal hypertension in a patient with primary splenic hemangiosarcoma. Clin Nucl Med 1990; 15:324.

69. Roth J, Brudler O, Henze E: Functional asplenia in malignant mastocytosis. J Nucl Med 1985; 26:1149.

70. Gross DJ, Braverman AJ, Koren G, et al: Functional asplenia in immunoblastic lymphoma. Arch Intern Med 1982; 142:2213.

71. Ammann AJ: Immunodeficiency diseases, in Stobo JD, Fudenberg HH (eds): Basic and Clinical Immunology, 5th ed, p 384. Los Altos, Lange Medical Publishers, 1984.

72. Reinherz EL, Rosen FS: New concepts of immunodeficiency. Am J Med 1981; 71:511.

73. WHO Report: Immunodeficiency. Clin Immunol Immunopathol 1979; 13:296.

74. van Houte AJ, Schuurman HJ, Huber J, et al: The periarteriolar lymphocyte sheath in immunodeficiency T- or B-lymphocyte area. Am J Clin Pathol 1990; 94:318.

75. Weston, J, Balfour BM, Tsohas W, et al: Splenic lesions in hypogammaglobulinaemia. Adv Exp Med Biol 1993; 329:437.

76. Neiman RS: Incidence and importance of splenic sarcoid-like granulomas. Arch Pathol Lab Med 1977; 101:518.

77. Edelstein AD, Miller A, Zimelman AP, et al: Adult severe combined immunodeficiency and sarcoid-like granulomas with hypersplenism. Am J Hematol 1978; 5:55.

78. Urmacher C, Nielsen S: The histopathology of the acquired immune deficiency syndrome. Pathol Ann 1985; 20:197.

79. Klatt EC, Meyer PR: Pathology of the spleen in the acquired immunodeficiency syndrome. Arch Pathol Lab Med 1987; 111:1050.

80. Niedt GW, Schinella RA: Acquired immunodeficiency syndrome: Clinicopathologic study of 56 autopsies. Arch Pathol 1985; 109:727.

81. Balfanz JR, Nesbit ME Jr, Jarvis C, et al: Overwhelming sepsis following splenectomy for trauma. J Pediatr 1988; 88:458.

82. Morris DH, Bulloch FD: The importance of the spleen in resistance to infection. Ann Surg 1919; 70:513.

83. King H, Shumaker HB Jr: Susceptibility to infection after splenectomy performed in infancy. Ann Surg 1952; 136:239.

84. Bisno AL: Hyposplenism and overwhelming pneumococcal infection: A reappraisal. Am J Med Sci 1971; 262:101.

85. Francke EL, Neu HC: Postsplenectomy infection. Surg Clin North Am 1981; 61:135.

86. Krivit W, Giebink GS, Leonard A: Overwhelming post-splenectomy infection. Surg Clin North Am 1979; 59:223.

87. O'Neal BJ, McDonald JC: The risk of sepsis in the asplenic adult. Ann Surg 1981; 194:775.

88. Singer DB: Post-splenectomy sepsis. Perspect Pediatr Pathol 1973; 1:285.

89. Walker W: Splenectomy during childhood in England and Wales. Br J Haematol 1974; 28:145.

90. Eraklis AJ, Kevy SV, Diamond LK, et al: Hazard of overwhelming infection after splenectomy in childhood. N Engl J Med 1967; 276:1225.

91. Gopal V, Bisno AL: Fulminant pneumococcal infections in "normal" asplenic hosts. Arch Intern Med 1977; 173:1526.

92. Hosea SW: Role of the spleen in pneumococcal infection. Lymphology 1983; 16:115.

93. Kitchens CS: The syndrome of post-splenectomy fulminant sepsis: Case report and review of the literature. Am J Med Sci 1977; 274:303.

94. Sullivan JL, Schiffman G, Miser J, et al: Immune response after splenectomy. Lancet 1978; 1:178.

95. Winkelstein JA: Splenectomy and infection. Arch Intern Med 1977; 137:1516.

96. Bisno AL, Freeman JC: The syndrome of asplenia, pneumococcal sepsis, and disseminated intravascular coagulation. Ann Intern Med 1970; 72:389.

97. Coonrod JD, Leach RP: Antigenemia in fulminant pneumococcemia. Ann Intern Med 1976; 84:561.

98. Rytel MW, Dee TH, Fersteinfeld JE, et al: Possible pathogenic role of capsular antigens in fulminant pneumococcal disease with disseminated intravascular coagulation (DIC). Am J Med 1974; 57:889.

99. Sekikawa T, Shatney CH: Septic sequelae after splenectomy for trauma in adults. Am J Surg 1983; 145:667.

100. Smith CH, Erlandson M, Schulman I, et al: Hazard of severe infections in splenectomized infants and children. Am J Med 1957; 22:390.

101. Evans D: Post-splenectomy sepsis 10 years or more after operation. J Clin Pathol 1985; 38:309.

102. Grinblat J, Bilboa Y: Overwhelming pneumococcal sepsis 25 years after splenectomy. Am J Med Sci 1975; 270:523.

103. Zarrabi MH, Rosner F: Serious infection in adults following splenectomy for trauma. Arch Intern Med 1984; 144:1421.

104. Meekes I, van der Staak F, van Oostrom C: Results of splenectomy performed on a group of 91 children. Eur J Ped Surg 1995; 5:19.

105. Singer DB: Post-splenectomy sepsis. Perspect Pediatr Pathol 1973; 1:285.

106. Holdsworth RJ, Neil GD, Irving AD, et al: Blood clearance and tissue distribution of ^{99}Tc-labelled pneumococci following splenectomy in rabbits. Br J Exp Path 1970; 70:669.

107. Spirer Z: The role of the spleen in immunity and infection: Adv Pediatr 1980; 27:55.

108. Neiman RS, Bischel MD, Lukes RJ: Hypersplenism in the uremic hemodialyzed patient: Pathology and proposed pathophysiologic mechanisms. Am J Clin Pathol 1973; 60:502.

109. Hosea SW, Burch CG, Brown EJ, et al: Impaired immune response of splenectomized patients to polyvalent pneumococcal vaccine. Lancet 1981; 1:804.

110. Schumacher MJ: Serum immunoglobulin and transferrin levels after childhood splenectomy. Arch Dis Child 1970; 45:114.

111. Llopis, MJP, Harms G, Hardonk MJ, et al: Human immune response to pneumococcal polysaccharides: Complement-mediated localization preferentially on CD21-positive splenic marginal zone B cells and follicular dendritic cells. J Allergy Clin Immunol 1996; 97:1015.

112. Vay Wyck DB: Overwhelming post-splenectomy infection (OPSI): The clinical syndrome. Lymphology 1983; 16:107.

113. Case Records of the Massachusetts General Hospital: Case 20-1983. N Engl J Med 1983; 308:1212.

114. Ammann AJ, Addiego J, Wara DW, et al: Polyvalent

pneumococcal-polysaccharide immunization of patients with sickle-cell anemia and patients with splenectomy. N Engl J Med 1977; 297:897.

115. Case Records of the Massachusetts General Hospital: Case 29-1986. N Engl J Med 1986; 315:241.

116. Chaudhuri AK, Hartley RB, Maddocks AC: Waterhouse-Friderichsen syndrome caused by DF-2 bacterium in a splectomized patient. J Clin Pathol 1981; 34:172.

117. Findling JW, Pohlmann GP, Rose HD: Fulminant gram-negative bacillemia (DF-2) following a dog bite in an asplenic woman. Am J Med 1980; 68:154.

118. Martone WJ, Zuehl RW, Minson GE, et al: Postsplenectomy sepsis with DF-2: Report of a case with isolation of the organism from the patient's dog. Ann Intern Med 1980; 93:457.

119. Rosner F, Zarrabi MH, Benach JL, et al: Babesiosis in splenectomized adults: Review of 22 reported cases. Am J Med 1984; 76:696.

120. Mellemkjaer L, Olsen JH, Linet MS, et al: Cancer risk after splenectomy. Cancer 1995; 75:577.

121. Robinette CD, Fraumeni JF Jr: Splenectomy and subsequent mortality in veterans of the 1939–45 war. Lancet 1977; 2:127.

Disorders of the White Pulp

II

5

REACTIVE LYMPHOID HYPERPLASIA

Splenic lymphoid tissue is affected by many physiologic and pathologic processes. Disorders associated with inactive or hypoplastic white pulp are discussed in Chapter 4. Reactive hyperplasia of splenic lymphoid tissue may present either with or without the formation of secondary germinal centers. These two types of presentation have been shown to represent different phases of the evolving response of lymphoid tissue to antigenic stimulation in experimental animals, and transitional patterns have been observed in human spleens.

REACTIVE LYMPHOID HYPERPLASIA WITHOUT GERMINAL CENTER FORMATION

This morphologic type of immune reaction has been referred to as the early activated immune reaction, "activated A,"[1] "immunoblastic hyperplasia,"[2] or "reactive nonfollicular hyperplasia."[3] Although this pattern of lymphoid proliferation is characteristic of many viral disorders[4-7] as well as of a variety of other conditions associated with systemic antigenic response, it is not as well recognized as the evolving activated reaction with secondary germinal center formation.[4]

Although the spleen is usually enlarged in patients with this reaction, the enlargement is frequently of modest degree and not palpable. The white pulp may not be greatly increased in size, and the spleen may be grossly unremarkable. On low-power microscopic examination, the architecture of the white pulp resembles that of the immunologically unstimulated state. Because germinal centers are usually not seen and the lymphoid follicles lack distinctive mantle zones, the white pulp may initially appear hypoplastic (Fig. 5–1). However, on closer examination the white pulp shows evidence of antigenic stimulation, characterized by the presence of lymphocytes in varying stages of transformation (Fig. 5–2). There is a mixture of small and large lymphocytes and immunoblasts. The immunoblasts are characterized by open chromatin, prominent nucleoli, and basophilic cytoplasm. Tingible body macrophages containing nuclear debris may be prominent (Fig. 5–3). There is often a proliferation of transformed lymphocytes and immunoblasts around the penicilliary arterioles as well (Fig. 5–4), and these cells may infiltrate the subendothelial zones of the trabecular veins, the trabeculae themselves, or the capsule (Fig. 5–5).[5] In some cases the proliferation may be extreme, extending throughout the red pulp and blurring the white pulp margins. This is characteristically observed in cases of infectious mononucleosis.[6, 7, 8] The occasional striking degree of immunoblastic proliferation in the red pulp as well as in the white pulp may be difficult to distinguish from immunoblastic lymphoma. This proliferation may also be difficult to distinguish on morphologic grounds from Hodgkin's disease, owing to the polymorphous cell population, which may include Reed-Sternberg–like cells (Fig. 5–6).[9-12] In infectious mononucleosis, venous thromboses and foci of hemorrhage may occur in the red pulp because of infiltration of the trabecular vessels by proliferating immunoblasts. Infiltration of the trabeculae by lymphoid cells may also cause dissolution of

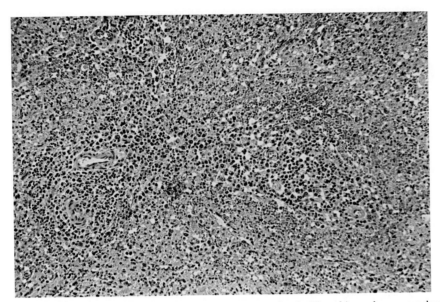

Figure 5–1. Early activated immune response in infectious mononucleosis. The white pulp appears hypoplastic and depleted of lymphoid elements.

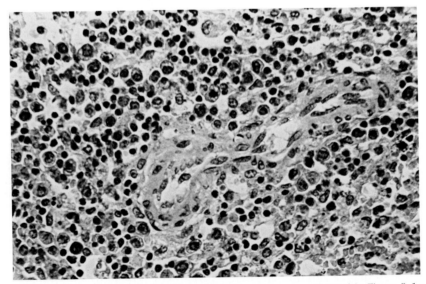

Figure 5–2. Higher-power examination of the white pulp in the same case as pictured in Figure 5–1 reveals that the lymphoid cells are transformed with numerous immunoblasts present.

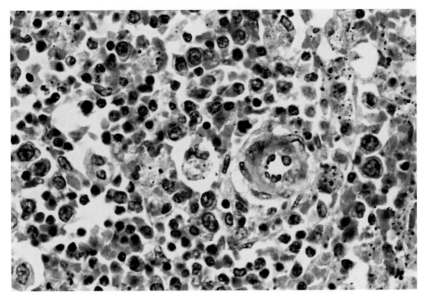

Figure 5–3. Splenic white pulp in infectious mononucleosis. Numerous phagocytic macrophages are present.

Figure 5–4. Early activated immune response. The penicilliary arteriole is surrounded by transformed lymphocytes and immunoblasts.

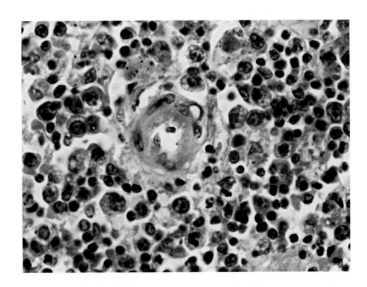

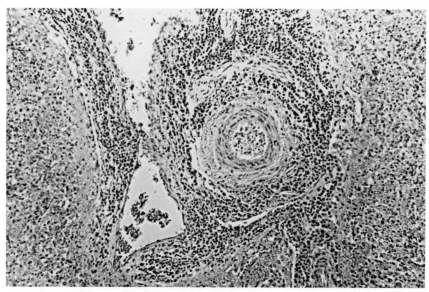

Figure 5–5. Trabecular and subendothelial infiltration of lymphocytes and immunoblasts in a case of infectious mononucleosis. This phenomenon predisposes the organ to rupture.

collagen, weakening the structural framework of the spleen and predisposing the spleen to rupture, which may occur 10 to 20 days after the onset of the viral infection.[13–16] This mechanism is also responsible for the splenic rupture that has been observed as a complication of other viral infections.[15–17]

The morphologic features of this form of immune reaction may occur in a wide variety of other viral infections, including those caused by the herpesviruses (Fig. 5–7). The "activated A" type of lymphoid hyperplasia was also noted in the spleen by Lukes[18] in a number of cases of hemorrhagic fever with renal syndrome (Korean hemorrhagic fever). This disorder is an acute febrile illness caused by *Hantavirus*[19] and is associated with hypotension and oliguria, followed by a diuretic phase. Pathologically, the illness is characterized by widespread capillary damage causing severe hemorrhagic manifestations, including splenic hematomas.[20]

Lymphoid reactions of this type may also occur in a wide variety of clinical settings associated with an altered (suppressed) immune system. Spleens from patients undergoing organ

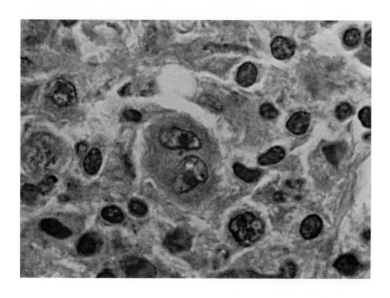

Figure 5–6. Early activated immune response; a binucleated plasmablast with inclusion-like nucleoli is present. Such cells may prompt an erroneous diagnosis of Hodgkin's disease.

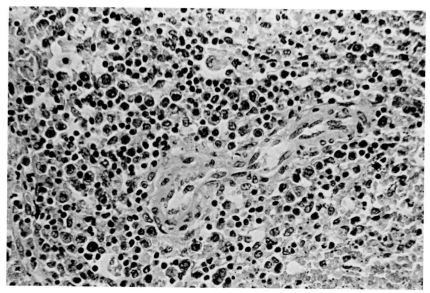

Figure 5–7. Disseminated herpes simplex. Small and large transformed lymphocytes proliferate around an arteriole of the white pulp.

transplant rejection and from patients having received antilymphocyte serum may show this type of lymphoid proliferation (Fig. 5–8) in combination with white pulp hypoplasia.[21] Similar findings may also be seen in the immune responses of very young children and elderly persons, both of whose immune systems are frequently incapable of reacting to antigenic stimuli as effectively as immunologically competent individuals.[4] This pattern of immune reaction was also described in a large autopsy series of patients with aplastic anemia[2] and in Japa-

nese atomic bomb casualties.[22] Spleens from patients with conditions involving chronic immunologic activation who are treated with corticosteroids may also show these features. We have observed this in cases of steroid-treated idiopathic thrombocytopenic purpura[23] and in autoimmune hemolytic anemia (Fig. 5–9),[4] in which steroid therapy suppresses or retards the immune response.[23] It has also been reported in patients with other autoimmune disorders, most notably rheumatoid arthritis, who were treated with methotrexate.[24-26] In these cases,

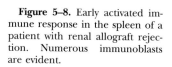

Figure 5–8. Early activated immune response in the spleen of a patient with renal allograft rejection. Numerous immunoblasts are evident.

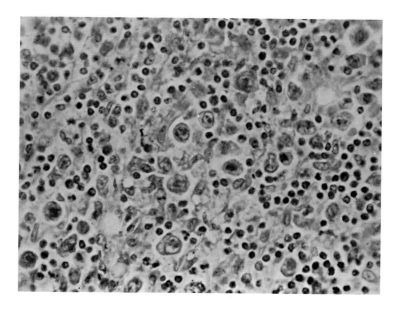

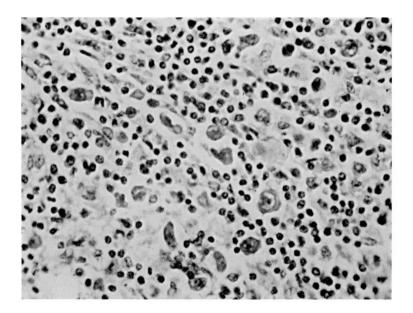

Figure 5–9. Early activated immune response in a patient with autoimmune hemolytic anemia treated with corticosteroids before splenectomy. The white pulp shows numerous immunoblasts and transformed lymphoid cells.

Epstein-Barr virus was implicated in the pathogenesis, and a morphologic resemblance to Hodgkin's disease was noted.

REACTIVE FOLLICULAR HYPERPLASIA

This form of reactive lymphoid hyperplasia, termed "evolving activated immune response," "activated B," or "reactive follicular hyperplasia," is characteristic of chronic immune reactions as well as many acute infectious processes.[1, 3, 4] This pattern of immune reaction occurs more frequently than that without germinal center formation, although the two patterns may overlap or occur simultaneously in the same patient. The presence of secondary germinal centers in the splenic white pulp is a normal finding in children and

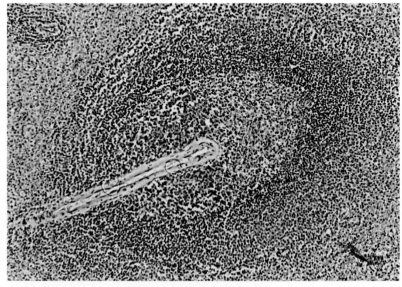

Figure 5–10. Evolving activated immune response in untreated idiopathic thrombocytopenic purpura. The malpighian corpuscle is composed of a tripartite germinal center, with a marginal zone of lymphocytes around the periphery, and a mantle zone of darker lymphocytes forming a corona around the center of the germinal follicle, which is composed of transformed lymphocytes.

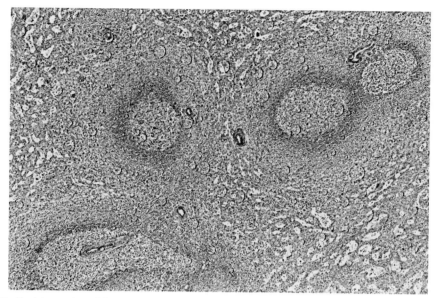

Figure 5–11. Evolving activated immune response in a case of chronic uremia. Note the widely expanded marginal zones in addition to the dark mantle zones and the central zones of transformed lymphocytes.

young adults. The spleen may be markedly enlarged in this form of immune reaction. The white pulp is expanded, and occasionally grossly visible nodules may be so large as to simulate malignant lymphoma (Color Plate 5). Microscopically, this pattern is characterized by follicular hyperplasia with partially or fully formed tripartite germinal centers (Fig. 5–10). At the height of the reaction, the follicles contain transformed lymphocytes, mitotic figures, and tingible body macrophages.[2, 4, 27, 28] The marginal zones are often widely expanded in more chronic cases (Fig. 5–11), and their fusion may result in grossly visible nodules. This phenomenon has been referred to by us as well as by others as splenic marginal zone hyperplasia.[29–32] It may be impossible, on morphologic grounds alone, to distinguish these cases from cases of so-called indolent marginal zone cell lymphoma (see Chapter 8) (Fig. 5–12). There is plasmacytosis of the red pulp, with proliferation of these cells around penicilliary arterioles (Fig. 5–13) and diffuse scattering in the cords of Billroth. The penicilliary

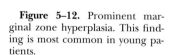

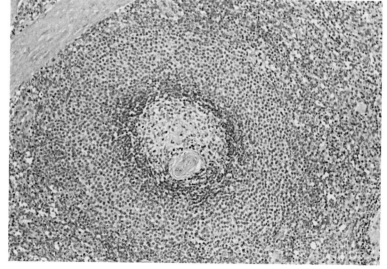

Figure 5–12. Prominent marginal zone hyperplasia. This finding is most common in young patients.

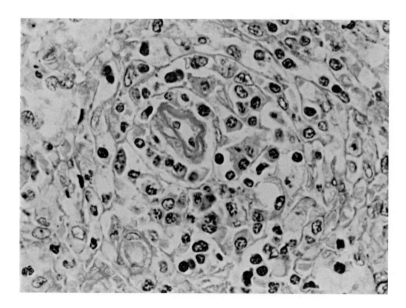

Figure 5–13. Evolving activated immune response. Note the plasmacytosis around the penicilliary arteriole.

arterioles may be prominent due to hyperplasia of the surrounding lymphoid sheaths, in contrast to the unstimulated state, in which they are often barely discernible.

The histologic features of reactive follicular hyperplasia may be seen in most bacterial infections and in themselves are not specific for a given organism. However, certain infections may be associated with characteristic morphologic findings. For example, the spleen in typhoid fever usually lacks a neutrophilic infiltrate and shows a proliferation of cordal macrophages with erythrophagocytosis, similar to the findings in other lymphoid organs. The organ is red because of the scarcity of neutrophils. Occasionally, focal necrosis may be seen, and rupture may be a rare complication.[33] Spleens from children with scarlet fever, diphtheria, or tularemia often contain foci of necrosis within germinal centers. We have also seen such foci of necrosis in the spleens of stillborn infants and neonates dying of overwhelming sepsis from a variety of causes (Fig. 5–14). Splenomegaly is common in patients with subacute bacterial endocarditis and may be an important diagnostic clue in a patient with fever and a cardiac murmur.[34–38] Immune complex deposition within splenic vessels has been considered, in part, to be responsible for the splenomegaly observed in these patients.[39] Septic emboli often result from infective vegetations on the tricuspid or mitral valve and may result in splenic infarction or rupture.[36, 40, 41]

Although follicular hyperplasia does not usually occur in most viral infections, some viral infections result in florid follicular hyperplasia. For example, this pattern is common in children with measles virus infection. Occasionally, spleens in patients with infectious mononucleosis may also show germinal center formation. In cases associated with AIDS, follicular hyperplasia as well as an increased number of plasma cells both in the white and in the red pulp is commonly observed.[42, 43] In advanced AIDS cases, splenic follicular lymphoid depletion with patchy hyalinization and decreased number of T lymphocytes around the periarterial lymphoid sheath is frequently noted. Another phenomenon noted in these cases is the strong expression of S-100 protein by a large number of cordal and intrasinusoidal macrophages.[43] This finding, which has not been associated with a demonstrable cause, must be distinguished from the moderate increase in the number of S-100 positive interdigitating cells typically found in early stages of most cases of AIDS.

Chronic autoimmune disorders are also usually associated with prominent reactive follicular hyperplasia and expanded marginal zones in the spleen.[3, 4] This pattern is characteristic of systemic lupus erythematosus (SLE) and the splenomegaly associated with rheumatoid arthritis and its related disorders, such as Felty syndrome (rheumatoid arthritis with neutropenia).[1, 4, 44, 45] This pattern is also typical of immune thrombocytopenic purpura[46–52] and autoimmune hemolytic anemia,[53] which are related to the production of antiplatelet and

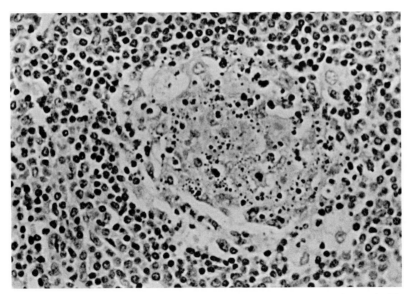

Figure 5–14. White pulp of the spleen of a neonate dying of overwhelming gram-negative sepsis. The germinal center is necrotic.

antierythrocyte antibodies, respectively. The spleen is important in these conditions both as a source of the antibodies, reflected by the follicular hyperplasia and plasmacytosis of the red pulp, and as a site of phagocytosis and destruction of antibody-coated cells.[54, 55] As discussed earlier, corticosteroid therapy alters the splenic morphology in these disorders. The white pulp of spleens from patients with steroid-treated chronic autoimmune disorders usually shows a dampened immune reaction, lacking the follicular hyperplasia characteristic of spleens obtained from untreated patients.[23] The evolving activated immune reaction has also been described in patients with chronic uremia undergoing hemodialysis. The antigenic stimulation in these cases is thought to be related to persistent stimulation by hepatitis-associated antigens from repeated blood transfusions.[29]

Secondary germinal center formation in the immune response usually regresses gradually as the source of antigenic stimulation subsides (Fig. 5–15).[3, 4] The germinal centers contract, and the marginal zone may become widened. Amorphous PAS-positive intercellular material may be seen within germinal centers (Fig. 5–16). Residual follicles containing hyalinized germinal centers, resembling the abnormal follicles seen in angiofollicular lymphoid hyperplasia (Castleman disease), may persist for long periods.[56–58]

LYMPHOID HYPERPLASIAS ASSOCIATED WITH SYSTEMIC AUTOIMMUNE DISEASES

This category includes a group of systemic autoimmune disorders characterized by the inappropriate and non–self-limited production of antibodies, often autoantibodies. SLE and rheumatoid arthritis (RA) are the most common of the systemic autoimmune disorders that involve the spleen. These conditions are associated with autoantibody production, particularly antinuclear antibody in SLE[59–61] and rheumatoid factor in RA.[62–64] Both disorders may also be associated with elevated serum immunoglobulin and autoimmune hemolytic anemia. Splenomegaly is found in approximately 20 percent of patients with SLE and 5 to 10 percent of patients with RA.[65] Hepatosplenomegaly and generalized lymphadenopathy are more common in juvenile rheumatoid arthritis (Still disease) than in the adult version. The degree of splenomegaly in the autoimmune disorders is usually moderate. Occasionally, however, the spleen may be markedly enlarged, particularly in rheumatoid arthritis associated with Felty syndrome, which is characterized by leukopenia and recurrent leg ulcers.[44] Splenomegaly has also been reported in Behçet syndrome (in which oral aphthous ulcers are associated with ulcers on the external genitalia), uveitis, and variable visceral manifestations.[66]

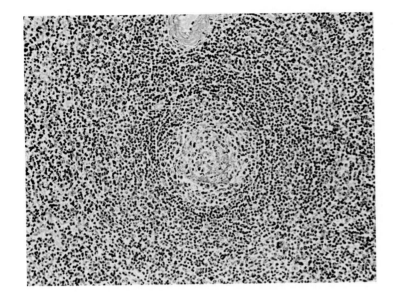

Figure 5–15. Evolving activated immune reaction; so-called chronic follicle in long-standing autoimmune hemolytic anemia.

Splenic morphology in the autoimmune disorders may be indistinguishable from other cases of reactive follicular hyperplasia. However, in our experience, the lymphoid proliferation often appears different from that seen in those reactions.[67] The splenic red pulp may contain an infiltrate of polyclonal plasma cells, plasmacytoid lymphocytes, and immunoblasts (Fig. 5–17).[44] The white pulp either shows follicular hyperplasia or, paradoxically, appears inactive. The immunoblastic proliferation may be a prominent feature in some cases. However, the red pulp infiltrate is usually limited to scattered mature plasma cells. The penicilliary arterioles in SLE may show a characteristic "onion skin" appearance resulting from concentric perivascular fibrosis. It is well known that patients with autoimmune diseases have an increased susceptibility to the development of malignant lymphomas.[68, 69] It has been postulated that the immunoblastic proliferations[70] (as well as the presence of light-chain restriction)[71] seen in Sjögren syndrome represent a transitional phase of evolution to lymphoma.[71] Whether this is generally true in autoimmune disorders is unknown.

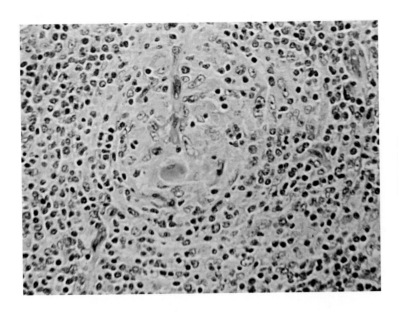

Figure 5–16. Amorphous material in germinal center in chronic immune reaction. This hyalinized material may persist for long periods and superficially resembles the chronic follicles in Castleman disease.

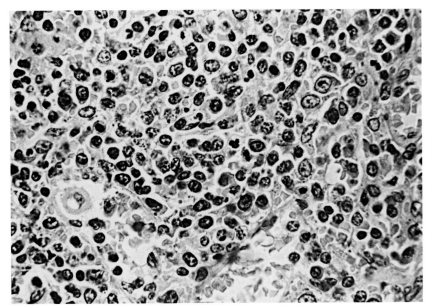

Figure 5–17. Splenic red pulp in SLE. The cords and sinuses contain numerous immunoblasts, plasma cells, and plasmacytoid lymphocytes.

ATYPICAL LYMPHOID HYPERPLASIA

This group of conditions includes angioimmunoblastic lymphadenopathy (AILD), or immunoblastic lymphadenopathy (IBL), and multicentric Castleman disease, which are usually associated with polyclonal hypergammaglobulinemia, although Castleman disease may rarely be associated with a monoclonal gammopathy. In addition, atypical lymphoid hyperplasia may also be observed in the presence of immunosuppression (both congenital and acquired), in patients with rheumatoid arthritis treated with methotrexate,[24–26] and in rare cases in which no obvious immunologic abnormality can be detected. The presence of numerous immunoblasts may cause confusion in distinguishing these lesions from malignant lymphomas and, in particular, Hodgkin's disease.[24–26]

Angioimmunoblastic Lymphadenopathy with Dysproteinemia or Immunoblastic Lymphadenopathy

Angioimmunoblastic lymphadenopathy[72, 73] or immunoblastic lymphadenopathy (represented by AILD/IBL)[74] was originally postulated to be a hyperimmune B-cell proliferation associated with a defect in immunoregulatory T cells, most probably a deficiency of T suppressor cells.[80] However, most cases are now considered to be a T-cell lymphoma and have been termed angioimmunoblastic T-cell lymphoma.[72, 73] Although the morphologic features were originally described in lymph nodes, splenomegaly is often present, and the splenic disease has been described.[72, 74–77]

Patients with AILD/IBL usually present with generalized lymphadenopathy and often have hepatosplenomegaly, fever, weight loss, and in some cases autoimmune hemolytic anemia and a maculopapular pruritic rash.[72, 74, 78] The peripheral blood may show lymphopenia or neutrophilic leukocytosis with eosinophilia. Lymph node biopsy reveals a characteristic morphologic triad including (1) diffuse replacement by a polymorphous lymphoid infiltrate, (2) a proliferation of small arborizing blood vessels, and (3) amorphous acidophilic interstitial material, shown by electron microscopy to be composed of cellular debris.[78, 79] The cellular infiltrate includes immunoblasts, plasma cells, and plasmacytoid lymphocytes.[72, 73] Eosinophils may be prominent. The polymorphic nature of the lesion may create difficulty in differentiating it from Hodgkin's disease, with which, in fact, it was confused for many years. The clinical course is usually progressive, with death resulting from fulminant infection, although occasional patients have died of supervening malignant lymphoma.[74, 80, 81–86] Rare instances of spontaneous regression have occurred.[77]

The majority of descriptions of the splenic form of AILD/IBL have been derived from autopsy cases. Occasionally, however, splenectomy is performed as a therapeutic measure in patients with severe hemolytic anemia. Neiman and coworkers[77] described two such cases in which the spleens weighed 620 g and 760 g. The cut surfaces of the organs showed a poorly defined nodularity distributed uniformly throughout the organ. Microscopically, one spleen showed nonspecific follicular hyperplasia of the white pulp. The second spleen showed an expansion of the white pulp by a polymorphous proliferation of lymphoid cells similar to that in involved lymph nodes (Fig. 5–18). The infiltrate included lymphoid cells at all stages of transformation and occasional plasma cells. The red pulp was heavily infiltrated by polyclonal plasma cells. Frizzera and associates[72] also described the morphologic findings in three cases which the spleen was removed. The splenic weights ranged from 230 to 910 g. The changes noted were predominantly in the marginal zones, where the cellular infiltrate was similar to that in lymph nodes, and were also found in focal aggregates in the red pulp. All spleens had an increase in concentric reticulin in the marginal zones and had prominent perifollicular fibrosis (Fig. 5–19). The white pulp in one case contained amorphous acidophilic material and loose aggregates of histiocytes within germinal centers. The second spleen showed the characteristic polymorphic infiltrate of AILD/IBL in the white pulp and infiltrating the red pulp; the third spleen showed nonspecific follicular hyperplasia. Although the white pulp has been noted to display prominent vascularity in some cases, the characteristic arborizing vascular proliferation that occurs in lymph nodes in AILD/IBL apparently does not occur in the spleen.[77]

The morphologic features of spleens obtained at autopsy are variable. In the series by Frizzera and colleagues,[72] three of eight spleens obtained at postmortem examination were morphologically similar to the surgical specimens in their series. The remainder showed marked lymphoid depletion and fibrosis of the white pulp, with plasma cell aggregates in the red pulp (Fig. 5–20). However, the majority of these patients had received chemotherapy. Lukes and Tindle[74] described the morphologic findings of 10 spleens obtained at autopsy, of which 5 showed a cellular proliferation recognizable as IBL. The degree of cellularity and fibrosis was variable. The end result of the disease, which may also reflect changes due to chemotherapy, appears to be generalized lymphoid depletion and fibrosis in the spleen as well as in lymph nodes.[77]

The lymphomas that occasionally arise in patients with AILD/IBL have usually been reported to be of the immunoblastic type, with plasmacytoid features in some cases. Nathwani and coworkers[83] reported their findings in 7

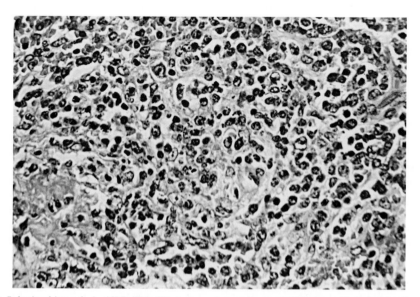

Figure 5–18. Splenic white pulp in AILD/IBL. There is a polymorphous proliferation of lymphoid cells and prominent interstitial amorphous material.

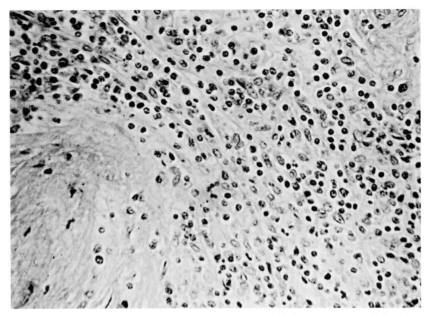

Figure 5–19. AILD/IBL. There is prominent perifollicular fibrosis in addition to a pleocytotic lymphocytic infiltrate.

surgical and 18 autopsy spleens obtained from patients with AILD and lymphoma. The lymphomas were all of the immunoblastic type. The spleens in all cases involved with lymphoma showed a miliary pattern grossly, resembling that of malignant lymphomas of small-cell type, without tumor masses. Microscopically, the tumor was seen as small nodules involving both the white and the red pulp.

This pattern of involvement is unusual for large cell lymphoma, which usually produces single or multiple tumor masses.

It is questionable whether AILD is a single disease. Several studies have suggested that AILD closely resembles cases of peripheral T-cell lymphoma with an AILD/IBL-like morphology. Reports in the Japanese literature have described a disorder termed "AILD-like

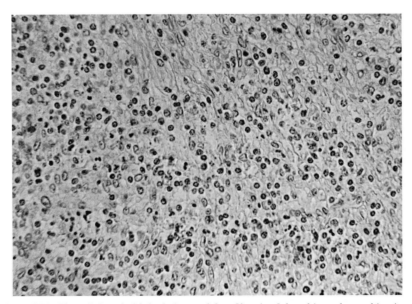

Figure 5–20. AILD/IBL. There is lymphoid depletion and fine fibrosis of the white pulp resulting in a blurring of the demarcation between red and white pulp.

T-cell lymphoma" in which the morphologic and clinical features simulated AILD/IBL.[76] O'Connor et al[75] found evidence of T-cell monoclonality in cases of AILD. In addition, Weiss and associates[87] described several cases of immunologically confirmed T-cell lymphomas with histologic resemblance to AILD/IBL. The pathognomonic feature in AILD/IBL-like lymphoma is the presence of multiple clusters of lymphoid cells with pale cytoplasm in varying number.[88] The cells that exhibit clear cytoplasm are of small, medium, or large size. The latter two cell types show readily identifiable nucleoli. The cytoplasm is abundant and clear to pale-staining. The proliferation of CD21-positive dendritic reticulum cells is also thought to be characteristic.[88]

Whenever possible, immunophenotypic and genotypic studies should be used to distinguish these disorders.[88] As to the immunophenotypic data, the results are variable. Most studies have shown a preponderance of T cells[87, 89–95]; some studies have shown a mixture of both T and B cells[89, 96, 97]; and a few have shown a preponderance of B cells.[77, 98] The genotypic data are similar to the phenotypic data.[91, 95, 98, 99] Clonal instability has also been frequently observed when serial biopsies are analyzed. In selected cases, the distinction between AILD/IBL malignant lymphoma arising in AILD/IBL and AILD/IBL-like malignancies may require a careful evaluation of morphology and immunophenotypic, genotypic, and cytogenetic data.

Castleman Disease

Castleman disease, or angiofollicular lymph node hyperplasia, typically involves lymph nodes, most commonly of the mediastinum.[56] Two histologic and two clinical subtypes of the disease have been described.[56–58] The hyaline-vascular type, which accounts for most cases, is characterized by atrophic lymphoid follicles surrounded by small lymphocytes in a concentric configuration.[56–58] Small vessels that are often hyalinized may be seen entering the follicles radially. This subtype is usually clinically localized and without associated constitutional symptoms.[56, 100] In 10 percent of cases, the lymph nodes show large reactive follicles and a striking interfollicular infiltrate of plasma cells. This subtype, called the plasma cell variant, may be clinically multicentric and is commonly associated with systemic symptoms, including fever, anemia, and hypergammaglobulinemia.[58, 100–103] Mild hepatosplenomegaly and generalized lymphadenopathy are frequently noted in this subtype, and rarely isolated splenomegaly may be the presenting feature.[104] The multicentric plasma cell variant of this disease has been recently associated with the presence of Kaposi sarcoma-associated herpesvirus[105, 106] and its virus-encoded interleukin-6–like activity.[107] This cytokine, a putative growth factor in multiple myeloma, is currently considered central to the pathophysiology of Castleman disease.[107–110] The relationship between the two subtypes of Castleman

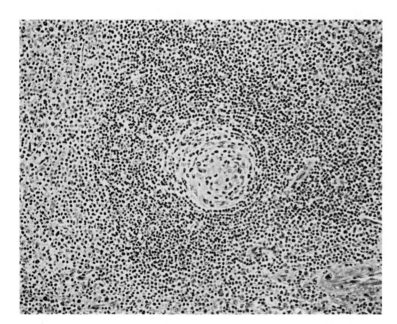

Figure 5–21. Multicentric Castleman disease in the spleen. The follicle of the malpighian corpuscle is atrophic with hyaline-vascular changes.

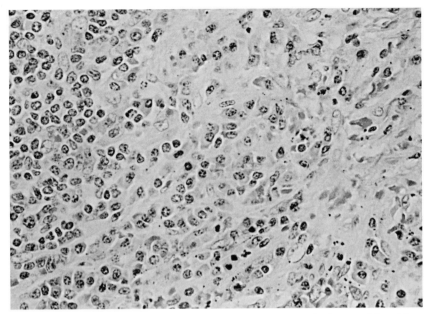

Figure 5–22. Multicentric Castleman disease. There is expansion of the marginal zone of the white pulp by fibrosis and plasmacytosis.

disease is unclear.[101] Despite the clinical and histologic difference between the localized and multicentric forms, in some cases they overlap.

The majority of the cases of multicentric Castleman disease involving the spleen are of the plasma cell type,[102, 111] although Gaba and coworkers[57] reported a case in which the morphology was more typical of that of the hyaline-vascular variant. That patient also had a polyclonal hypergammaglobulinemia and cold agglutinins. Weisenburger[111] reviewed seven cases of Castleman disease involving the spleen, five of which had the morphology of the plasma cell type. Splenic weights ranged from 155 to 664 g. The microscopic appearance was variable. Four cases of the plasma cell type showed atrophic follicles with hyaline-vascular germinal centers (Fig. 5–21), and one showed expansion of the marginal zones with plasma cells and fibrosis (Fig. 5–22), similar to three of four cases reported by Frizzera and associates.[102] The two cases in which the lymph node morphology was that of the hyaline-vascular type showed hyperplastic nodules of white pulp surrounded by dense fibrosis that coalesced to form macroscopic masses. All 11 cases in both studies showed a variable degree of plasmacytosis of the red pulp. These findings indicate the distinction between hyaline-vascular and plasma cell subtypes of Castleman

disease may be difficult and in some cases arbitrary.

REFERENCES

1. Lukes RJ: The pathology of the white pulp of the spleen, in Lennert K, Harms D (eds): Die Milz, p 130. Berlin, Springer-Verlag, 1970.
2. Burke JS: Surgical pathology of the spleen: An approach to the differential diagnosis of splenic lymphomas and leukemias—diseases of the white pulp. Am J Surg Pathol 1981; 5:551.
3. Burke JS: Diagnosis of lymphoma and lymphoid proliferation in the spleen, in Jaffe ES (ed): Surgical Pathology of the Lymph Nodes and Related Organs, 2nd ed, p 448. Philadelphia, WB Saunders Co, 1995.
4. Neiman RS, Orazi A: Spleen, in Damjanov I, Linder J (eds): Anderson's Pathology, 10th ed, p 1201. St. Louis, Mosby–Year Book, 1996.
5. Carter RL, Penman HG: Histopathology of infectious mononucleosis, in Carter RL, Penman HG (eds): Infectious Mononucleosis, p 146. Oxford, Blackwell Scientific, 1969.
6. Gowing NFC: Infectious mononucleosis: Histopathologic aspects. Pathol Ann 1975; 1:1.
7. Lukes RJ, Cox FH: Clinical and morphologic findings in thirty fatal cases of infectious mononucleosis. Am J Pathol 1958; 34:586.
8. Iijima T, Sumazaki R, Mori N, et al: A pathological and immunohistological case report of fatal infectious mononucleosis, Epstein-Barr virus infection, demonstrated by in situ and Southern blot hybridization. Virchows Arch 1992; 421:73.
9. Agliozzo CM, Reingold IM: Infectious mononucleosis simulating Hodgkin's disease: A patient with Reed-Sternberg cells. Am J Clin Pathol 1971; 56:730.

10. Gordon HW, McMahon NJ, Rosen RB: Reed-Sternberg cells in a patient with infectious mononucleosis. Lab Invest 1970; 22:498.

11. Lukes RJ, Tindle BH, Parker JW: Reed-Sternberg-like cells in infectious mononucleosis. Lancet 1969; 2:1003.

12. Tindle BH, Parker JW, Lukes RJ: "Reed-Sternberg cells" in infectious mononucleosis. Am J Clin Pathol 1972; 58:607.

13. Finch SC: Clinical signs and symptoms of infectious mononucleosis, in Carter RL, Penman HG (eds): Infectious Mononucleosis, p 19. Oxford, Blackwell Scientific, 1969.

14. Rawsthorne GB, Cole TP, Kyle RJ: Spontaneous rupture of the spleen in infectious mononucleosis. Br J Surg 1970; 57:396.

15. Smith EB, Custer RP: Rupture of the spleen in infectious mononucleosis: A clinicopathologic report of seven cases. Blood 1946; 1:317.

16. Rutkow IM: Rupture of the spleen in infectious mononucleosis: A critical review. Arch Surg 1978; 113:718.

17. Rogues AM, Dupon M, Cales V, et al: Spontaneous splenic rupture: An uncommon complication of cytomegalovirus infection. J Infect 1994; 29:83.

18. Lukes RJ: The pathology of thirty-nine fatal cases of epidemic hemorrhagic fever. Am J Med 1954; 16:639.

19. Hart CA, Bennett M: *Hantavirus:* an increasing problem? Ann Trop Med Parasitol 1994; 88:347.

20. Alexeyev OA, Morozov VG, Efremov AG, et al: A case of haemorrhagic fever with renal syndrome complicated by spleen haemorrhage. Scand J Infect Dis 1994; 26:491.

21. Slavin RE, Santos GW: The graft versus host reaction in man after bone marrow transplantation: Pathology, pathogenesis, clinical features and implications. Clin Immunol Immunopathol 1973; 1:472.

22. Liebow A, Warren S, DeCoursey E: Pathology of atomic bomb casualties. Am J Pathol 1949; 25:853.

23. Hassan NMR, Neiman RS: The pathology of the spleen in steroid-treated immune thrombocytopenic purpura. Am J Clin Pathol 1985; 84:433.

24. Kamel O, Weiss L, van de Rijn M, et al: Hodgkin's disease and lymphoproliferations resembling Hodgkin's disease in patients receiving long-term low-dose methotrexate therapy. Am J Surg Pathol 1996; 20:1279.

25. Kamel OW, van de Rijn M, Weiss LM, et al: Reversible Epstein-Barr virus–associated lymphomas during methotrexate therapy for rheumatoid arthritis and dermatomyositis. N Engl J Med 1993; 328:1317.

26. Kamel OW, van de Rijn M, Weiss LM, et al: Lymphoid neoplasms in patients with rheumatoid arthritis and dermatomyositis: Frequency of Epstein-Barr virus and other features associated with immunosuppression. Hum Pathol 1994; 25:638.

27. Millikin PD: Anatomy of germinal centers in human lymphoid tissue. Arch Pathol 1986; 82:499.

28. Millikin PD: The nodular white pulp of the human spleen. Arch Pathol 1969; 87:247.

29. Neiman RS, Bischel MD, Lukes RJ: Hypersplenism in the uremic hemodialyzed patient: Pathology and proposed pathophysiologic mechanisms. Am J Clin Pathol 1973; 60:502.

30. Fahri DC, Ashfaq R: Splenic pathology after traumatic injury. Immunopathol 1995; 105:474.

31. Harris S, Wilkins BS, Jones DB: Splenic marginal zone expansion in B-cell lymphomas of gastrointestinal mucosa–associated lymphoid tissue (malt) is reactive and does not represent homing of neoplastic lymphocytes. J Pathol 1996; 179:49.

32. Kroft SH, Singleton TP, Dahiya M, et al: Ruptured spleens with expanded marginal zones do not reveal occult B-cell clones. Mod Pathol 1997; 10:1214.

33. Videbaek A, Christensen BE, Jonsson V: The Spleen in Health and Disease, p 173. Chicago, Year Book Medical Publishers, 1982.

34. Buchbinder NA, Roberts WC: Left-sided valvular active infective endocarditis: A study of forty-five necropsy patients. Am J Med 1973; 53:20.

35. Delletier LL Jr, Petersdorf RG: Infective endocarditis: A review of 125 cases from the University of Washington Hospitals, 1963–1972. Medicine 1977; 56:287.

36. Baron JM, Weinshelbaum EI, Block GE: Splenic rupture associated with bacterial endocarditis and sickle cell trait. JAMA 1968; 205:102.

37. Chase RM Jr: Infective endocarditis today. Med Clin North Am 1973; 57:1383.

38. Lingeman CJ, Smith EB, Battersby JS, et al: Subacute bacterial endocarditis: Splenectomy in cases refractory to antibiotic therapy. Arch Intern Med 1956; 97:309.

39. Nast CC, Colodro IH, Cohen AH: Splenic immune deposits in bacterial endocarditis. Clin Immunol Immunopathol 1986; 40:209.

40. Vergne R, Selland B, Gobel FL, et al: Rupture of the spleen in infective endocarditis. Arch Intern Med 1975; 135:1265.

41. Wood WS, Hall B: Rupture of spleen in subacute bacterial endocarditis: Mycotic aneurysm of splenic artery and spontaneous rupture of spleen in subacute bacterial endocarditis. Arch Intern Med 1954; 93:633.

42. Klatt EC, Meyer PR: Pathology of the spleen in the acquired immunodeficiency syndrome. Arch Pathol Lab Med 1987; 111:1050.

43. Falk S, Muller H, Stutte H-J: The spleen in acquired immunodeficiency syndrome (AIDS). Pathol Res Pract 1988; 183:425.

44. Laszlo J, Jones R, Silberman HR, et al: Splenectomy for Felty's syndrome: Clinicopathological study of 27 patients. Arch Intern Med 1978; 138:597.

45. Louie JS, Pearson CM: Felty's syndrome. Semin Hematol 1971; 8:216.

46. Bowman HE, Pettit VD, Caldwell FT, et al: Morphology of the spleen in idiopathic thrombocytopenic purpura. Lab Invest 1955; 4:206.

47. Gugliotta L, Isacchi G, Guarini A, et al: Chronic idiopathic thrombocytopenic purpura (ITP): Site of platelet sequestration and results of splenectomy—a study of 197 patients. Scand J Haematol 1981; 26:40.

48. Hoffman R, Benz E Jr, Shattil S, et al: Immune thrombocytopenic purpura, neonatal alloimmune thrombocytopenia, and post-transfusion purpura, in Bussel J, Cines D (eds): Hematology, 2nd ed, p 1849. New York, Churchill Livingstone, 1995.

49. Karpatkin S: Autoimmune thrombocytopenic purpura. J Am Soc Hematol 1980; 56:329.

50. McMillan R: Chronic idiopathic thrombocytopenic purpura. N Engl J Med 1981; 304:1135.

51. McMillan R, Longmire RL, Yelenosky R, et al: Immunoglobulin synthesis in vitro by spleens from patients with idiopathic thrombocytopenic purpura. N Engl J Med 1972; 286:681.

52. Tavassoli M, McMillan R: Structure of the spleen in idiopathic thrombocytopenic purpura. Am J Clin Pathol 1975; 64:180.

53. Rappaport H, Crosby WH: Autoimmune hemolytic anemia. II. Morphologic observations and clinico-pathologic correlations. Am J Pathol 1957; 33:429.

54. Logue G: Felty's syndrome: Granulocyte-bound immunoglobulin G and splenectomy. Ann Intern Med 1976; 85:437.

55. McMillan R, Longmire RL, Yelenosky R, et al: Quantitation of platelet-binding IgG produced in vitro by spleens from patients with idiopathic thrombocytopenic purpura. N Engl J Med 1974; 291:812.

56. Castleman B, Iverson L, Menendez VP: Localized mediastinal lymph-node hyperplasia resembling thymoma. Cancer 1956; 9:822.

57. Gaba AR, Stein RS, Sweet DL, et al: Multicentric giant lymph node hyperplasia. Am J Clin Pathol 1978; 69:86.

58. Keller AR, Hochholzer L, Castleman B: Hyaline-vascular and plasma-cell types of giant lymph node hyperplasia of the mediastinum and other locations. Cancer 1972; 29:670.

59. Lorincz LL, Soltani K, Bernstein JE: Anti-nuclear antibodies. Int J Dermatol 1981; 20:401.

60. McCluskey RT: Evidence for an immune complex disorder in systemic lupus erythematosus. Am J Kid Dis 1982; 2:199.

61. Tan EM: Antinuclear antibodies in diagnosis and management. Hosp Pract 1983; 18:79.

62. Hay FC, Nineham LJ, Perumal R, et al: Intra-articular and circulating immune complexes and antiglobulins (IgG and IgM) in rheumatoid arthritis: Correlation with clinical features. Ann Rheum Dis 1979; 38:1.

63. Hollingsworth JW, Saykaly RJ: Systemic complications of rheumatoid arthritis. Med Clin North Am 1977; 61:217.

64. Ziff M: Immunopathogenesis of rheumatoid arthritis. Eur J Rheumatol Inflamm 1982; 5:469.

65. Weinstein IM: Lymph node enlargement and splenomegaly, in Williams WJ, Beutler E, Erslev AJ, et al (eds): Hematology, 3rd ed, p 937. New York, McGraw-Hill, 1983.

66. Kiernan TJ, Gillan J, Murray JP, et al: Behçet's disease and splenomegaly. Br Med J 1978; 2:1340.

67. Koo CH, Nathwani BN, Winberg CD, et al: Atypical lymphoplasmacytic and immunoblastic proliferation in lymph nodes of patients with autoimmune disease (autoimmune disease–associated lymphadenopathy). Medicine 1984; 63:274.

68. Kamel OW, van de Rijn M, Hanasono MM, et al: Immunosuppression-associated lymphoproliferative disorders in rheumatic patients. Leuk Lymphoma 1975; 16:363.

69. Santana V, Rose NR: Neoplastic lymphoproliferation in autoimmune disease: An update review. Clin Immunol Immunopathol 1992; 63:205.

70. Zulman J, Jaffe R, Talal N: Evidence that the malignant lymphoma of Sjögren's syndrome is a monoclonal B-cell neoplasm. N Engl J Med 1978; 299:1215.

71. Jordan RC, Pringle JH, Speight PM: High frequency of light chain restriction in labial gland biopsies of Sjögren's syndrome detected by in situ hybridization. J Pathol 1995; 177:35.

72. Frizzera G, Moran EM, Rappaport H: Angioimmunoblastic lymphadenopathy: Diagnosis and clinical course. Am J Med 1975; 59:803.

73. Frizzera G, Moran EM, Rappaport H: Angioimmunoblastic lymphadenopathy with dysproteinemia. Lancet 1974; 1:1070.

74. Lukes RJ, Tindle BH: Immunoblastic lymphadenopathy: A hyperimmune entity resembling Hodgkin's disease. N Engl J Med 1975; 291:1.

75. O'Connor NT, Crick JA, Wainscoat JS, et al: Evidence for monoclonal T-lymphocyte proliferation in angioimmunoblastic lymphadenopathy. J Clin Pathol 1986; 39:1229.

76. Shimoyama M, Minato K, Saito H, et al: Immunoblastic lymphadenopathy (IBL)–like T-cell lymphoma. Jpn J Clin Oncol 1979; 9:347.

77. Neiman RS, Dervan P, Haudenschild C, et al: Angioimmunoblastic lymphadenopathy: An ultrastructural and immunologic study with review of the literature. Cancer 1978; 41:507.

78. Lukes RJ, Tindle BH: Immunoblastic lymphadenopathy: A prelymphomatous state of immunoblastic sarcoma. Cancer Res 1978; 64:241.

79. Bluming AZ, Cohen HG, Saxon A: Angioimmunoblastic lymphadenopathy with dysproteinemia: A pathogenetic link between physiologic lymphoid proliferations and malignant lymphoma. Am J Med 1979; 67:421.

80. Kosmidis PA, Axelrod AR, Palacas C, et al: Angioimmunoblastic lymphadenopathy: A T-cell deficiency. Cancer 1978; 42:447.

81. Palutke M, Khilanani P, Weise R: Immunologic and electron microscopic characteristics of a case of immunoblastic lymphadenopathy. Am J Clin Pathol 1976; 65:929.

82. Rappaport H, Moran EM: Angioimmunoblastic (immunoblastic) lymphadenopathy. N Engl J Med 1975; 292:8.

83. Nathwani BN, Rappaport H, Moran EM, et al: Malignant lymphoma arising in angioimmunoblastic lymphadenopathy. Cancer 1978; 41:578.

84. Nathwani BN, Winberg CD, Bearman RM: Angioimmunoblastic lymphadenopathy with dysproteinemia and its progression to malignant lymphoma, in Jaffe ES (ed): Surgical Pathology of the Lymph Nodes and Related Organs, p 57. Philadelphia, WB Saunders Co, 1985.

85. Donhuijsen M, Donhuijsen-Ant R, Leder LD: Evolution of angioimmunoblastic lymphadenopathy. N Engl J Med 1977; 297:840.

86. Fisher RI, Jaffe ES, Braylan RC, et al: Immunoblastic lymphadenopathy: Evolution into a malignant lymphoma with plasmacytoid features. Am J Med 1976; 61:553.

87. Weiss LM, Strickler JG, Dorfman RF, et al: Clonal T-cell populations in angioimmunoblastic lymphadenopathy and angioimmunoblastic lymphadenopathy-like lymphoma. Am J Pathol 1986; 122:392.

88. Nathwani BN, Jaffe ES: Angioimmunoblastic lymphadenopathy (AILD) and AILD-like T-cell lymphomas, in Jaffe ES (ed): Surgical Pathology of the Lymph Nodes and Related Organs, p 390. Philadelphia, WB Saunders Co, 1995.

89. Namikawa R, Suchi T, Ueda R, et al: Phenotyping of proliferating lymphocytes in angioimmunoblastic lymphadenopathy and related lesions by the double immunoenzymatic staining technique. Am J Pathol 1987; 127:279.

90. Jaffe ES: Morphologic features, in Steinberg AD (moderator): Angioimmunoblastic lymphadenopathy with dysproteinemia. Ann Intern Med 1988; 108:577.

91. Weiss LM, Strickler JG, Dorfman RF, et al: Clonal T-cell populations in angioimmunoblastic lymphade-

nopathy and angioimmunoblastic lymphadenopathy-like lymphoma. Am J Pathol 1986; 122:392.

92. Watanabe S, Sato Y, Shimoyama M, et al: Immunoblastic lymphadenopathy, angioimmunoblastic lymphadenopathy, and IBL-like T-cell lymphoma: A spectrum of T-cell neoplasia. Cancer 1986; 58:2224.

93. Rudders RA, DeLellis R: Immunoblastic lymphadenopathy: A mixed proliferation of T and B lymphocytes. Am J Clin Pathol 1977; 68:518.

94. Ganesan TS, Dhaliwal HS, Dorreen MS, et al: Angioimmunoblastic lymphadenopathy: A clinical, immunological and molecular study. Br J Cancer 1987; 55:437.

95. Feller AC, Griesser H, Schilling CV, et al: Clonal gene rearrangement patterns correlate with immunophenotype and clinical parameters in patients with angioimmunoblastic lymphadenopathy. Am J Pathol 1988; 133:549.

96. Boros L, Bhaskar AG, D'Souza JP: Monoclonal evolution of angioimmunoblastic lymphadenopathy. Am J Clin Pathol 1981; 75:856.

97. Knecht H, Odermatt BF, Maurer R, et al: Diagnostic and prognostic value of monoclonal antibodies in immunophenotyping of angioimmunoblastic lymphadenopathy/lymphogranulomatosis X. Br J Haematol 1987; 67:19.

98. O'Conner NTJ, Crick JA, Wainscoat JS, et al: Evidence for monoclonal T-lymphocyte proliferation in angioimmunoblastic lymphadenopathy. J Clin Pathol 1986; 39:1229.

99. Griesser H, Feller AC, Lennert K, et al: Rearrangement of the B chain of the T-cell antigen receptor and immunoglobulin genes in lymphoproliferative disorders. J Clin Invest 1986; 78:1179.

100. Schnitzer B: Reactive lymphoid hyperplasia, in Jaffe ES (ed): Surgical Pathology of the Lymph Nodes and Related Organs, p 29. Philadelphia, WB Saunders Co, 1985.

101. Burgert EO, Gilchrist GS, Fairbanks VF, et al: Intra-abdominal angiofollicular lymph node hyperplasia (plasma cell variant) with an antierythropoietic factor. Mayo Clin Proc 1975; 50:542.

102. Frizzera G, Massarelli G, Banks PM, et al: A systemic lymphoproliferative disorder with morphologic features of Castleman's disease. Am J Surg Pathol 1983; 7:211.

103. Frizzera G: Castleman's disease: More questions than answers. Hum Pathol 1985; 16:202.

104. Levo Y, Behar AJ, Blum I, et al: A benign course of multicentric Castleman's disease with involvement of the spleen and bone marrow. Eur J Haematol 1987; 39:471.

105. Cesarman E, Knowles DM: Kaposi's sarcoma-associated herpesvirus: A lymphotropic human herpesvirus associated with Kaposi's sarcoma, primary effusion lymphoma, and multicentric Castleman's disease. Semin Diagn Pathol 1997; 14:54.

106. Gillison ML, Ambinder RF: Human herpesvirus-8. Curr Opin Oncol 1997; 9:440.

107. Parravicini C, Corbellino M, Paulli M, et al: Expression of a virus-derived cytokine, KSHV vIL-6, in HIV-seronegative Castleman's disease. Am J Pathol 1997; 151:1517.

108. Yoshizaki K, Matsuda T, Nishimoto N, et al: Pathogenic significance of interleukin-6 (IL-6/BSF2) in Castleman's disease. Blood 1989; 74:1360.

109. Brandt SJ, Bodine DM, Dunbar CE, et al: Dysregulated interleukin-6 expression produces a syndrome resembling Castleman's disease in mice. J Clin Invest 1990; 86:592.

110. Hsu SM, Xie SS, Hsu PL, et al: Interleukin-6, but not interleukin-4, is exprssed by Reed-Sternberg cells in Hodgkin's disease with or without histologic features of Castleman's disease. Am J Pathol 1992; 141:129.

111. Weisenburger DD: Multicentric angiofollicular lymph node hyperplasia: Pathology of the spleen. Am J Surg Pathol 1988; 12:176.

6

GRANULOMATOUS DISORDERS

Granulomatous disorders affecting the spleen may be divided into three subgroups: (1) lipogranulomas, (2) infectious granulomas, and (3) granulomas associated with presumed altered immune function (Table 6–1). Although some granulomas reflect involvement of the spleen as part of a systemic proc-

Table 6–1. Granulomatous Disorders of the Spleen

I. Lipogranulomas
II. Infectious granulomas
   A. Bacterial
      1. Catalase-producing organisms (chronic granulomatous disease)
      2. Mycobacterial infection
         a. Tuberculosis
         b. Leprosy
         c. Atypical mycobacteria
      3. Tularemia
      4. *Yersinia*
      5. Tertiary syphilis
      6. Brucellosis
   B. Fungal
      1. Histoplasmosis
      2. Blastomycosis
      3. Coccidioidomycosis
      4. Sporotrichosis
   C. Protozoal
      1. Toxoplasmosis
      2. *Pneumocystis carinii*
      3. Leishmaniasis (kala-azar)
   D. Schistosomiasis
III. Granulomas associated with altered immune function
      1. Sarcoidosis
      2. Hodgkin's disease
      3. Malignant lymphomas
      4. Chronic uremia
      5. Combined immunodeficiency
      6. Selective IgA deficiency

ess, the majority are isolated findings of little clinical significance.[1]

LIPOGRANULOMAS

Lipogranulomas are common in the spleen.[1–4] They may be found either at autopsy or incidentally in spleens removed for a variety of causes. They have been reported in 20 percent of surgically removed spleens[5] and 62 percent of autopsy specimens.[2] They are rarely found in the first 2 decades of life, and their incidence increases with age. Wiland and Smith[4] reported an increased incidence in males (64 percent) as compared with females (52 percent). Lipogranulomas occur in the white pulp. They are usually found adjacent to arterioles and are not seen within germinal centers (Fig. 6–1). The lipid droplets occur either as single large vacuoles or as numerous small ones within macrophages. There is rarely a conspicuous giant cell response, and there is no associated inflammatory cell infiltrate or fibrosis.

The cause of lipogranulomas is unclear. It was formerly postulated that they occurred more commonly in persons with disordered lipid metabolism, particularly diabetes mellitus.[6] However, Wiland and Smith[4] did not find an increased incidence in patients with diabetes and found no difference in incidence between treated and untreated diabetic patients. It has also been hypothesized that the lipid deposits are derived from exogenous lipids, particularly from ingestion of mineral oil.[2] Lipid globules have been found in the spleens of rats fed a high-cholesterol diet.[7] Lipid oil

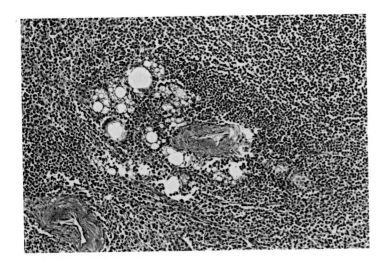

Figure 6–1. Splenic lipogranuloma. Lipogranulomas always occur in the white pulp and appear adjacent to arterioles.

droplets are also frequently found in humans in the lymph nodes in the porta hepatis.[8, 9] By mass spectrometry, these droplets have been shown to be deposits of saturated hydrocarbons with a composition typical of mineral oil. However, because lipogranulomas occur in spleens of patients who have never ingested mineral oil, this cannot be the source in all cases. Idiopathic lipogranulomatosis of the spleen associated with noncaseating granulomas of the liver has been reported in patients with acute febrile illness of undetermined origin.[10]

INFECTIOUS GRANULOMAS

Splenomegaly may be found in a variety of systemic infections, including those caused by protozoa, fungi, and bacteria. However, these disorders rarely produce grossly apparent masses, and the degree of splenic enlargement is usually modest. The histopathology of splenic granulomas produced by infectious agents is similar to that seen in other tissues of the body. They may be caseating, necrotizing, or noncaseating (sarcoidlike). Infectious granulomas occur randomly in the white and/ or red pulp and may be more frequent in the latter, in contrast to lipogranulomas and sarcoidal-type granulomas. In patients with immunosuppression caused either by an underlying disease, such as AIDS, or by therapy, granulomas are less well formed. The histiocytic proliferation in these cases may resemble Langerhans cell histiocytosis or lepromatous leprosy.

The spleen is usually modestly enlarged in miliary tuberculosis.[11–13] The typical pale yellow caseating granulomas usually measure approximately 1 to 2 mm, similar to the size of malpighian corpuscles (Fig. 6–2). Occasionally, however, very large caseous masses may result from coalescence of the lesions. Atypical mycobacterial infections may also produce necrotizing granulomas in the spleen.[3, 14] However, such infections usually occur in patients with compromised immune function, in whom the typical well-formed granulomas are rare. We have seen several spleens obtained at autopsy from patients with AIDS who died with disseminated *Mycobacterium avium-intracellulare* (see Chapter 4). These spleens showed sheets of foamy histiocytes containing numerous acid-fast bacilli without discrete granuloma formation. Leprosy has been reported as a cause of splenomegaly, resulting from multiple noncaseating granulomas containing the acid-fast bacilli *Mycobacterium leprae.*[1]

A miliary pattern of granulomas also occurs in disseminated fungal infections, including histoplasmosis, coccidioidomycosis, blastomycosis, and sporotrichosis, which are endemic in certain regions of the United States. In particular, disseminated histoplasmosis may produce splenomegaly with secondary hypersplenism (Fig. 6–3).[15, 16] The structure of the granulomas produced by these fungi is similar to that seen in other organs. In fulminant disseminated disease, well-formed epithelioid cell granulomas are not usually found, but instead there may be focal accumulations of macrophages containing numerous organisms (Fig. 6–4). We have seen cryptococcosis in the spleen of a patient with AIDS; the organ

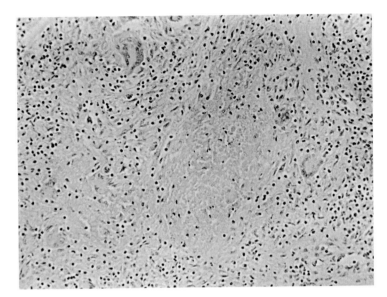

Figure 6–2. Splenic involvement in miliary tuberculosis showing caseating granulomas.

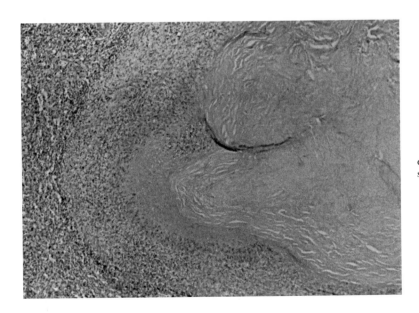

Figure 6–3. Splenic granuloma due to *Histoplasma capsulatum* showing central necrosis.

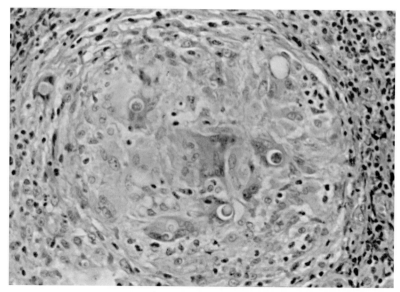

Figure 6–4. Splenic blastomycosis. Numerous macrophages containing organisms are present.

showed numerous macrophages without well-formed granulomas (Fig. 6–5).

Other organisms that uncommonly produce granulomas in the spleen include *Francisella tularensis* (tularemia) and *Yersinia pestis* (plague). These agents usually cause necrotizing granulomas similar to those described in lymph nodes. Splenomegaly with granulomatous inflammation may also be a feature of disseminated brucellosis.[17, 18] In the acute form of this disease there may be necrotizing lesions resembling abscesses or focal infarcts. However, more commonly there are healed calcific foci without active lesions. This is also true of healed histoplasmosis, particularly in spleens of patients from the Midwest, where histoplasmosis is endemic. We have seen two cases in which granulomas were present in the spleen in patients with diagnostic *Toxoplasma* titers. Splenic granulomas can also be found in patients with legionellosis.[19] Schistosoma granulomas may occasionally be found in the spleen, usually in the red pulp, as a reaction to eggs lodging in small vessels.[3, 11] However, splenomegaly in patients with schistosomiasis more commonly results from portal hypertension

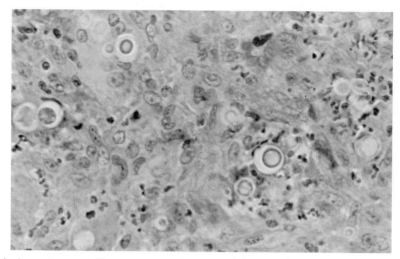

Figure 6–5. Splenic cryptococcosis. Numerous macrophages containing organisms are present, but well-formed granulomas are not apparent.

due to invasion of the portal venous system by *Schistosoma mansoni* or *S. japonicum*. Eosinophilic granulomas containing microfilariae have been reported in patients with loiasis.[20] Tertiary syphilis involving the spleen may produce large gummas, fibrocalcific nodules in which the spirochetes are rarely identified.[21, 22] Gummatous splenitis may rarely occur as an isolated manifestation of tertiary syphilis.[23] *Pneumocystis carinii* infection and kala-azar have also been reported as rare causes of granulomatous inflammation in the spleen.[11, 12, 24, 25] Noncaseating granulomas of the spleen may rarely also be observed in patients with infectious mononucleosis.[26]

Granulomatous reaction of the spleen is commonly observed in patients with chronic granulomatous disease (CGD) of childhood, a heterogeneous group of genetic defects that have in common the failure of neutrophils, monocytes, macrophages, and eosinophils to undergo a respiratory burst and generate superoxide. CGD is manifested clinically by recurrent bacterial and fungal infectious. Although the pattern of inheritance is variable, CGD is usually X-linked and affects male infants and young children.[27–32] In most if not all instances, the molecular heterogeneity of CGD can be organized into a classification scheme based on the oxidase component affected.[33] CGD is caused by defects in the activity (or activation) of NADPH oxidase,[34] which results in impaired destruction of catalase-positive bacteria by neutrophils. The enzymatic

defect results in failure of production of H_2O_2 by neutrophils during phagocytosis, although their ability to ingest bacteria is not compromised.[34–36] In the normal neutrophil, H_2O_2 accumulates within phagolysosomes and, with the aid of myeloperoxidase delivered from intracellular granules, kills the organisms. Certain bacteria, such as *Staphylococcus aureus*, elaborate the enzyme catalase that breaks down H_2O_2, inhibiting the H_2O_2 myeloperoxidase killing system. Normally the neutrophil produces enough H_2O_2 to exceed the inactivating capacity of these bacteria. However, in CGD the neutrophil does not produce H_2O_2, and that which is produced by the bacteria themselves is inactivated by catalase. Individuals with this disorder are therefore subject to recurrent infections with catalase-positive organisms, including *S. aureus* and most gram-negative bacilli.[37–39] Affected patients can resist catalase-negative organisms such as streptococcus and pneumococcus. The lesions found in children with CGD are characteristically granulomas with purulent necrotic centers (Fig. 6–6). Macrophages containing pigment resembling ceroid may also be noted in the spleens of these patients.[40]

Rarely, cat-scratch disease (CSD), an infection caused by a gram-negative bacillus currently known as *Bartonella henselae* (formerly *Rochalimaea henselae*),[41–43] presents with hepatosplenomegaly in the absence of identifiable cutaneous scratch lesions or superficial lymphadenopathy.[44, 45] This type of presentation oc-

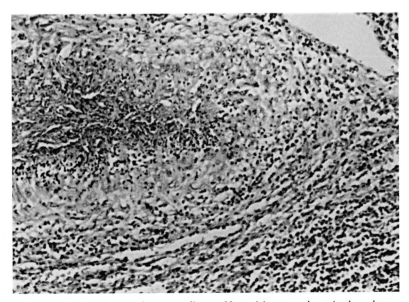

Figure 6–6. Chronic granulomatous disease. Necrotizing granuloma in the spleen.

curs in 10 percent of patients, usually children, and includes, in addition to hepatosplenic multifocal granulomas, Parinaud oculoglandular syndrome, meningoencephalitis, hematologic abnormalities, osteomyelitis, and fever of unknown origin.[46, 47] Typical necrotizing granulomas with central suppuration have been reported in the liver of these atypical CSD cases.[45–48] Abdominal ultrasonography and computed tomography show the presence of multifocal defects in the liver and spleen as well as frequent intra-abdominal lymphadenopathy.[49–51] The presence of antibody titers to *B. henselae* may be used to support the diagnosis of hepatosplenic CSD.[52–54] This microorganism can be demonstrated by Warthin-Starry staining in a proportion of the cases. An antibody reactive with *Rochalimaea quintana*, a closely related microorganism, can also be used to stain these bacilli.[55]

GRANULOMAS ASSOCIATED WITH ALTERED IMMUNE FUNCTION

Sarcoidal-type granulomas may be found in the spleen in a variety of disorders that appear to be associated with altered immune function. The prototype of this group is sarcoidosis[56] (Fig. 6–7). Although the spleen is commonly involved in this disorder, it is usually only mildly enlarged.[57–59] Clinically unsuspected splenic involvement is commonly found at autopsy. The granulomas are located in the white pulp in association with the arterial circulation (Fig. 6–8). Histologically, the granulomas are well formed and are composed of aggregates of epithelioid histiocytes with occasional Langerhans or foreign body–type giant cells. Although occasionally Schaumann bodies (laminated calcium concretions) or stellate-shaped asteroid bodies occur, these inclusions are uncommon.[1] The granulomas are noncaseating, although there may occasionally be central fibrinoid necrosis. Older granulomas may become hyalinized or fibrotic. The granulomas are usually small and may not be apparent grossly, but they may sometimes coalesce to produce small nodules. Although rarely of clinical significance, splenic involvement in sarcoidosis may lead to hypersplenism,[60, 61] and occasionally splenomegaly has been the presenting feature of the disease.[62] Several cases have been reported in which rapidly progressive splenomegaly was associated with anemia and severe hypercalcemia.[63]

Granulomas resembling those found in sarcoidosis were described in the spleens of patients with Hodgkin's disease by Kadin and colleagues[64] (Fig. 6–9). They were found in the spleens of 12.5 percent of untreated patients undergoing staging laparotomy. Granulomas were found less frequently in the liver or abdominal nodes and only occasionally in the bone marrow. None of the patients had evidence of disseminated sarcoidosis. Subsequent authors have reported similar frequencies.[65–67] Although these granulomas are occasionally found with concomitant splenic involvement by Hodgkin's disease, they are more commonly isolated findings. They are not a reaction to lymphangiogram dye because they may

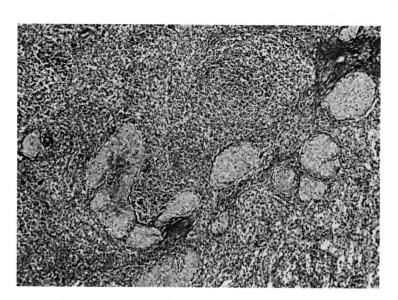

Figure 6–7. Sarcoidosis. The granulomas are located in the white pulp.

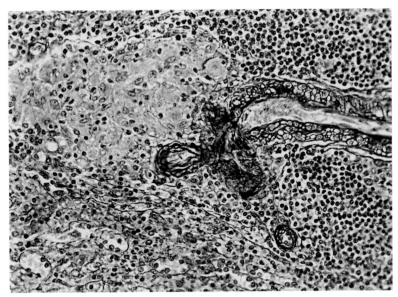

Figure 6–8. Sarcoid-type granuloma showing the association with the arteriolar circulation.

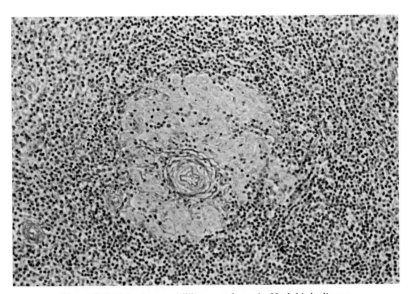

Figure 6–9. Splenic sarcoidlike granuloma in Hodgkin's disease.

occur in patients who have not had lymphangiography.[68] In a review of 412 spleens removed for a variety of disorders, Neiman found sarcoidal granulomas in 13 of 61 spleens (21 percent) obtained at staging laparotomy for Hodgkin's disease, including 8 with nodular sclerosis, 4 with mixed cellularity, and 1 with lymphocytic predominance subtype.[5] Concomitant Hodgkin's disease was found in only four of these spleens. The finding of isolated granulomas in spleens of patients with Hodgkin's disease does not alter the clinical stage of the disease or the treatment modality, although Sacks and associates[67] reported a somewhat improved prognosis in patients with splenic granulomas.

Splenic granulomas may be associated with non-Hodgkin's lymphomas, although less commonly than in Hodgkin's disease.[5, 69–71] Neiman and colleagues[72] reported such granulomas in the spleens of several patients with mantle cell lymphoma who presented with massive splenomegaly due to lymphomatous involvement (Fig. 6–10). Similar granulomas also occasionally occurred in the liver, lymph nodes, or bone marrow. Braylan and coworkers[69] reported three cases of lymphoma presenting with prominent splenomegaly in which extensive splenic granulomas nearly obscured the underlying malignant lymphoma. In these cases the granulomas were found in the marginal zones and red pulp and numbered as many as 50 per low-power field. Granulomas were also found in the lymph nodes and livers in these cases. The lymphoma was more easily recognized in abdominal lymph nodes and was described as being composed of atypical lymphocytes of small to intermediate size with a vaguely nodular pattern. In the spleen, the atypical lymphocytes replaced some of the follicles and were associated with some cleaved cells and occasional larger cells with prominent nucleoli. From the description, it seems likely that these cases represent additional examples of mantle cell lymphoma. In cases of Hodgkin's disease and non-Hodgkin's lymphomas, the granulomas may occur as isolated phenomena unassociated with foci of malignancy or may occur as part of the neoplastic focus. Bendix-Hansen and Bayer[73] also reported the presence of epithelioid granulomas in four patients with hairy cell leukemia. None of these cases showed granulomas in the bone marrow.

Splenic granulomas may also occur in patients with nonmalignant diseases. Neiman and colleagues[74] found granulomas in 3 of 28 spleens obtained from patients with chronic uremia who were undergoing hemodialysis (Fig. 6–11). Granulomas have been described

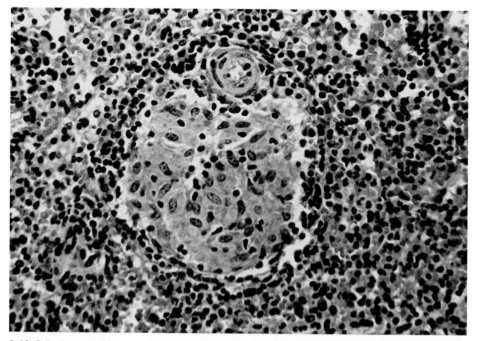

Figure 6–10. Splenic sarcoidlike granuloma in mantle cell lymphoma. The tumor cells surround the granuloma, which abuts a penicilliary arteriole.

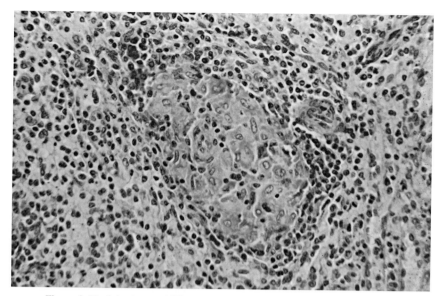

Figure 6–11. Splenic sarcoidlike granuloma in a patient with chronic uremia.

in the spleens of patients with severe combined immunodeficiency,[75] agammaglobulinemia,[76] and selective IgA deficiency (Fig. 6–12). Splenic granulomas have also been reported in other immunologic diseases such as extrinsic allergic alveolitis (Farmer lung)[77] and Wegener granulomatosis.[78]

The common factor in all these disorders associated with splenic sarcoidal-type granulomas appears to be deranged function of the immune system. In all instances we have stud-

ied, granulomas are located adjacent to the arterioles of the afferent limb of the splenic circulation, commonly in the marginal zones. Although occasionally they may also occur in the red pulp, they are almost always associated with penicilliary arterioles and therefore with the lymphatic sheath (see Figs. 6–7 through 6–12). Granulomas are not found free in the red pulp or within germinal centers. Their location in the white pulp near the arterial circulation, the zones of antigen trapping, sug-

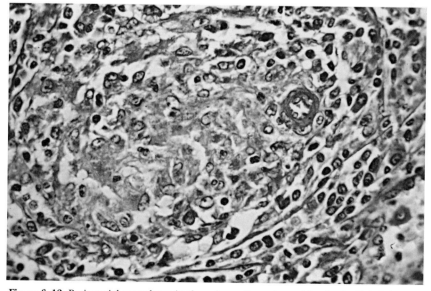

Figure 6–12. Periarterial granuloma in the spleen of a patient with selective IgA deficiency.

gests that they may be a response to a blood-borne antigen.[79, 80] The impaired immunity in these disorders appears to be related to T-cell dysfunction.[1, 5] Patients with sarcoidosis exhibit a depression of delayed hypersensitivity and increased levels of circulating antibodies, reflecting deficient cell-mediated immunity. However, functional studies of the lymphocytes from the lungs of patients with active disease have shown a marked increase in the number of T helper cells, although the ratio of helper to suppressor cells in the peripheral blood is decreased.[81–83] Suppressor T cells are found to be increased during the regression of the granulomas. The granulomas are believed to be caused by T-cell activation with lymphokine production. These as well as other cytokines are thought to be responsible for the observed accumulation, fusion, and epithelioid changes of macrophages. Polyclonal B-cell activation may be responsible for the observed T-cell dysfunction in these patients.[56]

Patients with Hodgkin's disease also have a similarly deficient T-cell function[84–91] associated with polyclonal B-cell activation that appears to be involved in the granuloma formation in these patients. Non-Hodgkin's lymphomas may also be associated with impaired immunologic function,[92, 93] and uremic patients also show impaired allograft rejection and delayed hypersensitivity,[94, 95] suggesting that a similar mechanism may be involved in the pathogenesis of sarcoidal granulomas in these conditions.

In some cases granulomas may be found in the spleen without an apparent underlying cause. Kuo and Rosai[96] reported 20 cases of granulomatous inflammation in the spleen in which patients presented with fever, weight loss, hepatosplenomegaly, and hypersplenism. The granulomas showed variable degrees of necrosis. Microorganisms were isolated in only three cases, including one each of *Histoplasma capsulatum, Sporotrichum schenkii,* and atypical mycobacterium. Granulomas were found in the liver and lymph nodes in all cases in which these organs were studied. Seven patients remained asymptomatic following splenectomy, whereas six showed persistent granulomatous inflammation in other organs. None of the patients developed a malignant lymphoma or Hodgkin's disease, although one developed systemic manifestations of sarcoidosis. Necrotizing splenic granulomas associated with febrile episodes have been described in two children in remission after treatment for acute

leukemia.[97] However, the presence of an infectious agent could not be documented in either child; and corticosteroid therapy was apparently curative. Because the disorder followed severe myelosuppression in both cases, it is possible that the granulomas were of infectious origin.

REFERENCES

1. Collins RD, Neiman RS: Granulomatous diseases of the spleen, in Joachim HL (ed): Pathology of Granulomas, p 189. New York, Raven Press, 1983.
2. Liber AF, Rose HG: Saturated hydrocarbons in follicular lipidosis of the spleen. Arch Pathol 1967; 83:116.
3. MacPherson AIS, Richmond J, Stuart AE: The Spleen, p 83. Springfield, Ill, Charles C Thomas, 1973.
4. Wiland OK, Smith EB: Lipid globules in the lymphoid follicles of the spleen. Arch Pathol 1957; 64:623.
5. Neiman RS: Incidence and importance of splenic sarcoid-like granulomas. Arch Pathol 1977; 101:518.
6. Klemperer P: The spleen, in Downey H (ed): Handbook of Hematology, p 1587. New York, Paul B. Hoeber, 1938.
7. Antischkow N: Ober experimentell erzeugte: Ablagerungen von anisotropen lipoidsubstanzen im der Milz und im knockenmark. Beitr Path Anat 1913; 57:201.
8. Boitnott JK, Margolis S: Mineral oil in human tissues. I. Detection of saturated hydrocarbons using thin-layer chromatography. Bull Johns Hopkins Hosp 1966; 118:402.
9. Boitnott JK, Margolis S: Mineral oil in human tissues. II. Oil droplets in lymph nodes of the porta hepatis. Bull Johns Hopkins Hosp 1966; 118:414.
10. Rubinstein A, Brenner S: Idiopathic lipogranulomatosis of spleen and periaortic lymph nodes with noncaseating granulomas of liver. Hum Pathol 1982; 13:1133.
11. Blaustein AU, Diggs LW: Pathology of the spleen, in Blaustein AU (ed): The Spleen, p 179. New York, McGraw-Hill, 1963.
12. Klemperer P: The pathologic anatomy of splenomegaly. Am J Clin Pathol 1936; 6:99.
13. Solomon HA, Doran WT: Primary tuberculosis of the spleen. N Y State J Med 1939; 39:1259.
14. Koenig MG, Collins RD, Heysell RM: Disseminated mycobacteriosis caused by Battey-type mycobacteria. Ann Intern Med 1966; 64:145.
15. Goodwin RA, Shapiro JL, Thurman GH, et al: Disseminated histoplasmosis: Clinical and pathologic correlations. Medicine 1980; 59:1.
16. Schwarz J, Silversman FN, Adriano SM, et al: The relation of splenic calcification to histoplasmosis. N Engl J Med 1955; 252:887.
17. Williams GD, Hara M: Active splenic granuloma as a source of recurrent brucellosis: Successful surgical treatment. Am J Surg 1967; 113:422.
18. Yow EM, Brennan JC, Nathan MH, et al: Calcified granulomata of the spleen in long-standing brucellar infection. Ann Intern Med 1961; 55:307.
19. Ibanez MA, Omar M, Mediavilla JD, et al: Legionellosis with a splenic granulomatous reaction. Med Clin (Barc) 1993; 100:438.
20. Burchard GD, Reimold-Jehle U, Burkle V, et al: Sple-

nectomy for suspected malignant lymphoma in two patients with loiasis. Clin Infect Dis 1996; 23:979.

21. Harmos O, Myers ME: Gummatous syphilitic splenomegaly. Am J Clin Pathol 1951; 21:737.

22. Mayo WJ: A review of 500 splenectomies with special reference to mortality and end results. Ann Surg 1928; 88:409.

23. Perez CM, Leon A, Oddo D, et al: Isolated gummatous splenitis. Clin Infect Dis 1995; 21:228.

24. Barnett RN, Hull JG, Vortel V, et al: *Pneumocystis carinii* in lymph nodes and spleen. Arch Pathol 1969; 88:175.

25. LeGolvan DP, Heidelberger KP: Disseminated granulomatous *Pneumocystis carinii* pneumonia. Arch Pathol 1973; 95:344.

26. Thomas DM, Akosa AB, Lampert IA: Granulomatous inflammation of the spleen in infectious mononucleosis. Histopathology 1990; 17:265.

27. Azimi PH, Bodenbender JG, Hintz RL, et al: Chronic granulomatous disease in three female siblings. JAMA 1968; 206:23.

28. Dupree E, Smith CW, McDougall NLT, et al: Undetected carrier state in chronic granulomatous disease. J Pediatr 1972; 81:77

29. Holmes B, Park BH, Malawista SE, et al: Chronic granulomatous disease in females: A deficiency of leukocyte glutathione peroxidase. N Engl J Med 1970; 283:217.

30. Mills EL, Rholl KS, Quie PG: X-linked inheritance in females with chronic granulomatous disease. J Clin Invest 1980; 66:332.

31. Quie PG, Kaplan EL, Page AR, et al: Defective polymorphonuclear leukocyte function and chronic granulomatous disease in two female children. N Engl J Med 1968; 278:976.

32. Windhorst DB, Page AR, Holmes B, et al: The pattern of genetic transmission of the leukocyte defect in fatal granulomatous disease of childhood. J Clin Invest 1968; 47:1026.

33 Curnutte JT: Disorders of phagocyte function, in Hoffman R, Benz EJ Jr, Shattil SJ, et al (eds): Hematology: Basic Principles and Practice, 2nd ed, p 792. New York, Churchill Livingstone, 1994.

34. Curnutte JT, Whitten DM, Babior BM: Defective superoxide production by granulocytes from patients with chronic granulomatous disease. N Engl J Med 1974; 290:593.

35. Hohn DC, Lehrer RI: NADPH oxidase deficiency in X-linked chronic granulomatous disease. J Clin Invest 1975; 55:707.

36. Karnovsky ML: Chronic granulomatous disease: Piece of a cellular and molecular puzzle. Fed Proc 1973; 32:1527.

37. Good RA, Quie PG, Windhorst DB: Fatal (chronic) granulomatous disease of childhood: A hereditary defect of leukocyte function. Semin Hematol 1968; 5:215.

38. Gray GR, Stamatovannopoulos G, Naiman SC: Neutrophil dysfunction, chronic granulomatous disease and nonspherocytic haemolytic anemia caused by complete deficiency of glucose-6-phosphate dehydrogenase. Lancet 1973; 2:530.

39. Johnston RB Jr, Baehner RL: Chronic granulomatous disease: Correlation between pathogenesis and clinical findings. Pediatrics 1971; 48:730.

40. Landing BH, Shirkey HS: A syndrome of recurrent infection and infiltration of viscera by pigmented lipid histiocytes. Pediatrics 1957; 20:431.

41. Goral S, Anderson B, Hager C, et al: Detection of *Rochalimaea henselae* DNA by polymerase chain reaction from suppurative nodes of children with cat-scratch disease. Pediatr Infec Dis J 1994; 13:994.

42. Bergmans AM, Groothedde JW, Schellekens JF, et al: Etiology of cat scratch disease: Comparison of polymerase chain reaction detection of *Bartonella* (formerly *Rochalimaea*) and *Afipia felis* DNA with serology and skin tests. J Infect Dis 1995; 171:916.

43. Szelc-Kelly CM, Goral S, Perez-Perez GI, et al: Serologic responses to *Bartonella* and *Afipia* antigens in patients with cat scratch disease. Pediatrics 1995; 96:1137.

44. Malatack JJ, Altman HA, Nard JA, et al: Cat-scratch disease without adenopathy. J Pediatr 1989; 114:101.

45. Delahoussaye PM, Osborne BM: Cat-scratch disease presenting as abdominal visceral granulomas. J Infec Dis 1990; 161:71.

46. Carithers HA: Cat-scratch disease: An overview based on a study of 1,200 patients. Am J Dis Child 1985; 139:1124.

47. Margileth AM: Cat scratch disease. Adv Pediatr Infec Dis 1993; 8:1.

48. Destuynder O, Vanlemmans P, Mboyo A, et al: Systemic cat scratch disease: Hepatic and splenic involvement about 3 pediatric cases. Eur J Pediatr Surg 1995; 5:365.

49. Lenoir AA, Storch GA, DeSchryver-Kecskemeti K, et al: Granulomatous hepatitis associated with cat scratch disease. Lancet 1988; 1:1132.

50. Rappaport DC, Cumming WA, Ros PR: Disseminated hepatic and splenic lesions in cat-scratch disease: Imaging features. Am J Roentgenol 1991; 156:122.

51. Larsen CE, Patrick LE: Abdominal (liver, spleen) and bone manifestations of cat scratch disease. Pediatr Radiol 1992; 22:353.

52. Golden SE: Hepatosplenic cat-scratch disease associated with elevated anti-*Rochalimaea* antibody titers. Pediatr Infec Dis J 1993; 12:868.

53. Doyle D, Eppes S, Klein J: Atypical cat-scratch disease: Diagnosis by a serologic test for *Rochalimaea* species. South Med J 1994; 87:485.

54. Tan TQ, Wagner ML, Kaplan SL: *Bartonella (Rochalimaea) henselae* hepatosplenic infection occurring simultaneously in two siblings. Clin Infec Dis 1996; 22:721.

55. Reed JA, Brigati DJ, Flynn SD, et al: Immunocytochemical identification of *Rochalimaea henselae* in bacillary (epithelioid) angiomatosis, parenchymal bacillary peliosis, and persistent fever with bacteremia. Am J Surg Pathol 1992; 16:650.

56. James DG, William WJ: Immunology of sarcoldosis. Am J Med 1982; 72:5.

57. Branson JH, Park JH: Sarcoidosis-hepatic involvement: Presentation of a case with fatal liver involvement, including autopsy findings and review of the evidence for sarcoid involvement of the liver as found in the literature. Ann Intern Med 1954; 40:111.

58. Ricker W, Clark M: Sarcoidosis: A clinicopathologic review of three hundred cases including twenty-two autopsies. Am J Clin Pathol 1949; 19:725.

59. Scadding JG: Sarcoidosis, p 22. London, Eyre and Spottiswoode, 1967.

60. Davis AE, Belber JP, Movitt ER: Association of hemolytic anemia with sarcoidosis. Blood 1954; 9:379.

61. West WO: Acquired hemolytic anemia secondary to Boeck's sarcoid: Report of a case and review of the literature. N Engl J Med 1958; 261:688.

62. Kay S: Sarcoidosis of the spleen: Report of four cases

with a twenty-three year follow-up in one case. Am J Pathol 1960; 26:427.

63. Nilsson BS, Hanngren A, Lins LE, et al: Acute phase of sarcoidosis with splenomegaly and hypercalcemia: Description of a case, including a report about splenectomy and the preparation and testing of a Kveim antigen from the spleen. Scand J Respir Dis 1978; 59:199.

64. Kadin ME, Donaldson SS, Dorfman RF: Isolated granulomas in Hodgkin's disease. N Engl J Med 1970; 283:859.

65. Brincker H: Sarcoid reactions and sarcoidosis in Hodgkin's disease and other malignant lymphomata. Br J Cancer 1972; 26:120.

66. O'Connell MJ, Schimpff SC, Kirschner RH, et al: Epithelioid granulomas in Hodgkin's disease: A favorable prognostic sign. JAMA 1975; 233:888.

67. Sacks EL, Donaldson SS, Gordon J, et al: Epithelioid granulomas associated with Hodgkin's disease: Clinical correlations in 55 previously untreated patients. Cancer 1978; 41:562.

68. Neiman RS: Current problems in the histopathologic diagnosis and classification of Hodgkin's disease. Pathol Ann 1978; 13:289.

69. Braylan RC, Long JC, Jaffe ES, et al: Malignant lymphoma obscured by concomitant extensive epithelioid granulomas: Report of three cases with similar clinicopathologic features. Cancer 1977; 39:1146.

70. Kim H, Dorfman RF: Morphological studies in untreated patients subjected to laparotomy for the staging of non-Hodgkin's lymphomas. Cancer 1974; 33:657.

71. Neiman RS, Sullivan AL, Jaffe R: Malignant lymphoma simulating leukemic reticuloendotheliosis: A clinicopathologic study of ten cases. Cancer 1979; 43:329.

72. Narang S, Wolf BC, Neiman RS: Malignant lymphoma presenting with prominent splenomegaly: A clinicopathologic study with special reference to intermediate cell lymphoma. Cancer 1985; 55:1948.

73. Bendix-Hansen K, Bayer KI: Granulomas of spleen and liver in hairy cell leukemia. APMIS 1984; 92:157.

74. Neiman RS, Bischel MD, Lukes RJ: Hypersplenism in the uremic hemodialyzed patient: Pathology and proposed pathophysiologic mechanisms. Am J Clin Pathol 1973; 60:502.

75. Edelstein AD, Miller A, Zimelman AP, et al: Adult severe combined immunodeficiency and sarcoid-like granulomas with hypersplenism. Am J Hematol 1973; 5:55.

76. Weston J, Balfour BM, Tsohas W, et al: Splenic lesions in hypogammaglobulinaemia. Adv Exp Med Biol 1993; 329:437.

77. Venho KK, Selroos O, Haahtela T, et al: Splenic granulomas in Farmer's lung disease: An extrapulmonary manifestation of extrinsic allergic alveolitis. Acta Med Scand 1992; 211:413.

78. Shah IA, Holstege A, Riede UN: Bioptic diagnosis of Wegener's granulomatosis in the absence of vasculitis and granulomas. Pathol Res Pract 1984; 178:407.

79. Klausner MH, Hirsch LJ, Leblond PF, et al: Contrasting splenic mechanisms in the blood clearance of red blood cells and colloidal particles. Blood 1975; 46:965.

80. Nossal GJV, Austin CM, Pye J, et al: Antigens in immunity. XII. Antigen trapping in the spleen. Int Arch Allergy Appl Immunol 1966; 29:368.

81. Crystal RG, Roberts WC, Hunninghake GW, et al: Pulmonary sarcoidosis: A disorder characterized and perpetuated by activated lung T-lymphocytes. Ann Intern Med 1981; 94:73.

82. Hunninghake GW, Crystal RG: Pulmonary sarcoidosis: A disorder mediated by excess helper T-lymphocyte activity at sites of disease activity. N Engl J Med 1981; 305:429.

83. Hunninghake GW, Gadek JE, Young RC, et al: Maintenance of granuloma formation in pulmonary sarcoidosis by T lymphocytes within lung. N Engl J Med 1980; 302:592.

84. Aisenberg AC: Studies of lymphocyte transfer reactions in Hodgkin's disease. J Clin Invest 1965; 44:555.

85. Bjorkholm M, Wedelin C, Holm G, et al: Immune status of untreated patients with Hodgkin's disease and prognosis. Cancer Treat Rep 1982; 66:701.

86. Brown RS, Haynes HA, Foley HT, et al: Hodgkin's disease: Immunologic, clinical and histologic features of 50 untreated patients. Ann Intern Med 1967; 67:291.

87. Chase MW: Delayed-type hypersensitivity and the immunology of Hodgkin's disease with a parallel examination of sarcoidosis. Cancer Res 1966; 26:1097.

88. Fisher RI: Implications of persistent T cell abnormalities for the etiology of Hodgkin's disease. Cancer Treat Rep 1982; 66:681.

89. Levy R, Kaplan HS: Impaired lymphocyte function in untreated Hodgkin's disease. N Engl J Med 1974; 298:181.

90. Schulof RS, Bockman RS, Garofalo JA, et al: Multivariate analysis of T-cell functional defects and circulating serum factors in Hodgkin's disease. Cancer 1981; 48:964.

91. Young RC, Corder MP, Berard CW, et al: Immune alterations in Hodgkin's disease: Effect of delayed hypersensitivity and lymphocyte transformation on course and survival. Arch Intern Med 1973; 131:446.

92. Miller DG: Immunological deficiency and malignant lymphoma. Cancer 1967; 20:579.

93. Miller DG: The immunologic capability of patients with lymphoma. Cancer Res 1968; 28:1441.

94. Merrill JP: The immunologic capability of uremic patients. Cancer Res 1968; 28:1449.

95. Wilson WEC, Kirkpatrick CH, Talmage DW: Suppression of immunologic responsiveness in uremia. Ann Intern Med 1965; 62:1.

96. Kuo T, Rosai J: Granulomatous inflammation in splenectomy specimens. Arch Pathol 1974; 98:261.

97. Walker DA, Howat AJ, Shannon RS, et al: Necrotizing granulomatous splenitis complicating leukemia in childhood. Cancer 1985; 56:371.

7

HODGKIN'S DISEASE

The spleen is the most common extranodal organ involved by Hodgkin's disease. Splenic involvement is found in approximately one third of patients undergoing staging laparotomy,[1, 2] and a similar incidence has been reported in an autopsy series.[3] However, primary splenic Hodgkin's disease is extremely rare, being reported even less commonly than primary splenic non-Hodgkin's lymphomas.[4-8] All histologic subtypes of Hodgkin's disease affect the spleen, although nodular sclerosis and mixed cellularity are the usual types noted. Kadin and coworkers,[1] in a review of spleens obtained at staging laparotomy from 117 patients with untreated Hodgkin's disease, found that nodular sclerosis involved the spleen most commonly (27 of 85 cases). However, mixed cellularity had a disproportionately higher incidence of involvement (12 of 19 cases). Splenic involvement in the lymphocyte-predominant subtype is rare, found in 2 of 13 patients in the series by Kadin and in only 1 of 35 cases reported by Trudel et al.[9] Lymphocyte depletion, an uncommon subtype of Hodgkin's disease, characteristically presents with subdiaphragmatic disease and affects the spleen in virtually all cases, although splenomegaly is frequently absent.[10] Hodgkin's disease is an infrequent cause of splenic rupture, although two cases of primary Hodgkin's disease are reported to have presented with rupture of the organ.[4, 8]

SPLENECTOMY IN HODGKIN'S DISEASE

Considerable controversy exists about the routine use of staging laparotomy and splenectomy in the management of patients with Hodgkin's disease. With the development of effective chemotherapy and more sophisticated noninvasive techniques such as computed tomography scans, the performance of staging laparotomies has decreased. In addition, there are risks associated with splenectomy. First, it has been associated with increased risk of developing secondary acute leukemia in patients treated with chemotherapy, especially alkylating agents.[11, 12] Second, there is the possibility of overwhelming postsplenectomy sepsis, although preoperative pneumococcal vaccination and improved surgical techniques during the last decade have greatly reduced the incidence of this complication.[13] In spite of these arguments against its use, surgical staging is still recommended for early-stage patients when the results influence the choice of treatment.[14, 15] In such cases, accurate assessment of splenic involvement by Hodgkin's disease requires splenectomy because clinical and radiologic evaluation of the spleen is often inaccurate.[16, 17] In a review of 443 cases, Sweet and associates[18] found that 81 of 125 spleens (65 percent) that were preoperatively believed to be involved were found to contain tumor when examined after splenectomy, whereas 100 of 318 (32 percent) thought to be free of disease were actually positive. The difficulty in accurate clinical evaluation results from the lack of correlation between splenic size and likelihood of involvement.[3, 19, 20] Normal splenic weight does not preclude involvement, and enlarged spleens are often uninvolved.[1, 3, 21] This fact was demonstrated in a study of 44 spleens obtained from untreated patients with Hodgkin's disease. Farrer-Brown and coworkers[22] found that the weights of uninvolved spleens ranged from 100 to 690 g, with a mean of 192 g, whereas involved spleens ranged from 77 to 780 g, with a mean of 304 g. That normal-sized spleens may be involved by Hodgkin's disease is a fact confirmed many times in our laboratory. In addition, ultrasonography, splenic scans, and computed tomography may not detect small foci of tumor, resulting in false-negative studies.[23-27] Splenic examination is therefore necessary if accurate staging is needed in circumstances in which management decisions depend on the accurate identification of splenic disease.[28]

There has been a movement to attempt to decrease the morbidity of staging laparotomy. Several authors have advocated partial splenectomy as a staging procedure in Hodgkin's disease,[29-33] particularly in children in whom splenectomy may produce overwhelming postsplenectomy sepsis. In our opinion, the high incidence of subtle focal involvement of the spleen in Hodgkin's disease makes partial splenectomy an unwise procedure, and we cannot advocate it. In addition, a great deal of interest has been generated by the recent possibility of performing abdominal lymphadenectomy and splenectomy by laparoscopy in patients with Hodgkin's disease.[34-36] This less invasive approach may result in shorter hospitalization and recovery time and less chance of pulmonary infections, while providing complete pathologic staging of subdiaphragmatic disease, and is currently being evaluated by a growing number of institutions.[37-40]

SPLENIC MORPHOLOGY

Hodgkin's disease produces either miliary nodules (Fig. 7–1) or, more frequently, solitary or multiple tumor masses in the spleen (Color Plate 6). Although splenic involvement is always evident grossly, it may be very subtle.[41] In some cases, the foci of tumor involvement may be few and very small, necessitating careful gross examination of thin slices of the spleen (Color Plate 7).[1, 11, 22, 42] Diebold and Temmin[20] have confirmed this observation by reporting that in 9 percent of 103 cases in which the spleen contained Hodgkin's disease, the only involvement was a single small lesion. We believe, therefore, that a meticulous search for lesions is mandatory before it can be confidently stated that the spleen is uninvolved in a given case of Hodgkin's disease.

Microscopically, the earliest lesions of Hodgkin's disease occur in the periarterial lymphoid sheath (PALS) or in the periphery of the white pulp in the region of the marginal zone (Fig. 7–2).[43] With more advanced disease the tumor expands to encroach on the lymphoid follicles and the red pulp. Tumor masses result from the coalescence of discrete white-pulp nodules. There is no apparent correlation between the histologic subtype of disease and the gross pattern of splenic involvement.

The criteria for the diagnosis of Hodgkin's disease in extranodal sites have not been for-

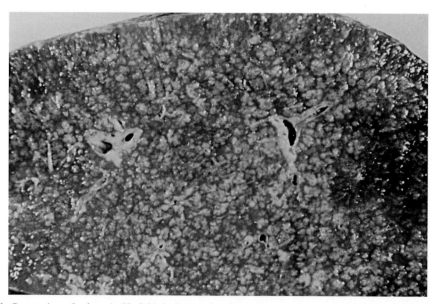

Figure 7–1. Cut section of spleen in Hodgkin's disease showing miliary pattern of involvement similar to that seen in malignant lymphomas of small lymphocytic type.

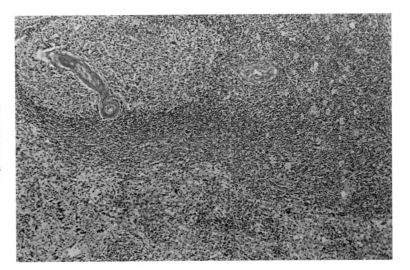

Figure 7–2. Microscopic focus of Hodgkin's disease in the spleen. The area of involvement in the upper right half of the picture is in the periarterial lymphoid sheath and contiguous to the secondary germinal center.

mally revised since the 1960s. In a patient with prior histologically documented nodal disease, these criteria are less stringent than those applied to tissues from patients without such a prior diagnosis.[41] Lukes[44] required that the general features of one of the histologic subtypes of Hodgkin's disease be found in a discrete focus, associated with one of the mononuclear or other variants of the Reed-Sternberg (RS) cell. The typical RS cell itself need not be found. In the absence of a prior histologic diagnosis, however, these atypical cells must be identified in the appropriate cellular environment. Although the presence of characteristic RS variants such as lacunar cells may allow subclassification of Hodgkin's disease in the spleen, such subtyping is often very difficult and need not be attempted in a previously confirmed case (Fig. 7–3). Extranodal Hodgkin's disease often cannot be subtyped histologically owing either to the lack of diagnostic RS variants such as L&H (popcorn cells) or lacunar cells or to the incomplete expression of the architectural alterations (e.g., birefringent sclerosis in nodular sclerosis) (Fig. 7–4). The difficulty of subclassification of Hodgkin's disease in the spleen is reflected in the study of Farrer-Brown and coworkers,[22] who reported

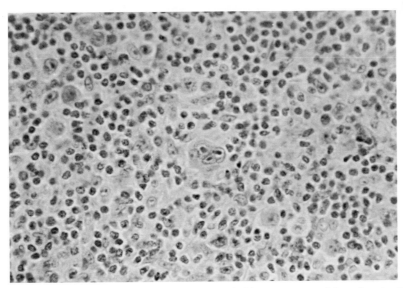

Figure 7–3. Focus of splenic Hodgkin's disease in patient with biopsy-proven nodular sclerosis. Although a Reed-Sternberg cell is present, lacunar cells are not found.

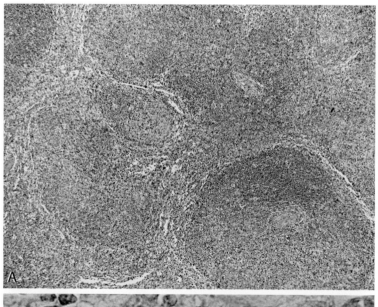

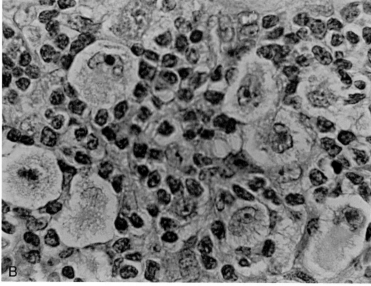

Figure 7–4. (A) Multiple nodules of involvement in the spleen of a patient with previously diagnosed nodular sclerosis. No fibrosis is seen. (B) High-power examination of an involved field, however, reveals numerous characteristic lacunar cells.

that the histologic subtype diagnosed in the spleen was the same as that of the previous diagnosis in the original lymph node biopsy in only 45 percent of cases. Five cases with initial diagnoses of either nodular sclerosis or mixed cellularity had the appearance of lymphocyte predominance in the spleen. In 27 percent of the cases, the spleens resembled lymphocyte-depletion subtype, and the initial node displayed another subtype. Other studies, however, have reported that the majority of cases retain their initial histologic subtype in subsequent biopsies, even in the course of relapse, suggesting that the apparent discordance be-

tween nodal and splenic morphology may reflect the difficulty in subtyping the disease in the spleen.[45, 46] The Ann Arbor Committee has emphasized that even the smallest amount of birefringent collagen and lacunar cells in combination should indicate nodular sclerosis Hodgkin's disease.[47] Furthermore, even if other histologic features are present, that is, a mixed cellularity background, the nodular sclerosis designation should prevail. We suggest that cases with focal disease lacking specific findings be called Hodgkin's disease NOS (not otherwise specified). In occasional cases, particularly those in which the histologic preparations are suboptimal, immunohistochemical studies can be helpful by showing an appropriate phenotype in cytologically atypical cells suspicious for RS cells. Although the phenotype of RS cells is a somewhat controversial topic, with the use of paraffin-reactive antibodies a consistent immunophenotype has been identified. In classic Hodgkin's disease (nodular sclerosis, mixed cellularity), RS cells express the myelomonocytic antigen CD15 (Leu-M1) and lymphoid activation antigen CD30 (Ki-1, Ber-H2) in the absence of leukocyte common antigen.[48–54] A second major paraffin-associated phenotype that is commonly observed in nodular lymphocyte-predominant Hodgkin's disease is the B-cell marker CD20 (L26), with CD45 positivity and absent CD15 expression.[55] RS cells in classic Hodgkin's disease may, however, express CD20 in a subset of cases,[56–58] and CD15 may be negative.[59] In view of the variable antigenic expression in RS cells, reliance on the results of comprehensive panels of antibodies is highly recommended. Molecular genetic investigations of Hodgkin's disease by Southern blot hybridization is compromised by the small number of tumor cells present in biopsy samples.[60–63] It is therefore not surprising that a germline configuration for both immunoglobulin and T-cell receptors is found in most cases. Recent studies[64] based on polymerase chain reaction have, however, discovered a B-cell derivation of RS cells in a variable proportion of case of classic Hodgkin's disease.[58, 65, 66] In addition, a strong association between the expression of B-cell markers and polymerase chain reaction evidence of immunoglobulin gene rearrangement in classic Hodgkin's disease has been reported by several groups, including ours.[58, 67, 68] However, others have found a percentage of cases with clonal rearrangements of T-cell receptor genes,[69] and T-cell antigen expression in RS cells has also been documented.[70] In view of these controversial results, it follows that genotyping alone does not especially help in separating cases of non-Hodgkin's lymphoma from Hodgkin's disease. The correct diagnosis may have to depend on the appropriate interpretation of the immunohistochemical and molecular data within the proper morphologic context.

Although the distinction between the nodular sclerosis and mixed cellularity subtypes of Hodgkin's disease may occasionally be impossible, the unique morphologic and immunologic characteristics of nodular lymphocyte-predominant Hodgkin's disease allow its distinction from the classic subtypes, at least in a proportion of cases.[71, 72] The presence of L&H cells that are CD45-positive, CD20-positive, and CD15-negative in a background of a nodular proliferation of small lymphocytes and epithelioid histiocytes are uniquely characteristic of lymphocyte-predominant Hodgkin's disease. This immunophenotypic profile is largely preserved in its rare occurrence in extranodal sites, including the spleen.[72] However, early involvement in lymphocyte-predominant Hodgkin's disease may be difficult to recognize because of the scarcity of characteristic L&H cells (Fig. 7–5). Lymphocyte-depletion Hodgkin's disease shows an overall decrease in white pulp cellularity and rarely produces significant splenomegaly or tumor masses (Fig. 7–6).[10] Although the sarcomatous variants of RS cells typical of this subtype allow subclassification in some cases, these cells may be rare, and the cellular depletion may result in acellular hyalinized foci, which are difficult to recognize as tumor involvement (Fig. 7–7). We believe that immunologic and immunogenetic studies are required to separate lymphocyte-depletion Hodgkin's disease from other high-grade tumors, especially anaplastic large-cell lymphoma.[73] We also believe that immunohistologic stains should be an integral part of the pathologic workup of all unusual lymphoid proliferations in extranodal sites in patients not known to have previously diagnosed nodal Hodgkin's disease.

Sarcoidal-type granulomas may be found in the spleens of patients with Hodgkin's disease (see Chapter 6).[41, 74–80] These granulomas may be related to the alterations in cell-mediated immunity commonly seen in patients with this disease. The granulomas are composed of tight clusters of epithelioid histiocytes, most commonly in the PALS in association with the splenic arterial circulation. Occasionally, granulomas may be evident grossly, mimicking a miliary pattern of tumor involvement. In the study by Kadin and colleagues,[74] such granulomas were found in 12.5 percent of spleens of previously untreated patients, and subsequent authors have reported similar frequencies. Although the granulomas may be found with concomitant splenic involvement by Hodgkin's disease, they are more commonly an isolated finding. They are not related to prior lymphangiography.[41] The presence of splenic granulomas in the absence of involvement by Hodgkin's disease does not alter the stage of the disease, although some studies have indicated

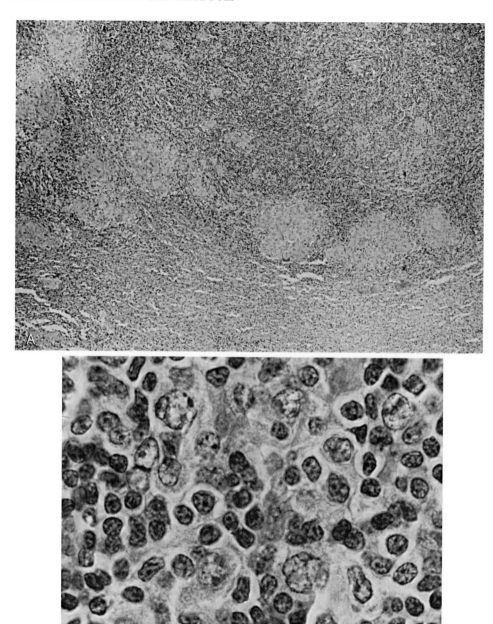

Figure 7–5. (A) A single focus of lymphocyte-predominant Hodgkin's disease in the spleen. Note the granulomatous reaction within the involved area. (B) Examination of the lymphoid infiltrate in this case revealed numerous L&H cells.

that the presence of such granulomas in the spleen is associated with an improved prognosis.[77, 78] Occasionally, the presence of these granulomas may cause diagnostic difficulties in microscopic examination, mimicking involvement with Hodgkin's disease, particularly the lymphocyte-predominant subtype.

Burke and Osborne[81] described a type of localized lymphoid hyperplasia in the spleen of four patients with Hodgkin's disease and two with non-Hodgkin's lymphomas that caused diagnostic difficulties. These solitary nodules ranged from 0.1 to 1.0 cm, suggesting involvement with lymphoma grossly. Microscopically, the authors found either focal aggregates of reactive germinal centers or a localized proliferation of lymphocytes, plasma cells, and immunoblasts. The latter cells were suggestive of

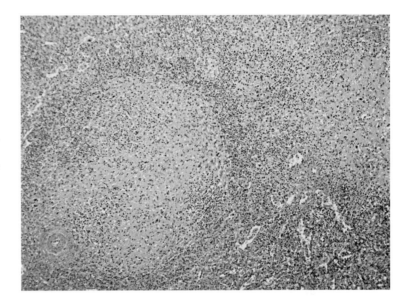

Figure 7–6. Lymphocyte-depletion Hodgkin's disease. The white pulp appears hypocellular and somewhat fibrotic.

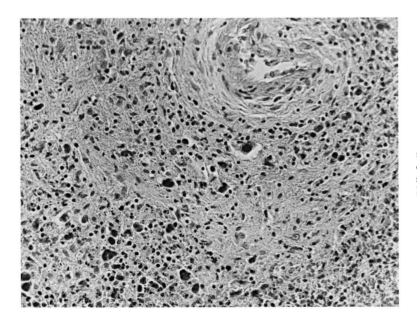

Figure 7–7. Lymphocyte-depletion Hodgkin's disease. There is overall depletion of lymphoid tissue. A few sarcomatous variants of Reed-Sternberg cells are present.

Hodgkin's disease. However, no truly diagnostic RS cells were found, and these nodules were considered to be benign reactive lesions.

SPLENIC INVOLVEMENT AND PROGNOSIS

The extent of Hodgkin's disease is described using the four-stage modified Ann Arbor System.[82, 83] Splenic involvement has therapeutic and prognostic implications, and several studies have indicated the spleen is a critical point in the dissemination of Hodgkin's disease.[16, 84–87] Hodgkin's disease is rarely found in the liver or bone marrow without disease in the spleen,[1, 88] and it has been postulated that splenic involvement reflects hematogenous dissemination.[18, 41] Involvement of the spleen, therefore, suggests that other prognostically unfavorable organs are at risk. Several authors have suggested that cases in which blood vessel invasion is identified in the spleen have the greatest incidence of disseminated disease, in particular extranodal involvement.[89]

Hoppe and coworkers[90, 91] reported that the extent of splenic involvement in patients with Hodgkin's disease was of prognostic significance. These investigators found that the presence of five or more grossly detectable splenic nodules was associated with a poor prognosis. However, the majority of investigators have reported that splenic involvement per se is not of prognostic significance, although the extent of abdominal disease does correlate with survival. Patients with abdominal disease limited to the upper abdomen (spleen and splenic hilar, celiac, and portal lymph nodes) have a prognosis similar to that of patients with stage II disease, whereas lower abdominal disease is associated with a poor prognosis.[92–94]

Splenectomy has not been shown to improve survival in Hodgkin's disease.[28] Occasionally, however, splenic involvement may lead to hypersplenism with resulting cytopenias. This is unusual and most often occurs as a late manifestation of the disease, indicating widespread dissemination. In such cases, splenectomy may be palliative, resulting in remission of the cytopenias.[95, 96]

As has been alluded to previously in this chapter, patients with Hodgkin's disease in whom splenectomy is performed have an increased susceptibility to infection.[3, 97] The risk is greater in patients who have received both total nodal irradiation and combination chemotherapy after splenectomy.[92, 98] Children with Hodgkin's disease are at highest risk.[99] Sepsis rarely occurs in adults who are treated less aggressively, i.e., receiving either radiation or chemotherapy alone.[98] The organisms most commonly involved in postsplenectomy infections are the encapsulated bacteria, particularly *Streptococcus pneumoniae* and *Haemophilus influenzae*, which are the organisms associated with fulminant infections in most asplenic states[100–102] (see Chapter 4).

IMMUNOLOGIC ABNORMALITIES

It has been known for some time that patients with Hodgkin's disease, even with asymptomatic localized disease, suffer from a selective yet well-documented impairment of their cell-mediated immunity.[103] The role of the spleen in this immunologic defect is unclear, despite the fact that the organ has been studied by numerous workers. Several studies have suggested that a serum factor, possibly produced by the spleen or by the foci of Hodgkin's disease in the spleen, is responsible for immunologic defects. Bieber and coworkers[104] demonstrated an E-rosette–inhibiting factor in extracts of spleens involved by Hodgkin's disease. In addition, Bjorkholm and colleagues[105] demonstrated a complement-dependent, cold-reactive lymphocytotoxic factor in the sera of 30 percent of Hodgkin's patients. This factor occurred more frequently in patients with bulky tumor involvement than in those with little tumor involvement of the spleen.

Several groups, using E-rosette formation of isolated splenic lymphocytes, have investigated the number and distribution of splenic lymphocytes in patients with Hodgkin's disease. Han and associates[106] found a reduction in splenic T cells, whereas Baroni and coworkers[107] found elevated numbers of T cells in the spleens. Other investigators have used monoclonal antibodies to study splenic lymphocytes and have also found conflicting evidence. Dorreen and associates[108] found the total T-cell number reduced, whereas Posner and colleagues[109] reported an equivalent increase in T cells in both involved and uninvolved spleens. Falk and colleagues[110] found an increased number of T lymphocytes, but only in spleens involved by Hodgkin's disease. All these studies must be interpreted with great caution because it is well known that the number of T lymphocytes and T subsets varies continually with time and with the age of the patient. However, recent studies have provided more convincing evidence that the distribution of T lymphocytes is altered in the spleens of patients with Hodgkin's disease. In particular, untreated patients with Hodgkin's disease have a decrease in CD4-positive peripheral blood T cells that is associated with the extent of disease.[111] A displacement of CD4-positive lymphocytes from the blood to peripheral lymphoid organs such as the spleen has been demonstrated.[112, 113] In spleens of patients with Hodgkin's disease, a high frequency of cytolytic CD4-positive lymphocytes has been observed, especially in those spleens involved by the disease.[114] A lectin binding site on the surface of cultured RS cells has been characterized.[115] This site binds to and stimulates T lymphocytes and is postulated to mutually activate and stimulate the growth and rosetting of RS cells and the CD4-positive T cells that surround them.[116] The observed lack of CD8-positive cytotoxic immune response against RS cells appears to be caused by the absence of HLA class I expression on these cells.[117] These studies strongly suggest that the observed T-lymphocyte changes in Hodgkin's disease may reflect a biologic response to the tumor that varies with different conditions related to patient immunity, such as the age and performance status, duration, and above all, extent of disease.

Defects in T-lymphocyte function have also been described in patients with Hodgkin's disease. These include a depressed response to T-cell mitogens,[103, 118] decreased capacity of T lymphocytes to respond in an autologous or syngeneic mixed lymphocyte response,[119] and decreased in vitro synthesis of interleukin-2 and interferon-gamma.[120] Some of these immune defects can be due to the direct or indirect effects of cytokines produced by the RS cells.[121]

Functional studies of lymphocytes in patients with Hodgkin's disease have also shown elevated natural killer cell activity in involved spleens.[122] B-cell number and function appear to be normal or more often increased in most patients with untreated Hodgkin's disease. There is increased IgG synthesis by uninvolved and minimally involved spleens of Hodgkin's disease patients similar to that of normal spleens after secondary antigenic stimulation.[123] Reactive follicular hyperplasia frequently observed in spleens obtained from patients with Hodgkin's disease is also consistent with the notion of a polycolonal B-lymphocyte

hyperactivity in this disease. The nature of the antigenic stimulus provoking this B-cell hyperactivity is at present unknown.

Alternations in macrophages and accessory cells have also been reported in patients with Hodgkin's disease.[121] These include decreased killing of *Candida* and excessive production of prostaglandin E_2.[124] Excessive synthesis of prostaglandins is considered to be responsible for the reduced T-lymphocyte blastogenesis and poor colony formation.[125–127] In spleens involved by Hodgkin's disease, a significant decrease in the number of cells reactive with selective monocyte/macrophage lineage associated monoclonal antibodies has also been observed.[110]

REFERENCES

1. Kadin ME, Glatstein E, Dorfman RF: Clinicopathologic studies of 117 untreated patients subjected to laparotomy for the staging of Hodgkin's disease. Cancer 1971; 27:1277.
2. Mauch PM, Kalish LA, Kadin M, et al: Patterns of presentation of Hodgkin disease. Cancer 1993; 71:2062.
3. Colby TV, Hoppe RT, Warnke RA: Hodgkin's disease at autopsy: 1972–1977. Cancer 1981; 47:1852.
4. Martinazzi M, Palatini M: A casual finding of primary splenic Hodgkin's disease in a case of traumatic rupture of the spleen. Tumori 1978; 64:639.
5. Kreamer BB, Osborne BM, Butler JJ: Primary splenic presentation of malignant lymphoma and related disorders. Cancer 1984; 54:1606.
6. Re G, Lambertina F, Bucchi ML, et al: Primary splenic Hodgkin's disease: Case report. Pathologica 1986; 78:635.
7. Zellers RA, Thibodeau SN, Banks PM: Primary splenic lymphocyte-depletion Hodgkin's disease. Am J Clin Pathol 1990; 94:453.
8. Brissette M, Dhru RD: Hodgkin's disease presenting as spontaneous splenic rupture. Arch Pathol Lab Med 1992; 116:1077.
9. Trudel M, Krikorian J, Neiman RS: Lymphocyte predominance in Hodgkin's disease: Clinical and morphologic heterogeneity. Cancer 1987; 59:99.
10. Neiman RS, Rosen PJ, Lukes RJ: Lymphocyte-depletion Hodgkin's disease: A clinicopathologic entity. N Engl J Med 1973; 288:751.
11. Rosenberg SA: Exploratory laparotomy and splenectomy for Hodgkin's disease: A commentary. J Clin Oncol 1988; 6:574.
12. Dietrich PY, Henry-Amar M, Cosset JM, et al: Second primary cancers in patients continuously disease-free from Hodgkin's disease: A protective role for the spleen? Blood 1994; 84:1209.
13. Jockovich M, Mendenhall NP, Sombeck MD, et al: Long-term complications of laparotomy in Hodgkin's disease. Ann Surg 1994; 219:615.
14. Mauch P, Somers R: Controversies in the use of diagnostic staging laparotomy and splenectomy in the management of Hodgkin's disease. Ann Oncol 1992; 4:41.

15. Marble KR, Deckers PJ, Kern KA: Changing role of splenectomy for hematologic disease. J Surg Oncol 1993; 52:169.

16. Glatstein E, Guernsey JM, Rosenberg SA, et al: The value of laparotomy and splenectomy in the staging of Hodgkin's disease. Cancer 1969; 24:709.

17. Glatstein E, Trueblood HW, Enright LP, et al: Surgical staging of abdominal involvement in unselected patients with Hodgkin's disease. Radiology 1970; 97:425.

18. Sweet DL Jr, Kinnealey A, Ultmann JE: Hodgkin's disease: Problems of staging. Cancer 1978; 42:957.

19. Askergren J, Bjorkholm M, Holm G: On the size and tumor involvement of the spleen in Hodgkin's disease. Acta Med Scand 1981; 209:217.

20. Diebold J, Temmin J: Etude anatomo-pathologique des prelevements effectus au cours de 250 laparotomies exploratrices pour maladie de Hodgkin. Ann Pathol 1980; 25:341.

21. Rosenberg SA, Boiron M, DeVita VT Jr, et al: Report of the committee on Hodgkin's disease staging procedures. Cancer Res 1971; 31:1862.

22. Farrer-Brown G, Bennett MH, Harrison CV, et al: The diagnosis of Hodgkin's disease in surgically excised spleens. J Clin Pathol 1972; 25:294.

23. Castellino RA: Imaging techniques for staging abdominal Hodgkin's disease. Cancer Treat Res 1982; 66:697.

24. Desforges JF, Rutherford CJ, Piro A: Hodgkin's disease. N Engl J Med 1979; 301:1212.

25. Milder MS, Larson SM, Bagley CM Jr, et al: Liver-spleen scan in Hodgkin's disease. Cancer 1973; 31:826.

26. Silverman S, DeNardo GL, Glatstein E, et al: Evaluation of the liver and spleen in Hodgkin's disease. II. The value of splenic scintigraphy. Am J Med 1972; 52:362.

27. Turner DA, Pinsky SM, Gottschalk A, et al: The use of gallium-67 scanning in the staging of Hodgkin's disease. Radiology 1972; 104:97.

28. Larson RA, Ultmann JE: The strategic role of laparotomy in staging Hodgkin's disease. Cancer Treat Rep 1982; 66:767.

29. Dearth JC, Gilchrist GS, Telander RI: Partial splenectomy for staging Hodgkin's disease: Risk of false-negative results. New Engl J Med 1978; 299:345.

30. Katz S, Schiller M: Partial splenectomy in staging laparotomy for Hodgkin's disease. Isr J Med Sci 1980; 16:669.

31. Roth H, Daum R, Bolkenius M: Partielle Milzresektion mit Fibrinklebung: Eine Alternative zur Splenektomie und Autotransplantation. Z Kinderchir 1982; 35:153.

32. Boles ET Jr, Haase GM, Hamoudi AB: Partial splenectomy in staging laparotomy for Hodgkin's disease: An alternative approach. J Pediatr Surg 1978; 13:581.

33. Hoekstra HJ, Tamminga RY, Timens W: Partial splenectomy in children: An alternative for splenectomy in the pathological staging of Hodgkin's disease. Annal Surg Oncol 1994; 1:480.

34. Arregui ME, Barteau J, Davis CJ: Laparoscopic splenectomy: Techniques and indications. Int Surg 1994; 79:335.

35. Robles AE, Andrews HG, Garberolgio C: Laparoscopic splenectomy: Present status and future outlook. Int Surg 1994; 79:332.

36. Childers JM, Balserak JC, Kent T, et al: Laparoscopic staging of Hodgkin's lymphoma. J Laparoendosc Surg 1993; 3:495.

37. Lefor AT, Flowers JL, Heyman MR: Laparoscopic staging of Hodgkin's disease. Surg Oncol 1993; 2:217.

38. Carroll BJ, Phillips EH, Semel CJ, et al: Laparoscopic splenectomy. Surg Endosc 1992; 6:183.

39. Emmermann A, Zornig C, Peiper M, et al: Laparoscopic splenectomy: Technique and results in a series of 27 cases. Surg Endosc 1995; 9:924.

40. Moores DC, McKee MA, Wang H, et al: Pediatric laparoscopic splenectomy. J Pediatr Surg 1995; 30:1201.

41. Neiman RS: Current problems in the histopathologic diagnosis and classification of Hodgkin's disease. Pathol Ann 1978; 2:289.

42. Desser PK, Moran EM, Ultmann JE: Staging of Hodgkin's disease and lymphoma. Med Clin North Am 1973; 57:479.

43. Wolf BC, Neiman RS: The histopathologic manifestations of the lymphoproliferative and myeloproliferative disorders involving the spleen, in Knowles DM (ed): Neoplastic Hematopathology. Baltimore, Williams & Wilkins, 1992.

44. Lukes RJ: Criteria for involvement of lymph nodes, bone marrow, spleen and liver in Hodgkin's disease. Cancer Res 1971; 31:1755.

45. Lukes RJ, Butler JJ: The pathology and nomenclature of Hodgkin's disease. Cancer Res 1966; 26:1063.

46. Strum SB, Rappaport H: Interrelations of the histologic subtypes of Hodgkin's disease. Arch Pathol 1971; 91:127.

47. Rappaport H, Berard CW, Butler JJ, et al: Report of the committee on histopathological criteria contributing to staging of Hodgkin's disease. Cancer Res 1971; 31:1864.

48. Hsu SM, Yang K, Jaffe ES: Phenotypic expression of Hodgkin's and Reed-Sternberg cells in Hodgkin's disease. Am J Pathol 1985; 118:209.

49. Dorfman FF, Gatter KC, Pulford KAF, et al: An evaluation of the utility of anti-granulocyte and anti-leukocyte monoclonal antibodies in the diagnosis of Hodgkin's disease. Am J Pathol 1986; 123:508.

50. Stein H, Uchanska-Ziegler B, Gerdes J, et al: Hodgkin and Sternberg-Reed cells contain antigens specific to late cells of granulopoiesis. Int J Cancer 1982; 29:283.

51. Falini B, Stein H, Pileri S, et al: Expression of lymphoid-associated antigens on Hodgkin's and Reed-Sternberg cells of Hodgkin's disease: An immunocytochemical study on lymph node cytospins using monoclonal antibodies. Histopathology 1987; 11:1229.

52. Chittal SM, Caveriviere P, Schwarting R, et al: Monoclonal antibodies in the diagnosis of Hodgkin's disease. Am J Surg Pathol 1988; 12:9.

53. Stauchen JA: Leucocyte-common antigen in the differential diagnosis of Hodgkin's disease. Hemat Oncol 1989; 7:149.

54. Strickler JG, Michie SA, Warnke RA, et al: The "syncytial variant" of nodular sclerosing Hodgkin's disease. Am J Surg Pathol 1986; 10:470.

55. Nicholas DS, Harris S, Wright DH: Lymphocyte predominance Hodgkin's disease: An immunohistochemical study. Histopathology 1990; 16:157.

56. Schmid C, Pan L, Diss T, et al: Expression of B-cell antigens by Hodgkin's and Reed-Sternberg cells in Hodgkin's disease. Am J Pathol 1991; 139:701.

57. Zukerberg LR, Collins AB, Ferry JA, et al: Coexpression of CD15 and CD20 by Reed-Sternberg cells in Hodgkin's disease. Am J Pathol 1991; 139:475.

58. Orazi A, Jiang B, Lee C-H, et al: Correlation between presence of clonal rearrangements of immunoglobulin heavy chain genes and B-cell antigen expression in Hodgkin's disease. Am J Clin Pathol 1995; 104:413.

59. Arber DA, Weiss LM: CD15: A review. Appl Immunohistochem 1993; 1:17.

60. Weiss LM, Strickler JG, Hu E, et al: Immunoglobulin gene rearrangements in Hodgkin's disease. Hum Pathol 1986; 17:1009.

61. Brinker MGL, Poppema S, Buys CH, et al: Clonal immunoglobulin gene rearrangements in tissues involved by Hodgkin's disease. Blood 1987; 70:186.

62. Sundeen J, Lipford E, Uppenkamp M, et al: Rearranged antigen receptor genes in Hodgkin's disease. Blood 1987; 70:96.

63. Raghavachar A, Binder T, Bartram CR: Immunoglobulin and T-cell receptor gene rearrangements in Hodgkin's disease. Cancer Res 1988; 48:3591.

64. Trainor KJ, Brisco MJ, Story CJ, et al: Monoclonality in B-lymphoproliferative disorders detected at the DNA level. Blood 1990; 75:2220.

65. Tamaru J-I, Hummel M, Zemlin M, et al: Hodgkin's disease with a B-cell phenotype often shows a VDJ rearrangement and somatic mutations in the V_H genes. Blood 1994; 84:708.

66. Kuppers R, Rajewsky K, Zhao M, et al: Hodgkin's disease: Hodgkin's and Reed-Sternberg cells picked from histological sections show clonal immunoglobulin gene rearrangements and appear to be derived from B cells at various stages of development. Proc Natl Acad Sci U S A 1994; 91:10962.

67. Kamel OW, Chang PP, Hsu FJ, et al: Clonal VDJ recombination of the immunoglobulin heavy chain gene by PCR in classical Hodgkin's disease. Am J Clin Pathol 1995; 104:419.

68. Manzanal A, Santon A, Oliva H, et al: Evaluation of clonal immunoglobulin heavy chain rearrangements in Hodgkin's disease using the polymerase chain reaction (PCR). Histopathology 1995; 27:21.

69. Griessler H, Feller AF, Mak TW, et al: Clonal rearrangements of T-cell receptor and immunoglobulin genes and immunophenotypic antigen expression in different subclasses of Hodgkin's disease. Int J Cancer 1987; 40:157.

70. Dallenbach FE, Stein H: Expression of T-cell-receptor beta chain in Reed-Sternberg cells. Lancet 1989; 2:828.

71. Siebert JD, Stuckey JH, Kurtin PJ, et al: Extranodal lymphocyte predominance Hodgkin's disease: Clinical and pathologic features. Am J Clin Pathol 1995; 103:485.

72. Chang KL, Kamel OW, Arber DA, et al: Pathologic features of nodular lymphocyte predominance Hodgkin's disease in extranodal sites. Am J Surg Pathol 1995; 19:1313.

73. Kant JA, Hubbard SM, Longo DL, et al: The pathologic and clinical heterogeneity of lymphocyte-depleted Hodgkin's disease. J Clin Oncol 1986; 4:284.

74. Kadin ME, Donaldson SS, Dorfman RF: Isolated granulomas in Hodgkin's disease. N Engl J Med 1970; 283:859.

75. Brincker H: Epithelioid-cell granulomas in Hodgkin's disease. Acta Pathol Microbiol Scand 1970; 78:19.

76. Brincker H: Sarcoid reactions and sarcoidosis in Hodgkin's disease and other malignant lymphomata. Br J Cancer 1972; 26:120.

77. O'Connell MJ, Schimpff SC, Kirschner RH, et al: Epithelioid granulomas in Hodgkin's disease: A favorable prognostic sign. JAMA 1975; 233:889.

78. Sacks EL, Donaldson SS, Gordon J, et al: Epithelioid granulomas associated with Hodgkin's disease: Clinical correlations in 55 previously untreated patients. Cancer 1978; 41:562.

79. Collins RD, Neiman RS: Granulomatous diseases of the spleen, in Joachim HL (ed): Pathology of Granulomas, p 189. New York, Raven Press, 1983.

80. Neiman RS: Incidence and importance of splenic sarcoid-like granulomas. Arch Pathol 1977; 101:518.

81. Burke JS, Osborne BM: Localized reactive lymphoid hyperplasia of the spleen simulating malignant lymphoma: A report of seven cases. Am J Surg Pathol 1983; 7:373.

82. Carbone PP, Kaplan HS, Musshoff K, et al: Report of the committee on Hodgkin's disease staging classification. Cancer Res 1971; 31:1860.

83. Rosenberg SA: Report of the committee on the staging of Hodgkin's disease. Cancer Res 1966; 26:1310.

84. Kaplan HS: On the natural history, treatment, and prognosis of Hodgkin's disease. Harvey Lect 1969; 64:215.

85. Kaplan HS, Dorfman RF, Nelsen TS, et al: Staging laparotomy and splenectomy in Hodgkin's disease: Analysis of indications and patterns of involvement in 285 consecutive unselected patients. Natl Cancer Inst Monogr 1973; 36:291.

86. Smithers DW: Spread of Hodgkin's disease. Lancet 1970; 1:1262.

87. Smithers DW, Lillicrop SC, Barnes A: Patterns of lymph node involvement in relation to hypotheses about the modes of spread of Hodgkin's disease. Cancer 1974; 34:1779.

88. Kaplan HS: Hodgkin's disease: Unfolding concepts concerning its nature, management, and prognosis. Cancer 1980; 45:2439.

89. Kirschner RH, Abt AB, O'Connell MJ, et al: Vascular invasion and hematogenous dissemination of Hodgkin's disease. Cancer 1974; 34:1159.

90. Hoppe RT, Cox RS, Rosenberg SA, et al: Prognostic factors in stage III Hodgkin's disease. Cancer Treat Rep 1982; 66:743.

91. Hoppe RT, Rosenberg SA, Kaplan HS, et al: Prognostic factors in pathological stage IIIA Hodgkin's disease. Cancer 1980; 46:1240.

92. Desser RK, Golomb HM, Ultmann JE, et al: Prognostic classification of Hodgkin's disease in pathologic stage III, based on anatomic considerations. Blood 1977; 49:883.

93. Levi JA, Wiernik PH: The therapeutic implications of splenic involvement in stage IIIA Hodgkin's disease. Cancer 1977; 39:2158.

94. Stein RS, Hilborn RM, Flexner JM, et al: Anatomical substages of stage III Hodgkin's disease: Implications for staging, therapy, and experimental design. Cancer 1978; 42:429.

95. Christensen BE, Hansen LK, Kristensen JK, et al: Splenectomy in haematology: Indications, results and complications in 41 cases. Scand J Haematol 1970; 7:247.

96. Crosby WH: Splenectomy in hematologic disorders. N Engl J Med 1972; 286:1252.

97. Aisenberg AC: The staging and treatment of Hodgkin's disease. N Engl J Med 1978; 299:1228.

98. Weitzman S, Aisenberg AC: Fulminant sepsis after the successful treatment of Hodgkin's disease. Am J Med 1977; 62:47.

99. Chilcote RR, Baehner RL, Hammond D, et al: Septicemia and meningitis in children splenectomized for Hodgkin's disease. N Engl J Med 1976; 295:798.

100. Nixon DW, Aisenberg AC: Fatal *Haemophilus influenzae* sepsis in an asymptomatic splenectomized Hodgkin's disease patient. Ann Intern Med 1972; 77:69.

101. Ravry M, Maldonado N, Vlez-Garcia E, et al: Serious infection after splenectomy for the staging of Hodgkin's disease. Ann Intern Med 1972; 77:11.

102. Stiver G, Sharrar R, Kendrick M: Bacterial risk in staging splenectomy. Ann Intern Med 1972; 76:670.

103. Levy RA, Kaplan HS: Impaired lymphocyte function in untreated Hodgkin's disease. N Engl J Med 1974; 290:181.

104. Bieber MM, Fuks Z, Kaplan HS: E-rosette inhibiting substance in Hodgkin's disease spleen extracts. Clin Exp Immun 1977; 29:369.

105. Bjorkholm M, Wedelin C, Holm G: Lymphocytotoxic serum factors and lymphocyte functions in untreated Hodgkin's disease. Cancer 1982; 50:2044.

106. Han T, Minowada J, Subramanian V: Splenic T and B lymphocytes and their mitogenic response in untreated Hodgkin's disease. Cancer 1980; 45:767.

107. Baroni CD, Ruco L, Uccini S: Tissue T-lymphocytes in untreated Hodgkin's disease: Morphologic and functional correlations in spleens and lymph nodes. Cancer 1982; 50:259.

108. Dorreen MS, Habeshaw JA, Wrigley PFM: Distribution of T-lymphocyte subsets in Hodgkin's disease characterized by monoclonal antibodies. Br J Cancer 1982; 45:491.

109. Posner MR, Reinhertz EL, Breard J, et al: Lymphoid subpopulations of peripheral blood and spleen in untreated Hodgkin's disease. Cancer 1981; 48:1170.

110. Falk S, Muller H, Stutte HJ: The spleen in Hodgkin's disease: An immunohistochemical study of lymphocyte subpopulations and macrophages. Histopathology 1988; 13:139.

111. Bjorkholm M, Holm G, Mellstedt H. Immunocompetence in patients with Hodgkin's disease, in Lacher MJ, Redman JR (eds): Consequences of Survival in Hodgkin's Disease, p 12. Philadelphia, Lea & Febiger, 1990.

112. Romagnani S, Del Prete GF, Maggi E, et al: Displacement of T lymphocytes with the "helper/inducer" phenotype from peripheral blood lymphoid organs in untreated patients with Hodgkin's disease. Scand J Haematol 1983; 31:305.

113. Grimfors G, Holm G, Mellstedt H, et al: Increased blood clearance of indium-111 oxine-labeled autologous CD4+ blood cells in untreated patients with Hodgkin's disease. Blood 1990; 76:583.

114. Maggi E, Parronchi P, Del Prete G, et al: Frequent T4-positive cells with cytolytic activity in spleens of patients with Hodgkin's disease (a clonal analysis). J Immunol 1986; 136:1516.

115. Paietta E, Stockert RJ, Morell AG, et al: Unique antigen of cultured Hodgkin's cells: A putative sialyltransferase. J Clin Invest 1986; 78:349.

116. Paietta E, Stockert RJ, McManus M, et al: Hodgkin's cell lectin: A lymphocyte adhesion molecule and mitogen. J Immunol 1989; 143:2850.

117. Poppema S, Visser L: Absence of HLA class I expression by Reed-Sternberg cells. Am J Pathol 1994; 145:37.

118. Romagnani S, Amadori A, Biti G, et al: In vitro lymphocyte response to phytomitogens in untreated and treated patients with Hodgkin's disease. Int Arch Allergy Appl Immunol 1976; 51:378.

119. Engleman EG, Benike CJ, Hoppe RT, et al: Autologous mixed lymphocyte reaction in patients with Hodgkin's disease: Evidence for a T-cell defect. J Clin Invest 1980; 66:149.

120. Ford RJ, Tsao J, Kouttab NM, et al: Association of an interleukin abnormality with the T-cell defect in Hodgkin's disease. Blood 1984; 64:386.

121. Kadin ME: Hodgkin's disease: Immunobiology and Pathogenesis, in Knowles DM (ed): Neoplastic Hematopathology, p 535. Baltimore, Williams & Wilkins, 1992.

122. Ruco LP, Procopio A, Uccini S: Natural killer activity in spleens and lymph nodes from patients with Hodgkin's disease. Cancer Res 1982; 42:2063.

123. Longmire RL, McMillan R, Yelenosky R, et al: In vitro splenic IgG synthesis in Hodgkin's disease. N Engl J Med 1973; 289:763.

124. Estevez ME, Ballart IJ, de Macedo MP, et al: Dysfunction of monocytes in Hodgkin's disease by excessive production of PGE-2 in long-term remission patients. Cancer 1988; 62:2128.

125. Goodwin JS, Messner RP, Bankhurst AD, et al: Prostaglandin-producing suppressor cells in Hodgkin's disease. N Engl J Med 1977; 297:963.

126. Schecter GS, Soehnlen F: Monocyte-mediated inhibition of lymphocyte blastogenesis in Hodgkin's disease. Blood 1978; 52:261.

127. Bockman RS: Stage-dependent reduction in T-colony formation in Hodgkin's disease: Coincidence with monocyte synthesis of prostaglandins. J Clin Invest 1980; 66:523.

8

LYMPHOMAS OF THE SPLEEN

Splenic involvement is frequent among patients with malignant lymphomas and may occur in three clinical settings. In the first and most common, the organ is involved as part of the patient's generalized disease. In the second and rarest presentation, termed "primary splenic lymphoma," the tumor is confined to the spleen or spleen and splenic hilar lymph nodes, with no involvement of other sites. In the third clinical setting, patients present with prominent and seemingly isolated splenomegaly but are found to have generalized disease on clinical workup and staging.

The vast majority of any of the malignant lymphomas that affect the spleen involve the white pulp. A variable degree of involvement of the red pulp may occur, however, particularly in patients with low-grade malignant lymphomas and those with leukemic dissemination. Isolated red pulp involvement has been reported in both B- and T-cell lymphomas, however, and appears characteristic in certain types of lymphoma that will be discussed later.

Lymphomatous involvement of the spleen may produce one of three gross patterns: miliary tumor nodules (Color Plate 8), single or multiple tumor masses (Color Plate 9), or, rarely, diffuse enlargement. Small-cell lymphomas, such as follicular lymphomas of the small cleaved and mixed cell types and mantle cell lymphoma, usually produce miliary nodules, but all types of large-cell lymphoma are almost always characterized by solitary or multiple tumor masses (Color Plate 10).

Most types of lymphomas produce a nodular pattern in the spleen, regardless of whether the growth pattern in involved lymph nodes is follicular (nodular) or diffuse; this is a result of the nodular character of the normal architecture of the white pulp. It is therefore inappropriate to classify lymphomas as follicular or diffuse on the basis of the pattern of splenic involvement.[1-3]

PRIMARY SPLENIC LYMPHOMA

Primary splenic lymphoma is rare, accounting for less than 1 percent of all lymphomas involving the organ. It is difficult to define the clinical and pathologic features of this entity because of differences in diagnostic criteria in the literature. Warnke et al[1] were able to identify 47 cases of primary splenic lymphomas fulfilling the most stringent diagnostic criteria (i.e., tumor confined to the spleen and splenic hilar lymph nodes).[4-16] The patients were all adults; a slight preponderance of males was noted. The most common presenting symptoms included left-sided abdominal pain and systemic symptoms such as fever, malaise, and weight loss. Two cases occurred in HIV-positive patients.[4, 9] The gross findings and the histologic characteristics were similar to those observed in spleens secondarily involved by malignant lymphoma. Of the 47 cases in their series, 30 cases were large-cell type, 15 were small-cell type (small lymphocytic, lymphoplasmacytoid, or mantle cell type), 1 was a mixed cell lymphoma of follicular center cell type, and 1 was small noncleaved cell type. When analyzed for cell lineage, a B-cell origin was found in most cases.[1] Of the 17 splenic lymphomas reported by Falk and Stutte[17] (which included cases with minimal extrasplenic involvement), 3 cases showed T-cell lineage. A case of primary splenic CD30-positive anaplastic large-cell lymphoma has also been described in an HIV-positive patient.[4]

The course of primary splenic lymphoma is

hard to predict because of the rarity of cases and the disparate histologic type. The overall survival rate is approximately 50 percent irrespective of the histologic type, although the different therapeutic regimens (chemotherapy, radiotherapy, or both) employed and the limited number of patients treated prevent any conclusive statement in this regard.[4–16]

SECONDARY SPLENIC INVOLVEMENT BY LYMPHOMA

Non-Hodgkin's lymphomas of different types involve the spleen with differing frequency (Table 8–1). Splenic involvement is particularly frequent in low-grade lymphomas.[1, 18] Liver involvement by lymphoma is rare in the absence of splenic disease.[19] Clinical assessment of the likelihood of splenic involvement by malignant lymphomas may be difficult. The weights of involved spleens vary widely.[19] Although tumor involvement usually results in palpable splenomegaly, Goffinet and coworkers[20] found that approximately one third of nonpalpable spleens was involved by lymphoma at staging laparotomy.

Small Lymphocytic Lymphoma

Splenic involvement is common in patients with small lymphocytic lymphoma (SLL), and prominent splenomegaly may occasionally be the presenting feature of this disorder.[21–26] Patients with SLL usually have stage IV disease at the time of presentation. SLL is cytologically

Table 8–1. Incidence of Secondary Splenic Involvement in Various Subtypes of Non-Hodgkin's Lymphoma

	Frequency of Involvement at Diagnosis
Small lymphocytic	Usually present
Lymphoplasmacytoid	Frequent
Mantle cell	Frequent
Follicular	Frequent
Large B cell	Frequent
Marginal zone cell (nodal)	Rare
Peripheral T cell	NA
Mycosis fungoides	Rare
Burkitt	Rare
Lymphoblastic	Rare
MALT	Rare

NA = reliable information not available

indistinguishable in the spleen, as well as in lymph nodes, from chronic lymphocytic leukemia (CLL).[27]

SLL usually produces grossly visible miliary nodules in the spleen due to irregular expansion of the white pulp, with only secondary red pulp involvement (Fig. 8–1).[28, 29] On occasion, particularly in cases with high numbers of circulating lymphocytes, the red pulp involvement may be so extensive as to completely mask the white pulp enlargement; such cases may be confused with red pulp disorders such as hairy cell leukemia (Fig. 8–2).[3] Because the clinical indications for splenectomy usually occur late in the course of CLL/SLL, it is usually observed that the white pulp nodules have coalesced, and red pulp infiltration is marked, which results in diffuse involvement that masks the nodular appearance on cross section. This pattern is unusual for other types of malignant lymphomas.[1, 3] The white pulp nodules in CLL/SLL are composed of a monotonous population of small lymphocytes with round nuclei, scanty cytoplasm, clumped chromatin, inconspicuous nucleoli, and rare or absent mitoses (Fig. 8–3). Cytologically, these nodules are indistinguishable from the white pulp of the immunologically unstimulated adult spleen. In some cases, there may be scattered large cells with vesicular nuclei and prominent nucleoli (prolymphocytes and paraimmunoblasts), similar to the cells of the pseudofollicular proliferation centers seen in lymph nodes, disturbing the monotony of the cell population.[28–31] Occasionally these larger cells may infiltrate the red pulp, resembling prolymphocytic leukemia.[3] Some cases show subendothelial infiltration of the trabecular veins.[23] The presence of numerous reactive epithelioid histiocytes has also been reported.[23, 32] The diagnosis of small lymphocytic lymphoma may be quite difficult on morphologic grounds alone in the early stages of splenic involvement and may require immunologic studies for confirmation. Examination of lymph nodes removed at the time of splenectomy, and in particular splenic hilar nodes, may also confirm the diagnosis of malignant lymphoma. Both SLL and CLL typically show low-density expression of surface immunoglobulins. The heavy chain is most commonly μ alone in SLL but μ plus δ in CLL. In addition, both express a variety of pan–B-cell markers as well as CD5, CD43, CD23, and L175, and lack expression of CD10. However, loss of CD5 expression has been reported in cases of SLL with extranodal presentation.[33]

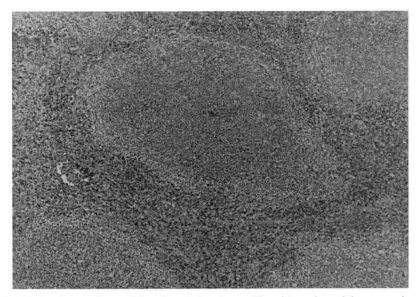

Figure 8–1. Splenic involvement by small lymphocytic lymphoma. The white pulp nodules encroach on one another. The intervening areas of red pulp are infiltrated by small lymphocytes.

Lymphoplasmacytic Lymphoma

Some cases of SLL show evidence of plasmacytoid differentiation, as evidenced by plasmacytoid cells and lymphocytes with intranuclear or cytoplasmic inclusions (Dutcher bodies, Russell bodies, or Mott cells). Tumors with these features have also been termed "lymphoplasmacytic lymphoma" (LPCL) or "immunocytoma."[27, 34–36] Although patients with this disorder are usually not leukemic, they often have marrow involvement at presentation.[27, 28, 36, 37] LPCL is frequently associated with a serum or urine paraprotein, or both, that is most frequently of the IgM type. The morphologic features of LPCL are characteristic of macroglobulinemia of Waldenström. However, not all patients with this morphologic picture and an IgM serum spike should be considered to have Waldenström macro-

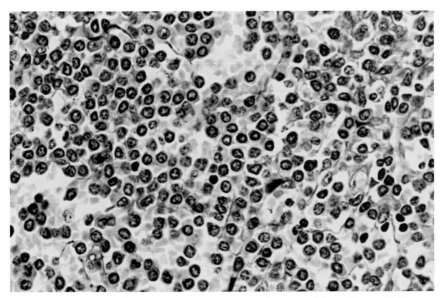

Figure 8–2. Small lymphocytic lymphoma. There is extensive involvement of the red pulp. Malignant cells infiltrate both cords and sinuses.

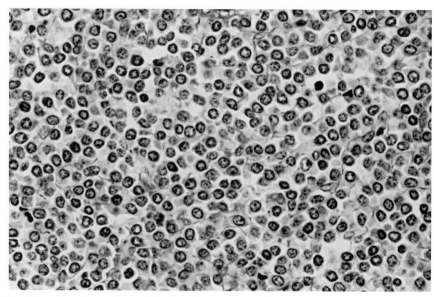

Figure 8–3. Small lymphocytic lymphoma. The lymphocytes are small with compact chromatin. Mitotic activity is low.

globulinemia, which we believe is a specific clinicopathologic entity.

The majority of cases of LPCL in the spleen are composed of uniformly distributed homogeneous mixtures of lymphocytes, plasmacytoid lymphocytes, and plasma cells (Fig. 8–4). Mast cells may be prominent, and hemosiderosis is often present as a consequence of the autoimmune hemolytic anemia that may be associated with the disorder. The neoplastic infiltrate of LPCL can sometimes be localized predominantly to the mantle zones of the malpighian follicles or show extension into the marginal zones and adjacent red pulp.[1, 38, 39] Some cases of LPCL present with prominent splenomegaly, minimal lymphadenopathy, and abnormal lymphocytes in the peripheral blood.[39–41] These cases represent a proportion of the cases included in the clinical entity termed "splenic lymphoma with villous lym-

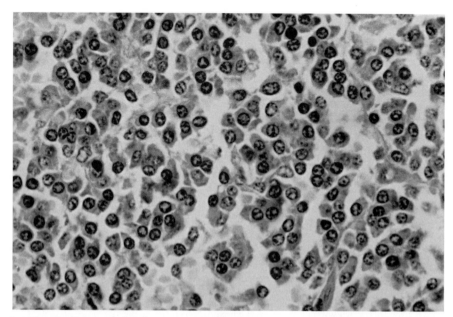

Figure 8–4. Lymphoplasmacytic lymphoma, or immunocytoma. The cells display evident plasmacytoid features.

phocytes." LPCL typically expresses surface and cytoplasmic μ heavy chain. Most cases also express CD25 and CD43 in addition to the usual B-cell markers, whereas less than half coexpress CD5. Approximately 10 to 20 percent express CD11c or CD23.[3, 36]

Mantle Cell Lymphoma

Mantle cell lymphoma (MCL) frequently involves the spleen.[25, 26, 42] Although MCL may present initially with clinically isolated splenomegaly, workup of these patients reveals that all are actually stage IV at the time of diagnosis, with bone marrow or liver involvement or both.[25, 26] The morphologic features of MCL in the spleen are similar to that seen in lymph nodes.[43–45] The white pulp is uniformly expanded, presenting a miliary pattern of involvement grossly similar to that of follicular small cleaved cell lymphoma and marginal zone lymphoma (Fig. 8–5). Tumor cells proliferate in widened mantle zones surrounding benign, often atrophic, germinal centers (Fig. 8–6) and secondarily infiltrate the red pulp.[25, 42] Some white pulp nodules may be surrounded by the non-neoplastic lymphocytes of the marginal zones, whereas others are composed of a homogeneous proliferation of tumor cells (Fig. 8–7). The residual germinal centers frequently contain PAS-positive hyalinelike extra-

cellular material. The nuclei of most of the tumor cells are neither round, as in small lymphocytic lymphoma, nor truly cleaved, as in small cleaved cell lymphoma, but have irregular nuclear contours (Fig. 8–8). However, lymphocytes with small round and small cleaved nuclei are present but do not constitute more than 30 percent of the tumor cells.[25, 44]

Involvement of the spleen by MCL is occasionally difficult to recognize.[25] Because of the residual germinal centers, the tumor nodules can easily be mistaken for reactive follicles. A useful criterion for the diagnosis of malignancy is the presence of small lymphoid cells infiltrating the red pulp. However, this is not always readily apparent. In some cases the diagnosis of lymphoma can be confirmed only by identifying involvement of lymph nodes (especially splenic hilar nodes) or bone marrow. In other cases, immunologic studies[25] or molecular analysis may be necessary to confirm the malignant nature of the lymphocytic proliferation in the spleen.[25] The tumor cells express bright surface immunoglobulin (IgM and usually also IgD), which is often of λ light chain type; strongly express B-cell–associated antigens and CD5, similar to CLL/SLL; but are CD23-negative.[36] The product of the cyclin D1 gene can be detected in the nuclei of the neoplastic cells by immunohistology; the presence of the gene product is useful in distinguishing MCL from other B-cell lymphoma.[46, 47]

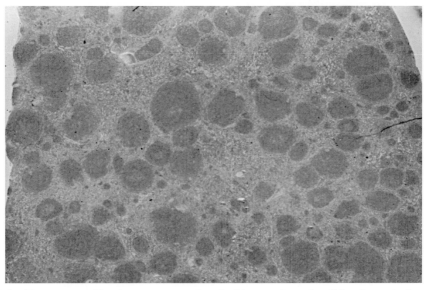

Figure 8–5. A miliary pattern of involvement, as seen here in this case of mantle cell lymphoma, is characteristic of all forms of low-grade B-cell lymphoma.

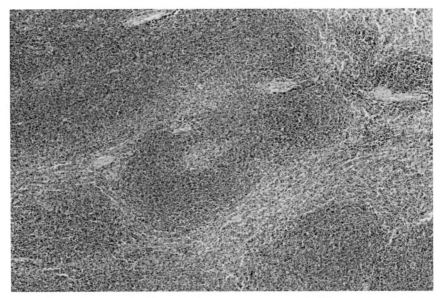

Figure 8–6. Mantle cell lymphoma. Mantle zones are expanded and surround atrophic germinal centers.

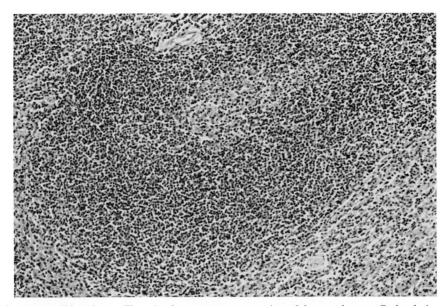

Figure 8–7. Mantle cell lymphoma. There is a homogeneous expansion of the mantle zone. Red pulp involvement can be seen at the lower right.

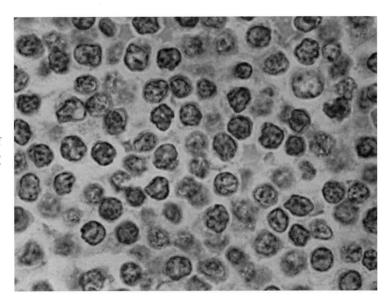

Figure 8–8. The lymphocytes of mantle cell lymphoma have irregular, although not truly cleaved, nuclear contours.

Follicular Lymphomas

Splenic involvement is common in follicular lymphomas, particularly in the small cleaved cell type, which is often disseminated at the time of diagnosis.[1, 21, 23, 26] Rarely, cases of follicular small cleaved cell lymphoma may present as isolated splenomegaly.[3, 22, 24, 25] Grossly, the spleen shows a miliary pattern (Fig. 8–9). There is a variable degree of red pulp involvement, and occasionally the white pulp nodules may coalesce to form small masses. Splenic involvement in these cases is also often difficult to recognize, owing to the uniform expansion of the malpighian corpuscles.[1, 2] However, in small cleaved cell lymphoma, the white pulp nodules are composed of a relatively monotonous population of small cleaved lymphocytes (Figs. 8–10, 8–11). Mixed small and large cell lymphomas may be more difficult to recognize in the early stages of splenic involvement because the admixture of cells results in a superficial resemblance to reactive germinal centers.[48] However, close examination reveals that

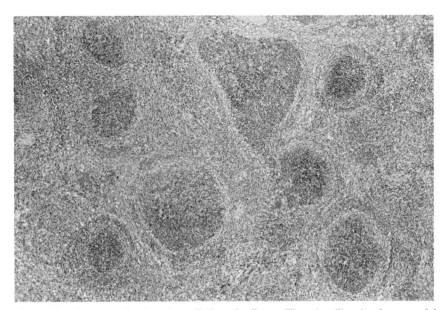

Figure 8–9. Malignant lymphoma, predominantly small cleaved cell type. There is miliary involvement of the white pulp.

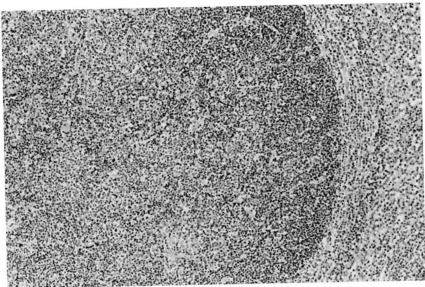

Figure 8–10. Malignant lymphoma, predominantly small cleaved cell type. As in Figure 8–9, a rim of marginal zone cells is evident.

the white pulp nodules are not tripartite as are reactive germinal centers; moreover, they contain a dimorphic cell population that includes cleaved cells rather than a range of cell types, and they usually lack the tingible body macrophages typical of reactive follicles. In addition, the red pulp does not display the plasmacytosis usually seen in reactive lymphoid hyperplasia and often contains smaller nodules composed of lymphoma cells. In difficult cases, subtle red pulp involvement can be effectively demonstrated by immunostaining with CD20 or other B-cell antibodies. In other cases, the diagnosis of lymphoma may depend on immunologic studies to demonstrate monoclonality and on BCL-2 expression.[1]

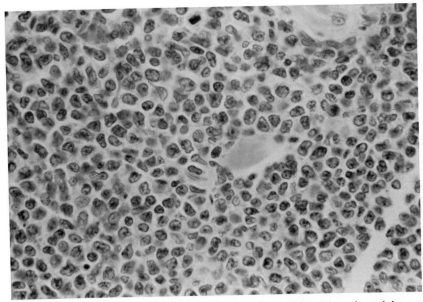

Figure 8–11. Malignant lymphoma, predominantly small cleaved cell type. The white pulp nodules are composed of a monotonous population of small cleaved lymphocytes.

Marginal Zone Lymphoma/Monocytoid B-Cell Lymphoma

Splenic involvement by nodal monocytoid B-cell lymphoma (MBCL) is rare.[49–51] When splenic involvement does occur, it is usually in cases with advanced disease and peripheral blood involvement.[52] However, splenomegaly may be the presenting feature.[53] The involvement is predominantly in the white pulp with a variable extension of the lymphoma cells into the red pulp. The white pulp often shows residual germinal centers and follicular mantles surrounded by pale cells with small nuclei, abundant cytoplasm, and distinct cell margins, expanding the marginal zone.[1, 3, 53] Although the lymphoma cells are cytologically similar to the cells of hairy cell leukemia, the two diseases show different patterns of splenic infiltration, and the tartrate-resistant acid phosphatase reaction in MBCL is negative.[36] Immunohistochemically, MBCL cells express B-cell markers, including KiB3 and DBA.44 and are typically CD11c-positive, CD5-negative, CD25-negative, and usually CD43-negative. Recent evidence has shown wide overlapping between low grade B-cell lymphomas of mucosal-associated lymphoid tissue (MALT) and MBCL in terms of morphology, immunophenotype,

and molecular features.[54] Although splenic marginal zone lymphoma also has some overlapping features with MBCL and MALT lymphomas, some of its specific findings justify a separate categorization.[54, 55] This is discussed later in this chapter.

Diffuse Large B-Cell Lymphomas

The incidence of secondary splenic involvement by malignant lymphomas of diffuse large B-cell types is less than the involvement by small cell lymphomas.[3, 21, 23, 26] Large cell lymphomas characteristically produce solitary or multiple tumor masses in the spleen (Fig. 8–12). These tumors do not necessarily tend to show a predilection for involvement of the white pulp. Their cytologic features are identical to those of involved lymph nodes.[56] Sclerosis has been observed in some cases.[23, 26] A predominant red pulp pattern of involvement and an increase in reactive erythrophagocytic histiocytes have also been observed (see Fig. 11–15).[26, 56] Some cases display predominant involvement of vascular sinuses (intravascular lymphoma) (Fig. 8–13). These cases must be distinguished from cases of malignant histiocytosis, peripheral T-cell lymphoma,[1, 56] and

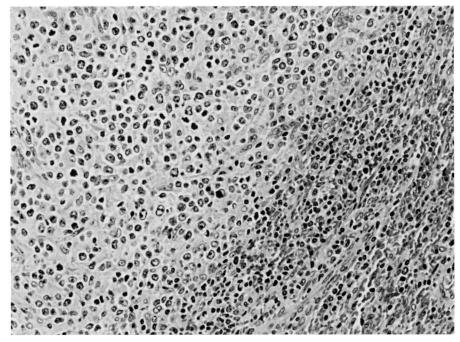

Figure 8–12. Malignant lymphoma, large-cell type. The tumor forms a large mass that compresses the surrounding splenic parenchyma.

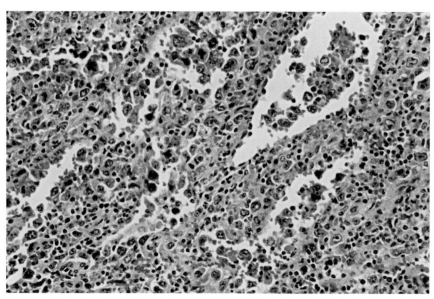

Figure 8–13. Malignant lymphoma, large-cell type (so-called intravascular lymphoma). Tumor cells infiltrate the cords of the red pulp but are also prominent in the sinuses.

poorly differentiated granulocytic sarcoma. In these cases, confirmation of the diagnosis of large cell lymphoma can be obtained by immunohistochemistry, which shows expression of lymphoid antigens and lack of histiocytic and myeloid reactivity in neoplastic cells. Further diagnostic difficulties may be encountered in cases in which diffuse large B-cell lymphoma is confined to the red pulp.[26, 57, 58] Betman et al[57] reported one such case in which the lymphoid infiltration was composed predominantly of small reactive T lymphocytes with occasional large atypical cells positive for B-cell antigens. This case seems to correspond to the morphologic variant of diffuse large B-cell lymphoma known as T-cell–rich B-cell lymphoma. This case also indicates that T-cell–rich B-cell lymphoma should be considered in the differential diagnosis in cases in which small T lymphocytes appear to predominate within the red pulp. Occasional large cell lymphomas may present as isolated splenomegaly. Although adjacent viscera and lymph nodes are frequently found to be involved in these cases, the lymphomas are not truly disseminated, in contrast to small cell lymphomas presenting in the spleen.

Lymphoblastic Lymphoma

Lymphoblastic lymphomas are neoplasms of precursor T or B cells, which are almost always terminal deoxynucleotidyl transferase (TdT)–positive. Most cases are of T-cell phenotype; one third, however, is of early pre–B cell or pre–B cell type, with CD10, CD19, and/or intracytoplasmic μ-heavy chain expression.[59] Lymphoblastic lymphoma usually affects adolescents and young adults, particularly males, but may be seen also in middle-aged patients.[60] This tumor is often associated with a mediastinal mass and bone marrow involvement, resulting in a leukemic phase early in the course of the disease. Lymphoblastic lymphoma has been considered the tissue manifestation of acute lymphoblastic leukemia of FAB L1 or L2 subtype, from which it is histologically indistinguishable.[61–63] The distinction is usually made clinically by taking into consideration the different pattern of presentation. Splenomegaly is more often associated with the diagnosis of acute lymphoblastic leukemia.[61, 62] The morphology of splenic involvement has not been well described. In early stages, the disease is localized adjacent to the white pulp, especially in the regions of the periarterial lymphoid sheath (PALS).[3] In the leukemic phase, diffuse red pulp involvement results in a homogeneous pattern with obliteration of the white pulp. The infiltrate is composed of cells with either convoluted or nonconvoluted nuclei, fine chromatin, scanty cytoplasm, and a high mitotic rate.

Lymphoblastic lymphoma can be easily confused with Burkitt lymphoma (BL)[62] and mantle cell lymphoma, blastoid variant,[64] particularly in suboptimal histologic preparations. However, BL is invariably a neoplasm of mature B-lineage, whereas the majority of lymphoblastic lymphomas are of T-cell origin. Paraffin-reactive B-cell antibodies may therefore help identify the former.[62] TdT, an antigen that can also be demonstrated in conventionally processed histology material,[65, 66] is positive in almost all cases of lymphoblastic lymphoma but negative in the other subtypes. In our experience, CD99 (013) may also help identify lymphoblastic lymphoma in paraffin sections.[67]

Burkitt Lymphoma

Involvement of the spleen is not common in BL.[3, 68, 69] Grogan and associates[70] reported splenic involvement in two patients, one of whom was leukemic; and Banks and colleagues[71] found splenic involvement in 10 of 17 cases of sporadic Burkitt tumor at autopsy. Banks et al noted that in some cases the tumor grew in a cohesive mass surrounding the spleen rather than infiltrating it. Two of the 10 cases had spleens that showed selective white pulp involvement, and 8 also showed involvement of the red pulp. Most cases have both red and white pulp involvement, although occasionally more selective involvement of the white pulp occurs, either in the malpighian corpuscles or in the marginal zones.[72] Immunohistochemistry can be used to separate BL from lymphoblastic malignancies.[65–67] In contrast to lymphoblastic lymphoma, BL is CD20-positive and CD99- and TdT-negative, and it expresses surface immunoglobulins. In difficult cases, molecular demonstration of *c-myc* rearrangement or cytogenetic analysis may be necessary to confirm the diagnosis.

In cases formerly classified as small noncleaved cell lymphoma, non-Burkitt-type cases more commonly show greater nuclear pleomorphism in tumor cells than in Burkitt cases and may display occasional multinucleated cells.[69, 73, 74] The nuclei often contain a single prominent nucleolus instead of the multiple nucleoli characteristic of Burkitt tumor.[74] These cases usually lack *c-myc* rearrangement and have frequent BCL-2 rearrangement, suggesting that these lesions are more closely related to large B-cell lymphomas of follicle center cell origin than to BL.[74] Features of splenic involvement in these cases have not been char-

acterized, but in two cases we have studied involvement was perisplenic and in the white pulp.

PERIPHERAL T-CELL LYMPHOMAS

Because of the relatively recent characterization of the peripheral T-cell lymphomas (PTCL) and their relative rarity in Western countries, there are few data characterizing the features of splenic involvement in these tumors. The patterns of splenic involvement by PTCL can be indistinguishable from those of large B-cell lymphoma.[75] However, in some cases, the tumor may be confined to the PALS and marginal zones.[3] Many of these tumors are pleomorphic; they were usually classified as diffuse mixed small and large cell or large cell immunoblastic type in the Working Formulation.[75] The Kiel classification, recognizing that peripheral T-cell lymphomas represent a heterogeneous group of disease entities, attempted to divide these malignancies into several categories. This subdivision has been criticized as poorly reproducible and of limited prognostic value. A better approach is to identify within the T-cell malignancies those lesions that represent distinct clinicopathologic entities, as recently advocated by several groups.[55]

Peripheral T-Cell Lymphoma, Unspecified

PTCL unspecified comprises up to 50 percent of the lymphomas previously classified as diffuse mixed small and large cell type and an unknown portion of cases classified as large cell immunoblastic type in the Working Formulation.[55] This group of PTCL typically contains a mixture of small and large atypical cells. The small lymphoid cells are characterized by irregular but noncleaved nuclei with condensed chromatin and largely inconspicuous nucleoli. In some cases the cells have abundant pale cytoplasm with somewhat more distinct nucleoli. The large cells of PTCL are more variable in their cytologic appearance, occasionally even resembling mononuclear Hodgkin cells. PTCL may also resemble Hodgkin's disease because of the presence of inflammatory cells such as plasma cells and eosinophils as well a variable degree of small vessel proliferation. The pattern of splenic involvement in PTCL has not been well characterized. In many cases, it appears that the proliferation is confined to the red pulp. It has been shown that a number of cases formerly called "malignant histiocytosis" are, in fact, tumors of peripheral T cells (see Chapter 11 and Fig. 11–15). In the description of PTCL by Waldron and coworkers,[76] three of six patients had massive splenomegaly. Brisbane and colleagues[77] described autopsy findings in one case in which the spleen showed coalescent masses as well as discrete involvement of the PALS. Weinberg and Pinkus[78] described an unusual variant of T-cell lymphoma composed of large multilobulated cells with splenic involvement in 2 of 10 cases, but they did not describe the splenic morphology. These cases may actually have been examples of anaplastic large cell lymphoma. Burke[3] reported several cases of immunologically confirmed T-immunoblastic lymphoma in which nodules were formed at the periphery of the white pulp and one case in which the red pulp was the predominant site of involvement. We have seen several such cases with differing types of involvement, some expanding the PALS diffusely, some producing discrete masses, and one mimicking the pattern of involvement seen in mycosis fungoides.

Lymphoepithelioid cell (Lennert) lymphoma[79-81] is a cytologic subtype of PTCL characterized by a high content of epithelioid histiocytes that may produce a characteristic but not specific splenic morphology. Early involvement usually occurs in the peripheral zones of follicles and the PALS, consistent with the T-cell origin of this lymphoma.[3] The epithelioid histiocytes tend to localize in a ringlike arrangement at the periphery of the white pulp, although they occasionally form clusters.[80, 82] Although originally thought to be characteristic for this type of lymphoma, the ringlike arrangement of epithelioid cells may be seen in other forms of lymphoma as well (Fig. 8–14). Lymphoepithelial cell lymphomas are aggressive tumors, similar to other PTCL. The majority of the patients have stage III or IV disease at the time of diagnosis. Patients often have a poor response to chemotherapy, and early relapse is common.[75]

Adult T-Cell Leukemia/Lymphoma (ATL)

These tumors are relatively common in Japan, where they are associated with a retrovirus termed "human T-cell leukemia/lymphoma virus" (HTLV-1), and have a clustering centered on the island of Kyushu in southwestern Japan.[83, 84] Ten to 15 percent of individuals in this area have antibodies to the virus, but only a small number develop malignancy, and then, in most cases, only after many years. Cases have also been reported in the South-

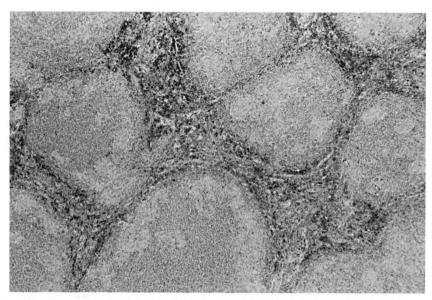

Figure 8–14. Malignant lymphoma, predominantly small cleaved cell type. Epithelioid histiocytes are present in all the nodules. These cells are occasionally seen in all forms of malignant lymphomas involving the spleen and are not unique to so-called Lennert lymphoma.

eastern United States, where a low incidence of HTLV serologic positivity has been documented, and in the Caribbean.[85-87] Most patients in the Western hemisphere are black. Patients present with characteristic generalized lymphadenopathy, hepatosplenomegaly, skin lesions, lytic bone lesions with hypercalcemia, and leukemic dissemination characterized by lymphoid cells with lobated nuclei in the peripheral blood.[88-90] The tumor cells are of mature CD4-positive T-cell phenotype. These lymphomas show a spectrum of cytologic findings, ranging from small lymphoid cells to mixed and pleomorphic variants. The pleomorphic type is most characteristic and is morphologically similar to peripheral T-cell lymphomas,[91-93] being composed of lymphoid cells of a wide range of sizes, including cells with marked nuclear irregularity and lobation, the so-called "floret cells." The course of the disease is usually biphasic, subacute, or chronic. Frequently there is a chronic phase of variable length, followed by a rapidly progressive terminal course. Although splenomegaly is often a feature of these lymphomas, the morphologic features of splenic involvement has not been described, and we have not seen such a case.

Mycosis Fungoides/Sézary Syndrome

Mycosis fungoides/Sézary syndrome (MF/SS) are neoplasms of CD4-positive T cells that have a characteristic morphologic feature in the skin. In MF, the bandlike infiltrate in the upper dermis is polymorphous, including small and large atypical lymphoid cells with irregular and folded nuclei, often accompanied by eosinophils, plasma cells, and histiocytes. The "mycosis cell" is a small hyperchromatic lymphoid cell with a lobulated and deeply clefted nucleus, which may be found within the epidermis in the characteristic Pautrier microabscesses. SS is a related condition in which a generalized exfoliative erythroderma is associated with a leukemia of Sézary cells, which have the same cytology as the cerebriform cells in the skin infiltrates of MF. When MF/SS disseminates into viscera, the infiltrate may show more pleomorphism, including bizarre and multinucleated Reed-Sternberg–like cells, and mycosis cells may be difficult to identify.[94]

MF is a chronic disorder that usually progresses rapidly once extracutaneous dissemination occurs. Lymph node involvement is a good predictor of visceral disease. Rappaport and Thomas[94] found extracutaneous lymphoma in 71 percent of autopsies, the most common viscera involved being the lung, spleen, and liver. Variakojis and coworkers[95] found splenic involvement in 4 of 13 patients who underwent staging laparotomy. The pattern of splenic involvement in MF is variable.[3, 94, 95] Some cases show a diffuse infiltrate in the red pulp, although in most cases the tumor produces irregular nodules in the red and white pulp (Fig. 8–15). Occasional cases, particularly in the early stage, show a predilection for the PALS, reflecting the T-cell homing of this lymphoma (Fig. 8–16).[96] The identification of diagnostic mycosis cells is helpful in recognizing this lymphoma in extracutaneous sites. However, these cells may be scarce. The polymorphous nature and the presence of Reed-Sternberg–like cells may create more than a superficial resemblance to Hodgkin's disease in the viscera. In difficult cases, immunohistochemistry can be helpful by demonstrating CD3 and other T-cell markers in the neoplastic cells.

MALIGNANT LYMPHOMAS PRESENTING WITH PROMINENT SPLENOMEGALY

The third of the clinical settings of malignant lymphoma of the spleen, that of presentation with significant splenomegaly and occult involvement of other organs, is the subject of the most recent study and controversy. It has been variously referred to as "malignant lymphoma presenting with massive splenomegaly," "primary splenic presentation of malignant lymphoma," "malignant lymphoma simulating hairy cell disease," "splenic lymphoma with villous lymphocytes," and "splenic marginal zone cell lymphoma," among others. We agree with the consensus that it is not one specific histopathologic or immunophenotypic type of malignant lymphoma but a syndrome that may be due to a variety of low- or intermediate-grade malignant lymphomas, probably all of B-cell type (Fig. 8–17).

Although the previous literature contains sporadic reports of malignant lymphoma with massive splenomegaly, Hickling[97] was probably the first to describe the entity in any detail. He reported four cases of what he termed "giant follicle lymphoma of the spleen" in 1960 and added a fifth case in 1964. Four of

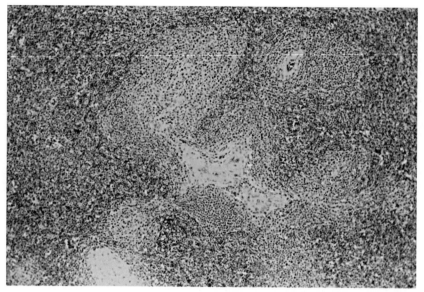

Figure 8–15. Mycosis fungoides. Early involvement involves predominantly the T-cell zones.

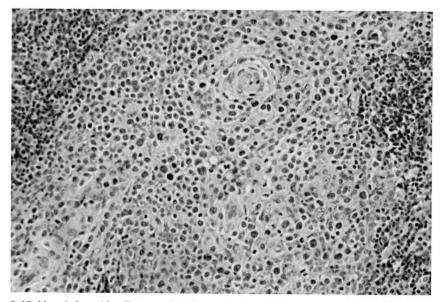

Figure 8–16. Mycosis fungoides. Tumor cells infiltrate the lymphoid tissue around the penicilliary arteriole.

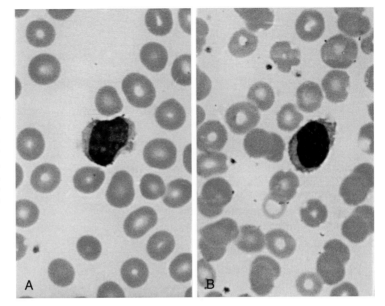

Figure 8–17. Villous lymphocytes in two cases of so-called splenic lymphoma with villous lymphocytes. (A) Shows a lymphocyte in a case of morphologically and immunologically confirmed marginal zone cell lymphoma. (B) Shows a lymphocyte in a case of morphologically and immunologically confirmed mantle cell lymphoma.

the five patients in his series were women, and all of them were middle-aged. All presented with striking splenomegaly and hypersplenism with inconspicuous clinical evidence of disease elsewhere. Two of the five patients had an absolute lymphocytosis, and all had morphologically abnormal lymphocytes present in blood smears. Pathologically confirmed marrow, liver, and splenic hilar nodal disease were present in each case. All patients had a miliary pattern of splenic white pulp involvement; photomicrographs published in the 1964 paper revealed expansion of both mantle and marginal zones. The disease appeared indolent, with marked clinical improvement following splenectomy. Hickling commented that the histology of the spleens was not the same in all cases and postulated that "different disease processes may cause giant follicle lymphoma" of the spleen.

Dacie et al[98] subsequently reported 10 cases of splenomegaly of unknown origin with peripheral blood cytopenias that they termed "non-tropical idiopathic splenomegaly" or "primary hypersplenism." Spleens in their series ranged from 575 to more than 5000 g. Five of the patients had autoimmune hemolytic anemia, and three had lymphocytosis of more than 20 percent in bone marrow smears. No other involvement was documented morphologically. Four of the 10 patients were noted to have developed "lymphocytic lymphoma" in a follow-up study published in 1978; and Dacie et al suggested that the cases

of lymphoma be termed "chronic lymphocytic lymphoma" (sic).[99] Analysis of the data in both papers and of the photomicrographs of the 10 spleens provided in the 1978 paper leads us to believe that only some of these cases were lymphomas, the others representing non-neoplastic immune reactions.

Several subsequent papers attempted to provide criteria for distinguishing malignant lymphomas presenting in the spleen from non-neoplastic lymphoid proliferations.[24, 100, 101] However, these studies were undertaken in the era antedating the modern immunologically supported classifications of lymphoma and in the absence of such ancillary studies as immunophenotyping, cytogenetics, and molecular techniques. The distinctions between benign and malignant lymphoid proliferations were inexact, relying on morphology alone or on clinical follow-up. Other studies[22, 23] did describe series of malignant lymphoid proliferations exclusively, but they included many cases of other neoplastic disorders, such as Hodgkin's disease and leukemias, and did not discriminate between the syndrome of malignant lymphoma presenting with prominent splenomegaly and true primary splenic lymphoma.

The first study describing an immunologically confirmed series of malignant lymphomas presenting with prominent splenomegaly was by Neiman and colleagues.[39] The preponderance of the 10 cases was in middle-aged or elderly women. All were originally considered to have hairy cell leukemia because of the clinical presentations, presence of atypical lymphoid cells in the peripheral blood, and a variable degree of tartrate-resistant acid phosphate activity in the lymphoid cells. All patients were noted to have occult, histologically confirmed dissemination of their disease, with marrow, liver, and nodal involvement. The tumors were all of B-cell type, with a varying degree of plasmacytoid morphologic features, monoclonal heavy or light chain expression, and/or serum paraprotein. Although some variation in morphology was observed in the cases in this series, all tumors were classified as small lymphocytic lymphoma, with or without plasmacytoid differentiation, mantle cell and marginal cell lymphomas not yet having been described.

In an updated and expanded study from the same institution in 1985, Narang et al[25] described 31 cases, classifying them according to Rapport, Lukes-Collins, and International Working Formulation subtypes. They noted that malignant lymphomas of small lymphocytic type (with and without plasmacytoid differentiation), small cleaved cell type, and mantle cell types were all represented. Spriano et al[40] subsequently reported eight similar cases. Because of the presence of a serum paraprotein and plasmacytoid features of the proliferating cells in all cases, they termed the disorder "splenomegalic immunocytoma."

In 1987 Melo and associates[41] published the first in a series of papers describing a group of patients with a disorder similar to that described by Neiman et al,[39] Spriano et al,[40] and Narang et al.[25] Emphasizing the morphologic features of the circulating lymphoid cells, they termed their cases "splenic lymphoma with villous lymphocytes" (SLVL).[41] Histologic examination of splenic tissues was similar to CLL and immunocytomas.[41, 102] SLVL occurs predominantly in elderly men who present with splenomegaly but with little or no lymphadenopathy. The disease usually runs an indolent course, splenectomy rather than chemotherapy being the most effective treatment, often resulting in long-standing control even in patients with bone marrow involvement.[103]

The circulating lymphoma cells in SLVL are usually larger than the lymphocytes in CLL. The nuclei are round or ovoid with a coarse chromatin pattern and a single small nucleolus. The nuclei are sometimes eccentrically placed. The cytoplasm is basophilic and usually abundant but may be scanty. The most important diagnostic feature is the presence of unevenly distributed short, thin villi often concentrated in one pole of the cell (see Fig. 8–17).[41] In nearly every case there is a variable proportion of plasmacytoid cells. The cells usually lack tartrate-resistant acid phosphatase reactivity. The bone marrow is involved in 75 percent of the cases.[104] The pattern of infiltration can be focal (interstitial or nodular) or focal and diffuse. A peculiar intravascular pattern has been recently described.[103] The pattern of splenic involvement was described earlier in this chapter. In SLVL there is never exclusive involvement of the red pulp as observed in hairy cell leukemia.[105] The immunophenotypic profile of SLVL is variable, with most cases resembling lymphoplasmacytoid lymphoma (Sig-positive, CD5-negative, CD23-negative).[104, 106] Molecular analysis shows lack of BCL-2 rearrangment[107]; some of the cases have shown the t(11;14) translocation, with rearrangement of the BCL-1 gene and increased expression of cyclin D1.[108]

Isaacson et al[109] reviewed the histopathology of 37 cases of SLVL from the original patient population from Catovsky's group. They concluded that SLVL is a histologically homogeneous entity, representing the leukemic variant of splenic marginal zone lymphoma.[110] They also suggested that, in the past, cases of splenic marginal zone cell lymphoma (SMZCL) may have been given different names (e.g., SLL, immunocytoma, mantle cell lymphoma).[109] This paper does not reflect the majority opinion among students of splenic lymphomas. As quoted by Isaacson et al in their paper, SLVL was discussed at a workshop of the Society of Hematopathology in Toronto in August 1993. It was the consensus at this workshop, in which the authors of this book participated, that SLVL is a clinical syndrome that may be caused by a variety of low- or intermediate-grade B-cell lymphomas including malignant lymphoma, small lymphocytic type with or without plasmacytoid differentiation; malignant lymphoma, follicular small cleaved cell type; and mantle cell lymphoma, as well marginal zone cell lymphoma. This opinion is supported by several recent studies indicating that SLVL cases display great variability in the expression of immunophenotypic markers and of cytogenetic and molecular genetic characteristics.[42, 111–117a] Recent evidence suggests that the leukemic cells in patients with SLVL have a remarkable morphologic and phenotypic fluctuation with time[116] due to their activation status. The disease has also been associated with the presence of persistent polyclonal B-cell proliferation as seen in patients with chronic malarial splenomegaly[118, 119] and has been associated with several autoimmune conditions.[120, 121] Moreover, in view of the uncertain characterization of SMZCL within the group of the marginal zone lymphomas,[113] it seems premature to accept the concept that SLVL and SMZCL are derived from the same cell type, especially while still awaiting confirmation of the appropriateness of the term "marginal zone lymphoma" for a low-grade B-cell lymphoma that displays overlapping characteristics with other well-established categories.

As mentioned previously, non-Hodgkin's lymphoma presenting with prominent splenomegaly appears to be a clinical syndrome but not a specific histologic entity. Almost any histologic type of lymphoma can present initially with a large spleen. Several types of low-grade B-cell lymphoma are, however, largely responsible for the bulk of cases with this clinical presentation, and they are discussed in this context in the following sections.

Small Lymphocytic Lymphoma and Lymphoplasmacytic Lymphoma

Prominent splenomegaly can be the presenting features in cases of small lymphocytic lymphoma and LPCL.[39–41] These latter cases have also been termed "splenomegalic immunocytoma." The gross and microscopic features are indistinguishable from cases in which the spleen is secondarily involved by nodal small lymphocytic malignancies. In the majority of cases, involvement of the marrow and the liver is observed. Serum M-protein is often detected. Lymphoplasmacytic lymphoma observed in spleen sections is consistent with the morphologic appearance of Waldenström macroglobulinemia in the bone marrow and appears to be the splenic manifestation of that disease. However, not all patients with LPCL have Waldenström macroglobulinemia.

A peculiar variant of LPCL, characterized by a nodular and diffuse proliferation of small lymphoid cells surrounded by a zonally distinct proliferation of large plasmacytoid cells, has also been reported to occur in the spleen (Fig. 8–18).[38] In one of these cases, the spleen was the only involved organ. The morphologic features of this variant of LPCL overlap greatly with those observed in SMZCL. In this latter disorder, a zonation phenomenon with concentration of the larger cells at the periphery of the neoplastic nodules as well as lymphoplasmacytoid differentiation has been described.

Splenomegalic SLL lymphoma, especially LPCL, may present with peripheral blood

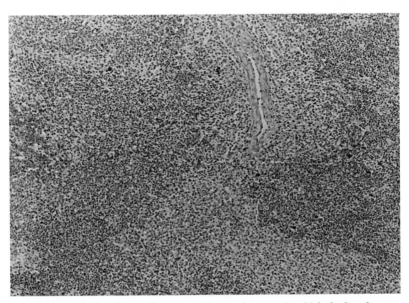

Figure 8–18. Lymphoplasmacytic lymphoma. Contrary to the usual pattern in which the lymphocytes and plasmacytoid are intermixed, this case illustrates a zonal distribution of the different cell types. The small lymphocytes, which appear darker in this photograph, occupy the malpighian corpuscles; the plasmacytoid cells, which appear lighter, are seen in the mantle and marginal zones and spill into the red pulp.

involvement with atypical lymphoid cells showing hairy appearance. This presentation may correspond to the clinical syndrome known as splenic lymphoma with circulating villous lymphocytes.

Mantle Cell Lymphoma

MCL has also been reported to present with massive splenomegaly.[25, 26, 42] The gross and histologic findings in cases with primary splenic presentation are indistinguishable from cases in which the spleen is involved as part of a diffuse disease (see previous section). Histologically and immunohistochemically, MCL can be distinguished from other low-grade B-cell lymphomas. However, it has been suggested that most of the splenic lymphoma cases previously reported as MCL or SLL are SMZCL.[109] We believe that these entities can and should be distinguished from SMZCL. In SMZCL, the typical compartmentalization of the white pulp and the characteristic polymorphic cellular composition are distinguishing features that are not found in the other subtypes. In addition, the strong CD5, IgM, IgD, and light chain expression; the presence of t(11;14); and the expression of PRAD-1 gene are characteristic findings in MCL that are not observed in SMZCL.[103, 122, 123] MCL may present with a leukemic phase.[124, 125] The cytologic features of the mantle cells in the peripheral blood and the characteristic MCL immunophenotype can be used to characterize these leukemic cells.[124] The peripheral blood cells have medium size, pleomorphic appearance, round or irregular nuclei, coarse chromatin, and fairly conspicuous nucleoli. Cytoplasmic villi may be noted in these cells (see Fig. 8–17). Leukemic MCL cases can at times be difficult to distinguish from CLL (mixed cell type), leukemic follicular lymphoma, and SMZCL with circulating villous lymphocytes. Immunophenotyping may be helpful in distinguishing these disorders because leukemic MCL cells do not have the typical phenotype observed in CLL or in follicular lymphoma.

Splenic Marginal Zone Cell Lymphoma

The marginal zone of the human splenic white pulp is a morphologically and immunologically distinct B-cell region.[126–129] Cells similar to splenic marginal zone lymphocytes have also been described in lymph nodes[129, 130] and in Peyer patches.[131] Marginal zone cells have been postulated to be the origin of extranodal MALT-type and nodal monocytoid B-cell lymphomas.[132–135] A number of cases of SMZCL have been reported.[109, 110, 113, 115, 136–143] Most patients present with splenomegaly, anemia, and weight loss. The bone marrow and liver are commonly involved. Rare cases with minimal or no splenomegaly and absent bone marrow or liver involvement have also been reported.[140, 143] In these latter cases, the neoplastic nodules closely resemble marginal zone hyperplasia (see Fig. 5–12) (Fig. 8–19). The course of SMZCL is reported to be indolent, and splenectomy may be followed by prolonged survival.[136, 139]

The cut surface of the spleen in SMZCL shows increased white pulp nodularity. Histologically, nodular involvement of the white pulp centered on preexisting follicles is observed (Fig. 8–20). Follicle centers are rarely identifiable, being often completely or partially replaced by small lymphocytes similar to mantle cells (Fig. 8–21). Toward the periphery of the neoplastic nodule, the small cells give way to larger cells with irregular nuclei and pale cytoplasm (Fig. 8–22). When residual follicle centers are identified, the medium-sized neoplastic cells are arranged into broad concentric strands around the germinal center (reactive or hyalinized), a pattern that may superficially resemble reactive marginal zone hyperplasia.[144–146] However, in marginal zone hyperplasia, lymphoid infiltration of the follicles is not observed. In addition, red pulp involvement is a common feature in SMZCL, which is not seen in reactive spleens.

Bone marrow involvement in SMZCL has been reported as focal, interstitial, or nodular, and rarely paratrabecular or diffuse.[110, 136, 138, 140] Follicular centers are only rarely observed.[110] An intrasinusoidal pattern of involvement has also been observed in some cases.[105, 147] Immunohistochemically, the lymphoma cells express various B-cell markers, surface immunoglobulin (usually IgM [± IgD]), and BCL-2, but not CD5, CD10, CD23, CD11c, or CD43. CD72 (DBA.44) is positive in a minority of cases. Molecular analysis shows lack of BCL-1 or BCL-2 rearrangement.[148]

It has been suggested that SMZCL overlaps with extranodal (MALT-type) and nodal (monocytoid) marginal zone B-cell lymphoma. However, SMZCL differs clinically from those other lymphomas by virtue of its dissemination

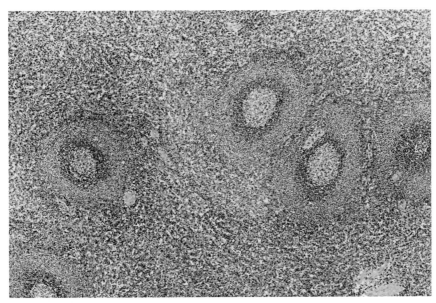

Figure 8–19. So-called indolent splenic marginal zone cell lymphoma. The neoplastic nodules resemble marginal zone hyperplasia (see also Figure 5–12).

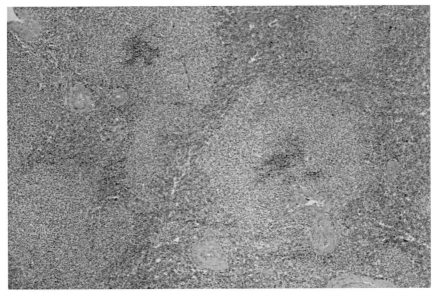

Figure 8–20. Splenic marginal zone cell lymphoma. Expanded marginal zones proliferate around the atrophic follicles. The dark cells in the centers of the nodules represent residual mantle cells.

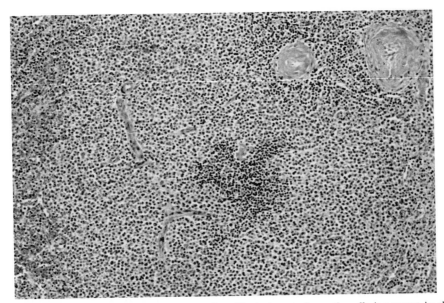

Figure 8–21. Splenic marginal zone cell lymphoma. A residual cluster of mantle cells is present in the center of the nodule.

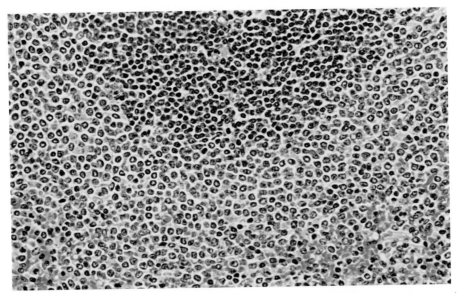

Figure 8–22. Splenic marginal zone cell lymphoma. The tripartite nature of the nodule simulates a reactive process. The neoplastic cells contain more cytoplasm than the mantle cells in the dark zone above.

at presentation. In addition, the histologic and immunohistochemical findings are only partially overlapping.[110, 113, 136] The so-called marginal zone pattern, i.e., the presence of a distinct outer layer of neoplastic lymphocytes encircling reactive follicles and the preservation of the normal periarterial lymphoid cuffs, described in spleens involved by monocytoid B-cell lymphoma is not observed in SMZCL.[1, 3, 53] Also, the selective replacement of germinal centers by neoplastic lymphocytes (follicular colonization), which is considered to be a prominent feature of MALT-type lymphomas, is usually absent in SMZCL. Differences in selected antigen expression have also been reported between these three lymphoma subtypes.[54, 110] Monocytoid B-cell lymphoma in particular shows much closer similarities with hairy cell leukemia (cytologic findings and CD11c and DBA.44 reactivity) than with SMZCL or MALT-type lymphomas. The low incidence of trisomy 3 in SMZCL cases also suggests that this neoplastic process may be genetically distinct from other types of marginal zone cell lymphomas.[117]

From this discussion, it appears that the appropriateness of the term "marginal zone lymphoma" for all of these splenic lymphomas is questionable. Most of the cases associated with circulating villous lymphocytes have a lymphoplasmacytoid appearance and an IgM gammopathy.[109] The presence of larger cells with plasmacytoid features at the periphery of the malpighian corpuscles within the marginal zone area responsible for the observed margination is another feature that SMZCL and LPCL have in common. It may be more appropriate to consider such cases as examples of low-grade peripheral B-cell lymphoma, lymphoplasmacytic, with distribution to splenic marginal zone areas.

Hepatosplenic T-Cell Lymphoma

Hepatosplenic T-cell lymphoma (HTCL) is a distinct clinical entity within the clinical spectrum of peripheral T-cell lymphomas.[149–153] It typically occurs in young adults, more frequently males, and is associated with a poor prognosis. The presenting symptoms include fever, weight loss, hepatosplenomegaly, and variable cytopenias. This tumor overlaps to a certain degree with a rare type of T-cell lymphoma that also involves the spleen, termed "erythrophagocytic T-gamma lymphoma."[154]

In this latter disorder, the tumor cells show erythrophagocytic activity as well as CD16 (FcRI receptor) expression, features that have not been observed in the HTCL cases reported to date. Splenic involvement in both conditions is similar. Macroscopically, the spleen is enlarged, usually weighing 3000 g or more, with a homogeneous cut surface and loss of white pulp markings. Histologically, the neoplastic cells diffusely infiltrate the red pulp cords and conspicuously fill the sinuses (Fig. 8–23). The lymphoid cells are medium-sized and have oval or folded nuclei, with chromatin less condensed than that of small lymphocytes and a moderate amount of pale cytoplasm (Fig. 8–24). Although erythrophagocytosis may be noted, the cells may not show the degree of erythrophagocytosis seen in erythrophagocytic T-gamma lymphoma (Fig. 8–25). The histologic appearance of the spleen may mimic hairy cell leukemia.[153] However, blood lakes are not seen in HTCL. In addition, the immunophenotypic differences are distinctive. The main feature of liver and bone marrow involvement, similar to that in the spleen, is an intrasinusoidal distribution of the neoplastic cells. Abdominal lymph node involvement has been observed in one HTCL case in which the lymph node showed partial infiltration by similar lymphoid cells arranged in an interfollicular and sinusoidal pattern. The neoplastic cells stain with various pan–T-cell markers including CD3. CD56 is also often positive. Most cases characteristically express the gamma/delta T-cell receptor,[149, 150, 153] although some cases also express the alpha/beta receptor.[151] Most cases show clonal rearrangement of the gamma or delta chain of the T-cell receptor gene, whereas the beta-chain T-cell receptor gene may be either germline or rearranged.[149, 152] Recent evidence has suggested that HTCL is associated with the presence of isochromosome 7_q10 in tumor cells.[153, 155] The spleen normally contains a high frequency of gamma/delta T cells as compared with other lymphoid organs.[156] This distinctive involvement probably represents the neoplastic counterpart of the splenic red pulp gamma/delta T-cell component that maintains its preferential homing to the original splenic microenvironment.

Hepatosplenic B-Cell Lymphoma

Several investigators have shown that hepatitis C virus (HCV) infection may be related to

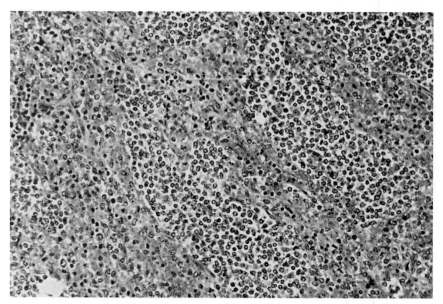

Figure 8–23. Hepatosplenic T-cell lymphoma. The tumor cells infiltrate cords and sinuses of the red pulp. Note the striking sinusoidal involvement.

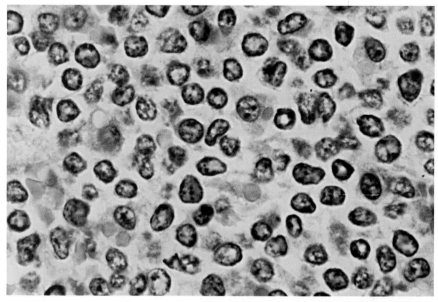

Figure 8–24. Hepatosplenic T-cell lymphoma. The tumor cells are intermediate in size.

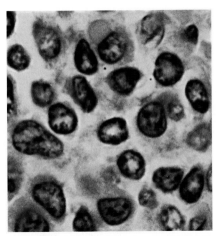

Figure 8–25. Erythroplagocytic T-gamma lymphoma. The infiltrate in the splenic red pulp resembles that of hepatosplenic T-cell lymphoma. However, erythrophagocytosis is present (top).

the pathogenesis of different types of B-cell malignancies such as Waldenström macroglobulinemia,[157] non-Hodgkin's lymphoma,[158, 159] and mixed cryoglobulinemia.[157, 160] Among the HCV-associated lymphomas, several cases have been diagnosed as primary hepatosplenic B-cell lymphomas.[161–165] Most cases are of large cell type. The direct causal relationship between the occurrence of hepatosplenic B-cell lymphoma and chronic HCV infection is unclear; a relation with chronic hepatitis has been suggested. A pathogenetically similar relationship between persistent infection and local development of B-cell malignancy has been demonstrated in cases of gastric MALT lymphomas.[166, 167]

SPLENECTOMY IN MALIGNANT LYMPHOMAS

The role of diagnostic splenectomy in patients with malignant lymphoma is less controversial than is therapeutic splenectomy. In cases of true primary splenic lymphoma as well as in many cases of lymphomas with massive splenomegaly, splenectomy is the only practical means to establish a diagnosis. In addition, in the latter group, splenectomy is an effective therapy for the cytopenias that are usually present. The role of therapeutic splenectomy in patients with confirmed malignant lymphomas, however, is controversial. In some cases hypersplenism may necessitate splenectomy. This may occur with any lymphoma that pro-

duces significant splenomegaly. In addition, small lymphocytic lymphoma may be associated with autoimmune thrombocytopenia or anemia. Hypersplenism tends to occur earlier in the course of malignant lymphomas than in Hodgkin's disease, and splenectomy may have a more significant palliative role.[168–171] Kehoe and coworkers,[172] in a review of 46 cases, found that patients whose cytopenias did not respond to splenectomy tended to have larger spleens and lower platelet counts. Kehoe and colleagues suggested that palliative splenectomy should be considered earlier in the course of the disease. These authors found that patients who responded to splenectomy by amelioration of cytopenias had a 5-year survival rate of 40 percent, whereas all nonresponders died within 36 months. Adler and associates[173] studied 50 patients with advanced disease who had failed to respond to splenic irradiation or corticosteroids, or both, and found only eight complete failures to splenectomy, although the mean duration of remission was only 7 months. The responders in their series had an increased tolerance to further chemotherapy and a decreased need for transfusions. Failure to demonstrate splenic sequestration of radio-isotope-labeled erythrocytes did not preclude a response to splenectomy in the study. Other investigators have also reported a better tolerance to chemotherapy following splenectomy.[174] Brodsky et al[175] found that splenectomy was effective only in selected cases of non-Hodgkin's lymphomas. Splenectomy in non-Hodgkin's lymphomas is a potentially dangerous procedure. The most frequent complications include bleeding and sepsis, which occur most frequently in patients with spleens weighing more than 2000 g.[176]

Staging laparotomy is not usually performed in patients with non-Hodgkin's lymphoma. Veronesi and colleagues[177] found that staging laparotomy changed the clinical stage in 27 percent of cases and revealed occult splenic disease in 12 percent. However, therapeutic regimens for the malignant lymphomas are not as crucially dependent on stage as is the treatment of Hodgkin's disease, in which documentation of splenic involvement may alter the therapeutic regimen.

REFERENCES

1. Lymphomas of the spleen, in Warnke RA, Weiss LM, Chan JKC, et al (eds): Atlas of Tumor Pathology:

Tumors of the Lymph Nodes and Spleen, 3rd series, fascicle 14, p 411. Washington, DC, Armed Forces Institute of Pathology, 1995.

2. Wolf BC, Neiman RS: The histopathologic manifestations of the lymphoproliferative and myeloproliferative disorders involving the spleen, in Knowles DM (ed): Neoplastic Hematopathology. Baltimore, Williams & Wilkins, 1992.

3. Burke JS: Diagnosis of lymphoma and lymphoid proliferations in the spleen, in Jaffe ES (ed): Surgical Pathology of the Lymph Nodes and Related Organs, 2nd ed, p 448. Philadelphia, WB Saunders, 1995.

4. Bellany CO, Krajewski AJ: Primary splenic large cell anaplastic lymphoma associated with HIV infection. Histopathology 1994; 24:481.

5. Brox A, Bishinsky JI, Berry G: Primary non-Hodgkin lymphoma of the spleen. Am J Hematol 1991; 38:95.

6. Brox A, Shustik C: Non-Hodgkin's lymphoma of the spleen. Leuk Lymphoma 1993; 11:165.

7. Das Gupta T, Coombes B, Brasfeld RD: Primary malignant neoplasms of the spleen. Surg Gynecol Obstet 1965; 120:947.

8. Falk S, Karhoff M, Takeshita M, et al: Primary pleomorphic T-cell lymphoma of the spleen. Histopathology 1990; 16:191.

9. Fausel R, Sun NC, Klein S: Splenic rupture in HIV-infected patient with primary splenic lymphoma. Cancer 1990; 66:2414.

10. Hara K, Ito M, Shimizu K, et al: Three cases of primary splenic lymphoma: Case report and review of the Japanese literature. Acta Pathol Jpn 1985; 35:419.

11. Harris NL, Aisenberg AC, Meyer JE, et al: Diffuse large cell (histiocytic) lymphoma of the spleen: Clinical and pathologic characteristics of ten cases. Cancer 1984; 54:2460.

12. Ishihara T, Takahashi M, Uchino F, et al: A filiform large cell lymphoma of the spleen: A case report with immunohistochemical and electron microscopic study. Ultrastruct Pathol 1990; 14:193.

13. Kobrich U, Falk S, Karhoff M, et al: Primary large cell lymphoma of the splenic sinuses: A variant of angiotropic B-cell lymphoma (neoplastic angioendotheliomatosis)? Hum Pathol 1992; 23:1184.

14. Montanaro A, Patten R: Primary splenic malignant lymphoma, histiocytic type, with sclerosis. Cancer 1979; 43:329.

15. Spier CM, Kjeldsberg CR, Eyre HJ, et al: Malignant lymphoma with primary presentation in the spleen: A study of 20 patients. Arch Pathol Lab Med 1985; 109:1076.

16. Weide R, Gorg C, Pfluger KH, et al: Concomitant primary low grade non-Hodgkin's lymphoma of the spleen and breast carcinoma. Leuk Lymphoma 1992; 7:337.

17. Falk S, Stutte JH: Primary malignant lymphomas of the spleen: A morphologic and immunohistochemical analysis of 17 cases. Cancer 1990; 66:2612.

18. Kim H, Dorfman RF: Morphological studies of 84 untreated patients subjected to laparotomy for the staging of non-Hodgkin's lymphomas. Cancer 1974; 33:657.

19. Lotz MJ, Chabner B, DeVita VT, et al: Pathological staging of 100 consecutive untreated patients with non-Hodgkin's lymphomas. Cancer 1976; 37:266.

20. Goffinet DR, Warnke R, Dunnick NR, et al: Clinical and surgical (laparotomy) evaluation of patients with non-Hodgkin's lymphomas. Cancer Treat Rep 1977; 61:981.

21. National Cancer Institute–Sponsored Study of Classifications of Non-Hodgkin's Lymphomas: Summary and description of a working formulation for clinical usage: The Non-Hodgkin's Lymphoma Pathologic Classification Project. Cancer 1982; 49:2112.

22. Ahmann DL, Kiely JM, Harrison EG Jr, et al: Malignant lymphoma of the spleen: A review of 49 cases in which the diagnosis was made at splenectomy. Cancer 1966; 19:461.

23. Kraemer BB, Osborne BM, Butler JJ: Primary splenic presentation of malignant lymphoma: A study of 49 cases. Cancer 1984; 54:1606.

24. Long JC, Aisenberg AC: Malignant lymphoma diagnosed at splenectomy and idiopathic splenomegaly. Cancer 1974; 33:1054.

25. Narang S, Wolf BC, Neiman RS: Malignant lymphoma presenting with prominent splenomegaly: A clinicopathologic study with special reference to intermediate cell lymphoma. Cancer 1985; 55:1948.

26. Arber DA, Rappaport H, Weiss LM: Non-Hodgkin's lymphoproliferative disorders involving the spleen. Mod Pathol 1997; 10:18.

27. Pangalis GA, Nathwani BN, Rappaport H: Malignant lymphoma well-differentiated lymphocytic: Its relationship with chronic lymphocytic leukemia and macroglobulinemia of Waldenstrom. Cancer 1977; 39:999.

28. Evans HL, Butler JJ, Youness EL: Malignant lymphoma, small lymphocytic type: A clinicopathologic study of 84 cases with suggested criteria for intermediate lymphocytic lymphoma. Cancer 1978; 41:1440.

29. Rappaport H: Tumors of the Hematopoietic System, in Atlas of Tumor Pathology, section 3, fascicle 8, p 28. Washington, DC, Armed Forces Institute of Pathology, 1966.

30. Dick F, Maca R: The lymph node in chronic lymphocytic leukemia. Cancer 1978; 41:283.

31. Lennert K, Mohri N, Stein H, et al: The histopathology of malignant lymphoma. Br J Haematol 1975; 31:193.

32. Braylan RC, Long JC, Jaffe ES, et al: Malignant lymphoma obscured by concomitant extensive epithelioid granulomas: Report of three cases with similar clinicopathologic features. Cancer 1977; 39:1146.

33. Sundeen JT, Longo DL, Jaffe ES: CD5 expression in B-cell small lymphocytic malignancies: Correlations with clinical presentation and sites of disease. Am J Surg Pathol 1992; 16:130.

34. Lukes R, Collins R: New approaches to the classification of the lymphomata. Br J Cancer 1975; 31:1.

35. Dutcher T, Fahey J: Immunocytochemical demonstration of intranuclear localization of 18 S-gamma macroglobulin in macroglobulinemia of Waldenstrom. Proc Soc Exp Biol Med 1960; 103:452.

36. Lymphocytic and diffuse small cleaved cell lymphomas, in Warnke RA, Weiss LM, Chan JKC, et al (eds): Atlas of Tumor Pathology: Tumors of the Lymph Nodes and Spleen, 3rd series, fascicle 14, p 119. Washington, DC, Armed Forces Institute of Pathology, 1995.

37. Dick FR: Small lymphocytic malignancies and related immunoproliferative disorders, in Jaffe ES (ed): Surgical Pathology of the Lymph Nodes and Related Organs, 2nd ed, p 205. Philadelphia, WB Saunders, 1995.

38. Alberti VN, Neiman RS: Lymphoplasmacytic lymphoma: A clinicopathologic study of a previously unrecognized composite variant. Cancer 1984; 53:1103.

39. Neiman RS, Sullivan AL, Jaffe R, et al: Malignant lymphoma simulating leukemic reticuloendotheliosis. Cancer 1979; 43:329.

40. Spriano P, Barosi G, Invernizzi R, et al: Splenomegalic immunocytoma with circulating hairy cells: Report of eight cases and revision of the literature. Haematologica 1986; 71:25.

41. Melo JV, Hedge U, Parreira A, et al: Splenic B-cell lymphoma with circulating villous lymphocytes: Differential diagnosis of B-cell leukaemias with large spleens. J Clin Pathol 1987; 40:642.

42. Pittaluga S, Verhoef G, Criel A, et al: "Small" B-cell non-Hodgkin's lymphomas with splenomegaly at presentation are either mantle cell lymphoma or marginal zone cell lymphoma. Am J Surg Pathol 1996; 20:211.

43. Weisenburger DD, Nathwani BN, Diamond LW, et al: Malignant lymphoma intermediate lymphocytic type: A clinicopathologic study of 42 cases. Cancer 1981; 48:1415.

44. Weisenburger DD, Linder J, Daley DT, et al: Intermediate lymphocytic lymphoma: An immunohistologic study with comparison to other lymphocytic lymphomas. Hum Pathol 1987; 18:781.

45. Weisenburger DD, Kim H, Rappaport H: Mantle-zone lymphoma: A follicular variant of intermediate lymphocytic lymphoma. Cancer 1982; 49:1429.

46. Yang WI, Zukerberg LR, Motokura T, et al: Cyclin D1 (Bcl-1, PRAD1) protein expression in low-grade B-cell lymphomas and reactive hyperplasia. Am J Pathol 1994; 145:86.

47. Zukerberg LR, Yang WI, Arnold A: Cyclin D1 expression in non-Hodgkin's lymphomas: Detection by immunohistochemistry. Am J Clin Pathol 1995; 103:756.

48. Lukes RJ, Parker JW, Taylor CR, et al: Immunologic approach to non-Hodgkin's lymphomas and related leukemias: Analysis of the results of multiparameter studies of 425 cases. Semin Hematol 1978; 15:322.

49. Sheibani K, Burke JS, Swartz WG, et al: Monocytoid B-cell lymphoma: Clinicopathologic study of 21 cases of a unique type of low-grade lymphoma. Cancer 1988; 62:1531.

50. Agnarsson BA, Kadin ME: An unusual B-cell lymphoma simulating hairy cell leukemia. Am J Clin Pathol 1987; 88:752.

51. Ngan B-Y, Warnke RA, Wilson M, et al: Monocytoid B-cell lymphoma: A study of 36 cases. Hum Pathol 1991; 22:409.

52. Traweek ST, Sheibani K: Monocytoid B-cell lymphoma: The biologic and clinical implications of peripheral blood involvement. Am J Clin Pathol 1992; 97:591.

53. Vasef M, Katzin WE: Monocytoid B-cell lymphoma with a distinctive clinical presentation. Hum Pathol 1993; 24:558.

54. Mollejo M, Menarguez J, Cristobal E, et al: Monocytoid B cells: A comparative clinical pathological study of their distribution in different types of low-grade lymphomas. Am J Surg Pathol 1994; 18:1131.

55. Harris NL, Jaffe ES, Stein H, et al: A revised European-American classification of lymphoid neoplasms: A proposal from the International Lymphoma Study Group. Blood 1994; 84:1361.

56. Stroup RM, Burke JS, Sheibani K, et al: Splenic involvement by aggressive malignant lymphomas of B-cell and T-cell types: A morphologic and immunophenotypic study. Cancer 1992; 69:413.

57. Betman HF, Vardiman JW, Lau J: T-cell–rich B-cell lymphoma of the spleen. Am J Surg Pathol 1994; 18:324.

58. Faravelli A, Gambini S, Perego D, et al: Splenic lymphoma: Unusual case with exclusive red pulp involvement. Pathologica 1995; 87:692.

59. Cossman J, Chosed TM, Fisher RI, et al: Diversity of immunologic phenotypes of lymphoblastic lymphomas. Cancer Res 1983; 43:4486.

60. Barcos MP, Lukes RJ: Malignant lymphoma of convoluted lymphocytes: A new entity of possible T-cell type, in Sinks LF, Godden JO (eds): Conflicts in Childhood Cancer: An evaluation of Current Management, vol 4, p 147. New York, Alan R. Liss, 1975.

61. Nathwani BN, Kim H, Rappaport H: Malignant lymphoma, lymphoblastic. Cancer 1976; 38:964.

62. Brownell MD, Sheibani K, Battifora H, et al: Distinction between undifferentiated (small noncleaved) and lymphoblastic lymphoma: An immunohistologic study on paraffin-embedded, fixed tissue sections. Am J Surg Pathol 1987; 11:779.

63. Picozzi VJ, Coleman CN: Lymphoblastic lymphoma. Semin Oncol 1990; 17:96.

64. Lardelli P, Bookman MA, Sundeen J, et al: Lymphocytic lymphoma of intermediate differentiation: Morphologic and immunophenotypic spectrum and clinical correlations. Am J Surg Pathol 1990; 14:752.

65. Orazi A, Cattoretti G, John K, et al: Terminal deoxynucleotidyl transferase staining of malignant lymphomas in paraffin sections. Mod Pathol 1994; 7:582.

66. Orazi A, Cotton J, Cattoretti G, et al: Terminal deoxynucleotidyl transferase staining in acute leukemia and normal bone marrow in routinely processed paraffin sections. Am J Clin Pathol 1994; 102:640.

67. Robertson PB, Neiman RS, Worapongpaiboon S, et al: 013 (CD99) positivity in hematologic proliferations correlates with TdT positivity. Mod Pathol 1997; 10:277.

68. Arseneau JC, Canellos GP, Banks PM, et al: American Burkitt's lymphoma: a clinicopathologic study of 30 cases. I. Clinical features related to prolonged survival. Am J Med 1975; 58:314.

69. Pavlova A, Parker J, Taylor C, et al: Small noncleaved follicular center cell lymphoma: Burkitt's and non-Burkitt's variants in the U.S. Cancer 1987; 59:1892.

70. Grogan TM, Warnke RA, Kaplan HS: A comparative study of Burkitt's and non-Burkitt's "undifferentiated" malignant lymphoma: Immunologic, cytochemical, ultrastructural, histopathologic, clinical, and cell culture features. Cancer 1982; 49:1817.

71. Banks PM, Arseneau JC, Gralnick HR, et al: American Burkitt's lymphoma: A clinicopathologic study of 30 cases. II. Pathologic correlations. Am J Med 1975; 58:322.

72. Mann RB, Jaffe ES, Braylan RC, et al: Nonendemic Burkitt's lymphoma: A B-cell tumor related to germinal centers. N Engl J Med 1976; 295:685.

73. Miliauskas JR, Berard CW, Young RC, et al: Undifferentiated non-Hodgkin's lymphomas (Burkitt's and non-Burkitt's type): The relevance of making this histologic distinction. Cancer 1982; 50:2115.

74. Medeiros JL: Intermediate and high grade diffuse non-Hodgkin's lymphomas in the working formulation, in Jaffe ES (ed): Surgical Pathology of the Lymph Nodes and Related Organs, 2nd ed, p 283. Philadelphia, WB Saunders, 1995.

75. Jaffe ES: Post-thymic lymphoid neoplasia, in Jaffe ES (ed): Surgical Pathology of the Lymph Nodes and

Related Organs, 2nd ed, p 344. Philadelphia, WB Saunders, 1995.

76. Waldron JA, Leech JH, Glick AD, et al: Malignant lymphoma of peripheral T-lymphocyte origin: Immunologic, pathologic, and clinical features in six patients. Cancer 1977; 40:1604.

77. Brisbane JU, Berman LD, Neiman RS: Peripheral T-cell lymphoma: A clinicopathologic study of nine cases. Am J Clin Pathol 1983; 79:285.

78. Weinberg DS, Pinkus GS: Non-Hodgkin's lymphoma of large multilobated cell type: A clinicopathologic study of ten cases. Am J Clin Pathol 1981; 76:190.

79. Lennert K, Mestdagh J: Lymphogranulomatosen mit konstant hohem epithelioid zell gehalt. Virchows Arch 1968; 344:1.

80. Burke JS, Butler JJ: Malignant lymphoma with a high content of epithelioid histiocytes (Lennert's lymphoma). Am J Clin Pathol 1976; 66:1.

81. Kim H, Jacobs C, Warnke RA, et al: Malignant lymphoma with a high content of epithelioid histiocytes: A distinct clinicopathologic entity and a form of so-called "Lennert's lymphoma." Cancer 1978; 41:620.

82. Klein MA, Jaffe R, Neiman RS: "Lennert's lymphoma" with transformation to malignant lymphoma, histiocytic type (immunoblastic sarcoma). Am J Clin Pathol 1977; 68:601.

83. Gallo RC, de The GB, Ito Y: Kyoto workshop on some specific recent advances in tumor virology. Cancer Res 1981; 41:4738.

84. Uchiyama T, Yodoi J, Sagawa K, et al: Adult T-cell leukemia: Clinical and hematologic features of 16 cases. Blood 1977; 50:481.

85. Blattner WA, Kalyanaraman VS, Robert-Guroff M, et al: The human-type C retrovirus, HTLV, in blacks from the Caribbean region and relationship to adult T-cell leukemia/lymphoma. Int J Cancer 1982; 30:257.

86. Catovsky D, Rose M, Goolden AWG, et al: Adult T-cell lymphoma/leukemia in blacks from the West Indies. Lancet 1982; 1:639.

87. Jaffe ES, Blattner WA, Blayney DW, et al: The pathologic spectrum of adult T-cell leukemia/lymphoma in the United States: Human T-cell leukemia/lymphoma virus-associated lymphoid malignancies. Am J Surg Pathol 1984; 8:263.

88. Blayney DW, Jaffe ES, Blattner WA, et al: The human T-cell leukemia/lymphoma virus (HTLV) associated with American adult T-cell leukemia/lymphoma (ATL). Blood 1983; 62:401.

89. Blayney DW, Jaffe ES, Fisher RI, et al: The human T-cell leukemia/lymphoma virus (HTLV), lymphoma, lytic bone lesions, and hypercalcemia. Ann Intern Med 1983; 98:144.

90. Grossman B, Schecter GP, Horton JE, et al: Hypercalcemia associated with T-cell lymphoma/leukemia. Am J Clin Pathol 1981; 75:149.

91. Hanaoka M: Progress in adult T-cell leukemia research. Acta Pathol Jpn 1982; 31:171.

92. Kikuchi M, Mitsui T, Matsui N, et al: T-cell malignancies in adults: Histopathological studies of lymph nodes in 110 patients. Jpn J Clin Oncol 1979; 9:407.

93. Suchi T, Tajima K: Peripheral T-cell malignancy as a problem in lymphoma classification. Jpn J Clin Oncol 1979; 9:443.

94. Rappaport H, Thomas LB: Mycosis fungoides: The pathology of extracutaneous involvement. Cancer 1974; 34:1198.

95. Variakojis D, Rosas-Uribe A, Rappaport H: Mycosis fungoides: Pathologic findings in staging laparotomies. Cancer 1974; 33:1589.

96. Thomas LB, Rappaport H: Mycosis fungoides and its relationship to other malignant lymphomas, in Rebuck JW, Berard CW, Abell MR (eds): The Reticuloendothelial System, International Academy of Pathology Monograph No. 16, p 243. Baltimore, Williams & Wilkins, 1975.

97. Hickling RA: Giant follicle lymphoma of the spleen: Recovery after splenectomy. Br Med J 1960; 1:1464.

98. Dacie JV, Brain MC, Harrison CV, et al: "Non-tropical idiopathic splenomegaly" (primary hypersplenism): A review of ten cases and their relationship to malignant lymphomas. Br J Haematol 1969; 17:317.

99. Dacie JV, Galton DA, Gordon-Smith EC, et al: Nontropical "idiopathic splenomegaly": A follow-up study of ten patients described in 1969. Br J Haematol 1978; 38:185.

100. Skarin AT, Davey RF, Moloney WC: Lymphosarcoma of the spleen: Results of diagnostic splenectomy in 11 patients. Arch Intern Med 1971; 127:259.

101. Davey FR, Karin AT, Moloney WC: Pathology of splenic lymphoma. Am J Clin Pathol 1973; 59:95.

102. Melo JV, Robinson DS, Gregory C, et al: Splenic B-cell lymphoma with "villous" lymphocytes in the peripheral blood: A disorder distinct from hairy cell leukemia. Leukemia 1987; 1:294.

103. Mulligan SP, Catovsky D: Splenic lymphoma with villous lymphocytes. Leuk Lymphoma 1992; 6:97.

104. Lymphomas of the spleen, in Warnke RA, Weiss LM, Chan JKC, et al (eds): Atlas of Tumor Pathology: Tumors of the Lymph Nodes and Spleen, 3rd series, fascicle 14, p 427. Washington, DC, Armed Forces Institute of Pathology, 1995.

105. Labouyrie E, Marit G, Vial J, et al: Intrasinusoidal bone marrow involvement by splenic lymphoma with villous lymphocytes: A helpful immunohistologic feature. Mod Pathol 1997; 10:1015.

106. Matutes E, Morilla R, Owusu-Ankomah K, et al: The immunophenotype of splenic lymphoma with villous lymphocytes and its relevance to the differential diagnosis with other B-cell disorders. Blood 1994; 83:1558.

107. Dyer MJ, Zani VJ, Lu WZ, et al: BCL2 translocations in leukemias of mature B cells. Blood 1994; 83:3682.

108. Jadayel D, Matutes E, Dyer MJ, et al: Splenic lymphoma with villous lymphocytes: Analysis of BCL-1 rearrangements and expression of the cyclin D1 gene. Blood 1994; 83:3664.

109. Isaacson PG, Matutes E, Burke M, et al: The histopathology of splenic lymphoma with villous lymphocytes. Blood 1994; 84:3828.

110. Schmid C, Kirkham N, Diss T, et al: Splenic marginal zone cell lymphoma. Am J Surg Pathol 1992; 16:455.

111. Oscier DG, Matutes E, Gardiner A: Cytogenetic studies in splenic lymphoma with villous lymphocytes. Br J Haematol 1993; 85:487.

112. Sun T, Susin M, Brody J, et al: Splenic lymphoma with circulating villous lymphocytes: Report of seven cases and review of the literature. Am J Hematol 1994; 45:39.

113. Wade JPA, Wilkins BS, Wright DH: Low-grade B-cell lymphomas of the splenic marginal zone: A clinicopathological and immunohistochemical study of 14 cases. Histopathology 1995; 27:129.

114. Sun T, Dittmar K, Koduru P, et al: Relationship between hairy cell leukemia variant and splenic lymphoma with villous lymphocytes: Presentation of a new concept. Am J Hematol 1996; 51:282.

115. Swerdlow SH, Zukerberg LR, Yang W-I, et al: The morphologic spectrum of non-Hodgkin's lymphomas with BCL1/cyclin D1 gene rearrangements. Am J Surg Pathol 1996; 20:627.

116. Dargent JL, Delville JP, Kornreich A, et al: Morphologic and phenotypic changes of the leukemic cells in a case of marginal zone B-cell lymphoma. Annal Hematol 1997; 74:149.

117. Brynes RK, Almaguer PD, Leathery KE, et al: Numerical cytogenetic abnormalities of chromosomes 3, 7, and 12 in marginal zone B-cell lymphomas. Mod Pathol 1996; 9:995.

117a. Piris MA, Mollejo M, Campo E, et al: A marginal zone pattern may be found in different varieties of non-Hodgkin's lymphoma: The morphology and immunohistology of splenic involvement by B-cell lymphomas simulating splenic marginal zone lymphoma. Histopathol 1998; 33:230.

118. Bates I, Bedu-Addo G, Rutherford TR, et al: Circulating villous lymphocytes: A link between hyperreactive malarial splenomegaly and splenic lymphoma. Trans R Soc Trop Med Hyg 1997; 91:171.

119. Bates I, Bedu-Ado G: Chronic malaria and splenic lymphoma: Clues to understanding lymphoma evolution. Leukemia 1997; 11:2162.

120. de Figueiredo M, Lima M, Macedo G, et al: Association of splenic lymphoma with villous lymphocytes and primary biliary cirrhosis in a man. Sangre 1996: 41:262.

121. Murakami H, Irisawa H, Saitoh T, et al: Immunological abnormalities in splenic marginal zone cell lymphoma. Am J Hematol 1997; 56:173.

122. Vasef MA, Medeiros LJ, Koo C, et al: Cyclin D1 immunohistochemical staining is useful in distinguishing mantle cell lymphoma from other low-grade B-cell neoplasms in bone marrow. Am J Clin Pathol 1997; 108:302.

123. Wu CD, Jackson CL, Medeiros LJ: Splenic marginal zone cell lymphoma: An immunophenotypic and molecular study of five cases. Am J Clin Pathol 1996; 105:277.

124. De Oliveira MS, Jaffe ES, Catovsky D: Leukaemic phase of mantle zone (intermediate) lymphoma: Its characterization in 11 cases. J Clin Pathol 1989; 42:962.

125. Criel A, Pittaluga S, Verhoef G, et al: Small B cell NHL and their leukemic counterpart: Differences in subtyping and assessment of leukemic spread. Leukemia 1996; 10:848.

126. Gray D, Kumararatne DS, Lortan J, et al: Relation of intra-splenic migration of marginal zone B cells to antigen localization on follicular dendritic cells. Immunology 1984; 52:659.

127. Hsu SM: Phenotypic expression of B lymphocytes. III. Marginal zone B cells in the spleen are characterized by the expression of Tac and alkaline phosphatase. J Immunol 1985; 135:123.

128. MacLennan ICM, Liu YJ, Oldfield S, et al: The evolution of B-cell clones. Curr Top Microbiol Immunol 1990; 159:37.

129. van Krieken JHJM, von Schilling C, Kluin M, et al: Splenic marginal zone lymphocytes and related cells in the lymph node: A morphologic and immunohistochemical study. Hum Pathol 1989; 20:320.

130. Van den Oord JJ, De Wolf-Peeters C, Desmet VJ: The marginal zone in the human reactive lymph node. Am J Clin Pathol 1986; 86:475.

131. Spencer J, Finn T, Pulford KAF, et al: The human gut contains a novel population of B lymphocytes which resemble marginal zone cells. Clin Exp Immunol 1985; 62:607.

132. Myhre MJ, Isaacson PG: Primary B cell gastric lymphoma: A reassessment of its histogenesis. J Pathol 1987; 152:1.

133. Smith-Ravin J, Spencer J, Beverley PCL, et al: Characterization of two monoclonal antibodies (UCL4D12 and UCL3D3) that discriminate between human mantle zone and marginal zone B cells. Clin Exp Immunol 1990; 82:181.

134. Spencer J, Diss TC, Isaacson PG: A study of the properties of a low-grade mucosal B-cell lymphoma using a monoclonal antibody specific for the tumor immunoglobulin. J Pathol 1990; 160:231.

135. Isaacson PG, Spencer J: The biology of low grade MALT lymphoma. J Clin Pathol 1995; 48:395.

136. Mollejo M, Menarguez J, Lloret E, et al: Splenic marginal zone lymphoma: A distinctive type of low-grade B-cell lymphoma—a clinicopathological study of 13 cases. Am J Surg Pathol 1995; 19:1146.

137. Palutke M, Eisenberg L, Narang S, et al: B lymphocytic lymphoma (large cell) of possible splenic marginal zone origin presenting with prominent splenomegaly and unusual cordal red pulp distribution. Cancer 1988; 62:593.

138. Cousar JB, McKee LC, Greco FA, et al: Report of an unusual B-cell lymphoma, probably arising from the perifollicular cells (marginal zone) of the spleen. Lab Invest 1980; 42; 109A.

139. Sendelbach KM, Pugh WC, Rodriguez J, et al: Splenic marginal zone lymphoma (MGZL): Clinical and pathologic characteristics of 11 cases. Mod Pathol 1994; 7:120A.

140. Rosso R, Neiman RS, Paulli M, et al: Splenic marginal zone cell lymphoma: Report of an indolent variant without massive splenomegaly presumably representing an early phase of the disease. Hum Pathol 1995; 26:39.

141. Dierlamm J, Pittaluga S, Wlodarska I, et al: Marginal zone B-cell lymphomas of different sites share similar cytogenetic and morphologic features. Blood 1996; 87:299.

142. Mollejo M, Lloret E, Menarguez J, et al: Lymph node involvement by splenic marginal zone lymphoma: Morphological and immunohistochemical features. Am J Surg Pathol 1997; 21:772.

143. Dunphy CH, Bee C, McDonald JW, et al: Incidental early detection of a splenic marginal zone lymphoma by polymerase chain reaction analysis of paraffin-embedded tissue. Arch Pathol Lab Med 1998; 122:84.

144. Harris S, Wilkins BS, Jones DB: Splenic marginal zone expansion in B-cell lymphomas of gastrointestinal mucosa-associated lymphoid tissue (MALT) is reactive and does not represent homing of neoplastic lymphocytes. J Pathol 1996; 179:49.

145. Farhi DC, Ashfaq R: Splenic pathology after traumatic injury. Am J Clin Pathol 1996; 105:474.

146. Kroft SH, Singleton TP, Dahiya M, et al: Ruptured spleens with expanded marginal zones do not reveal occult B-cell clones. Mod Pathol 1997; 10:1214.

147. Franco V, Florena AM, Campesi G: Intrasinusoidal bone marrow infiltration: A possible hallmark of splenic lymphoma. Histopathology 1996; 29:571.

148. Lymphomas of the spleen, in Warnke RA, Weiss LM, Chan JKC, et al (eds): Atlas of Tumor Pathology: Tumors of the Lymph Nodes and Spleen, 3rd series, fascicle 14, p 429. Washington, DC, Armed Forces Institute of Pathology, 1995.

149. Farcet JP, Gaulard P, Marolleau JP, et al: Hepato-splenic T-cell lymphoma: Sinusal/sinusoidal localization of malignant cells expressing the T-cell receptor gamma delta. Blood 1990; 75:2213.

150. Cooke CB, Greiner T, Raffeld M, et al: Gamma delta T-cell lymphoma, a distinct clinicopathologic entity. Mod Pathol 1994; 7:106A.

151. Krishnan J, Goodman Z, Frizzera G: Primary hepatic sinusoidal presentation of malignant T-cell lymphoma. Mod Pathol 1992; 5:81A.

152. Sun T, Brody J, Susin M, et al: Extranodal T-cell lymphoma mimicking malignant histiocytosis. Am J Hematol 1990; 35:269.

153. Wong KF, Chan JK, Matutes E, et al: Hepatosplenic gamma delta T-cell lymphoma: A distinctive aggressive lymphoma type. Am J Surg Pathol 1995; 6:718

154. Kadin ME, Kamoun M, Lamberg J: Erythrophago-cytic T-gamma lymphoma: A clinicopathologic entity resembling malignant histiocytosis. N Engl J Med 1981; 304:648.

155. Francois A, Lesesve J-F, Stamatoullas A, et al: Hepatosplenic gamma/delta T-cell lymphoma: A report of two cases in immunocompromised patients, associated with isochromosome 7q. Am J Surg Pathol 1997; 2:781.

156. Bordessoule D, Gaulard P, Mason DY: Preferential localization of human lymphocytes bearing T-cell receptors to the red pulp of the spleen. J Clin Pathol 1990; 43:461.

157. Santini GF, Crovatto M, Modolo ML, et al: Waldenström macroglobulinemia: A role of HCV infection? Blood 1993; 82:2932.

158. Ferri C, Caracciolo F, Zignego AL, et al: Hepatitis C virus infection in patients with non-Hodgkin's lymphoma. Br J Haematol 1994; 88:392.

159. Pozzato G, Mazzaro C, Crovatto M, et al: Low-grade malignant lymphoma, hepatitis C virus infection, and mixed cryoglobulinemia. Blood 1994; 84:3047.

160. Mussini C, Ghini M, Mascia MT, et al: Monoclonal gammopathies and hepatitis C virus infection. Blood 1995; 85:1144.

161. Murakami Y, Hotei H, Tsumura H, et al: A case of primary splenic malignant lymphoma and a review of 98 cases reported in Japan. J Jpn Soc Clin Surg 1988; 49:716.

162. Naschitz JE, Zuckerman E, Elias N, et al: Primary hepatosplenic lymphoma of the B-cell variety in a patient with hepatitis C liver cirrhosis. Am J Gastroenterol 1994; 89:1915.

163. De Vita S, Sansonno D, Dolcetti R, et al: Hepatitis C virus within a malignant lymphoma lesion in the course of type II mixed cryoglobulinemia. Blood 1995; 86:1887.

164. Izumi T, Sasaki R, Miura Y, et al: Primary hepatosplenic lymphoma: Association with hepatitis C virus infection. Blood 1996; 87:5380.

165. Izumi T, Sasaki R, Tsunoda S, et al: B cell malignancy and hepatitis C virus infection. Leukemia 1997; 11:516.

166. Wotherspoon AC, Ortiz-Hidalgo C, Falzon MR, et al: *Helicobacter pylori*-associated gastritis and primary B-cell gastric lymphoma. Lancet 1991; 338:1175.

167. Hussel T, Isaacson PG, Crabtree JE, et al: The response of cells from low-grade B-cell gastric lymphomas of mucosa-associated lymphoid tissue to *Helicobacter pylori*. Lancet 1993; 342:571.

168. Gill PG, Souter RG, Morris PJ: Splenectomy for hypersplenism in malignant lymphomas. Br J Surg 1981; 68:29.

169. Morris PJ: Splenectomy for haematological cytopenias in patients with malignant lymphomas. Lancet 1975; 2:250.

170. O'Brien PH, Hartz WH Jr, Derlacki D, et al: Splenectomy for hypersplenism in malignant lymphoma. Arch Surg 1970; 101:348.

171. Schwartz SI, Bernard RP, Adams JT, et al: Splenectomy for hematologic disorders. Arch Surg 1970; 101:338.

172. Kehoe JE, Daly JM, Straus DJ, et al: Value of splenectomy in non-Hodgkin's lymphoma. Cancer 1985; 55:1256.

173. Adler S, Stutzman L, Sokal JE, et al: Splenectomy for hematologic depression in lymphocytic lymphoma and leukemia. Cancer 1975; 35:521.

174. Nies BA, Creger WP: Tolerance of chemotherapy following splenectomy for leukopenia or thrombocytopenia in patients with malignant lymphomas. Cancer 1967; 20:558.

175. Brodsky J, Abcar A, Styler M: Splenectomy for non-Hodgkin's lymphoma. Am J Clin Oncol 1996; 19:558.

176. Horowitz J, Smith JL, Weber TK, et al: Postoperative complications after splenectomy for hematologic malignancies. Ann Surg 1996; 223:290.

177. Veronesi U, Musumegi R, Pizzetti F, et al: The value of staging laparotomy in non-Hodgkin's lymphomas (with emphasis on the histiocytic type). Cancer 1974; 33:446.

9

PLASMA CELL DYSCRASIAS AND RELATED DISORDERS

The plasma cell dyscrasias or paraproteinemias, are a clinically and morphologically heterogeneous group of systemic disorders of the lymphoid system that are usually associated with monoclonal immunoglobulin production. They are abnormal because the immunoglobulin production occurs in the absence of a definable antigenic stimulation, and because they are not self-limited.[1] Some of the conditions in this group appear morphologically benign, and others show histologic features of malignancy. In contrast to many of the malignant lymphomas and to Hodgkin's disease, the dysproteinemias frequently affect both the red and the white pulp of the spleen, with a predominance of red pulp involvement in many cases.

A common finding in these proliferations is the presence of morphologic evidence of immunoglobulin accumulation, including plasma cells with single (Russell bodies) or multiple cytoplasmic globules (Mott cells); plasmacytoid lymphocytes with intranuclear periodic acid–Schiff (PAS)–positive immunoglobulin inclusions (Dutcher bodies) and, occasionally, amyloid deposition. Mott cells and Russell bodies may be seen in both benign and malignant proliferations, although they are rarely abundant in the latter. Dutcher bodies represent intranuclear invaginations of cytoplasmic immunoglobulin, usually IgM.[2] The PAS positivity is believed to result from the high hexose content of the immunoglobulin, IgM and IgA staining more intensely than IgG. Dutcher bodies may also occasionally occur in benign proliferations.

The plasma cell dyscrasias are characterized by the presence of a monoclonal, or rarely biclonal, paraprotein (M band) in the serum or urine or both. The morphologically benign lesions associated with monoclonal paraproteins include primary amyloidosis and IgG heavy chain disease and some cases of IgM heavy chain disease. The morphologically malignant-appearing lesions include multiple myeloma, Waldenström macroglobulinemia, and plasma cell leukemia. Many types of malignant lymphomas of B-cell origin, particularly small lymphocytic lymphoma/chronic lymphocytic leukemia, may be associated with monoclonal gammopathy[3, 4] and are discussed in Chapter 8. The plasma cell dyscrasias that do not result in morphologic alterations in the spleen, such as solitary plasmacytomas and the so-called "benign monoclonal gammopathies of uncertain significance," are beyond the scope of this book.

PRIMARY AMYLOIDOSIS

We have chosen to include primary amyloidosis in this chapter because many cases of systemic amyloidosis are associated with paraproteinemia and because of our experience that they frequently are associated with monoclonal plasmacytosis in lymphoreticular organs, both when involved and uninvolved by amyloid deposits.[5, 6]

Primary and multiple myeloma-related amyloidosis is commonly associated with monoclonal paraproteins.[7–10] The amyloid fibrils are structurally homologous to portions of the immunoglobulin light chain, most commonly the variable region of the λ light chain known as amyloid/AL protein.[7, 11–13] In contrast, the

137

amyloid fibrils in cases of amyloidosis secondary to chronic inflammatory disorders are related to a nonimmunoglobulin serum protein.[7, 14] Patients with secondary amyloidosis rarely have a circulating paraprotein but may have polyclonal hypergammaglobulinemia and polyclonal plasmacytosis.[5]

Although both types of amyloidosis may involve the spleen, amyloid deposits are more common in the secondary form. They may be subtle and not cause splenic enlargement, or they may produce prominent splenomegaly. Two patterns of amyloid deposition may be seen grossly.[15] That pattern referred to as the "sago spleen" results from nodular deposition of amyloid in the white pulp (Fig. 9–1). In contrast, the "lardaceous" spleen results from amyloid deposition in the sinuses of the red pulp (Fig. 9–2). The spleen in such cases appears homogeneous and waxy (Color Plate 11). Electron microscopic studies have indicated that amyloid in the follicles in the sago type of amyloidosis initially surrounds small nests of cells, forming deposits that eventually fuse to replace the white pulp. In contrast, involvement of the red pulp usually results from amyloid deposition in apposition to the sinus walls and in the walls of small blood vessels. Extensive amyloid deposition in the red pulp may be a cause of functional hyposplenism, and fulminant sepsis caused by *Pneumococcus*, *Pseudomonas*, and *Staphylococcus* has been reported as a complication in such patients with this disease.[16–18] Destruction of the phagocytic potential of the red pulp by the replacement of cordal macrophages by amyloid deposits is thought to be the mechanism by which hyposplenism occurs in these cases. The white pulp in both primary and secondary amyloidosis often contains numerous morphologically normal-appearing plasma cells that are predominantly mature and lymphocytes with plasmacytoid features (Fig. 9–3). In most cases of primary amyloidosis that we have studied, immunohistochemical stains have demonstrated light-chain restriction in these cells, most often of the lambda type.[5]

Special stains such as Congo red or thioflavine T should be used to confirm the presence of amyloid. Immunohistochemical methods that use antibodies against different types of amyloid-related proteins (AL, AA, prealbumin, beta$_2$-microglobulin) are helpful in distinguishing primary, secondary, senile, familial, and dialysis-associated amyloidosis.[19–21]

Although splenic amyloidosis is almost always seen in patients with systemic disease, Chen and associates[22] reported a case of an isolated amyloid tumor of the spleen in a patient with a history of a malignant lymphoma of the palate.

HEAVY CHAIN DISEASES

Splenic involvement may be a feature of both γ and μ heavy chain disease. Patients with these disorders usually have a serum

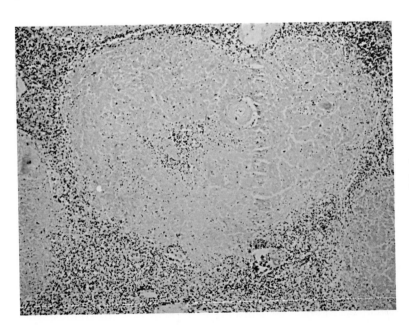

Figure 9–1. Splenic amyloidosis. This "sago spleen" is the result of nodular deposits of amyloid in the white pulp.

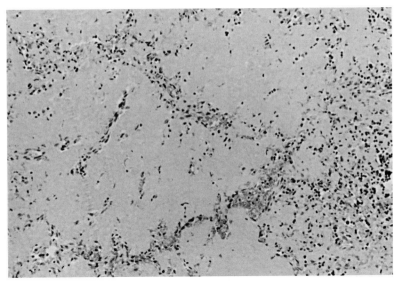

Figure 9–2. Splenic amyloidosis, "lardaceous" type. The amyloid deposition is in the red pulp, obscuring the normal cordal-sinusoidal relationship.

paraprotein, which consists of an intact but structurally abnormal heavy chain.[23, 24] These abnormal immunoglobulin forms tend to polymerize, producing variably sized immunoglobulin molecules with different net charges.[25–27] This diversity of immunoglobulin molecules may cause difficulties in detecting them by serum protein electrophoresis. Normal or broad bands rather than a characteristic "spike" may be observed. The diagnosis is made by showing that serum protein reacts on immunoelectrophoresis with antisera to heavy chains, but not to light chains.[28] Immunohistochemistry can be used to reveal isolated intracytoplasmic heavy chains without the additional presence of light or other heavy chain staining.

α Heavy chain disease, included in the spectrum of immunoproliferative small intestinal diseases, is limited to the intestine, mesenteric lymph nodes and, less commonly, respiratory tract[29, 30] and is not considered here.

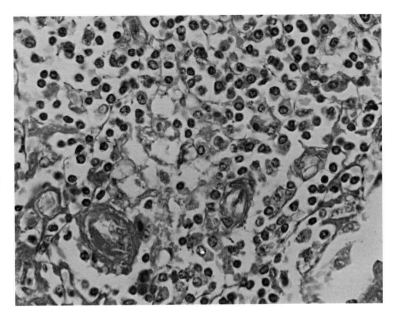

Figure 9–3. Splenic white pulp in primary amyloidosis. Numerous plasma cells and plasmacytoid lymphocytes are present. Immunohistologic stains revealed monoclonal λ light chains in the plasma cells and plasmacytoid lymphocytes.

γ Heavy chain (Franklin) disease has the clinical features of a systemic lymphomalike disorder, including hepatosplenomegaly and generalized lymphadenopathy.[24, 31] Characteristically, Waldeyer ring is involved.[32–40] Fever, Coombs positive hemolytic anemia, sinusitis, and erythema of the uvula and palate are frequent findings.[33, 35] In most cases, involvement is characterized by a diffuse infiltrate of lymphocytes and atypical plasma cells. However, not all cases show similar morphology,[24, 31] and there is no specific pathognomonic histopathology for this disease.[36] Eosinophils are often numerous, and immunoblasts may be seen. It may be difficult to differentiate this disorder histologically from an atypical immune reaction (Fig. 9–4). The infiltrate may be in either the red or white pulp. A similar infiltrate may be found in the bone marrow, although the marrow may show only nonspecific findings such as mild eosinophilia.[33, 34] Plasma cells and plasmacytoid lymphocytes are sometimes seen in the peripheral blood.[34] These cells sometimes herald transformation to plasma cell leukemia.

In contrast to γ heavy chain disease, μ heavy chain disease usually presents as a slowly progressive disorder that clinically and pathologically resembles chronic lymphocytic leukemia.[37–41] Hepatosplenomegaly is common, but peripheral lymphadenopathy is rare. Patients typically have hypogammaglobulinemia. Although μ chains do not occur in the urine,

Bence-Jones light chains, usually consisting of κ light chains, occur in about half the cases. Light chains are still produced in μ heavy chain disease, but they are not readily incorporated into intact immunoglobulins because of heavy chain structural anomalies. Immunoelectrophoresis reveals reactivity to anti-μ in polymers of different sizes. The spleen, bone marrow, and other organs contain an infiltrate of plasma cells that have vacuolated cytoplasm and numerous Russell bodies. In other cases the infiltrate is more polymorphous, including lymphocytes and immunoblasts as well as the typically vacuolated plasma cells that are a useful diagnostic feature.

Occasionally, immunoblastic proliferations in the spleen may be associated with a monoclonal gammopathy. These poorly understood conditions may include immunoblastic proliferations resembling angioimmunoblastic lymphadenopathy. An example we have seen was a spleen that was removed for trauma in an otherwise healthy young male. The white pulp contained numerous plasma cells with Dutcher and Russell bodies and Mott cells. Work-up of the patient revealed a monoclonal paraprotein of the IgA κ type without other evidence of hematologic disease.

MULTIPLE MYELOMA

The spleen is rarely involved in multiple myeloma. When it is, it is most often involved

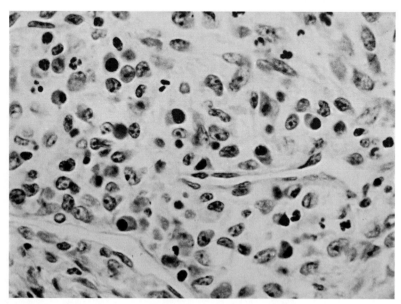

Figure 9–4. Gamma heavy-chain (Franklin) disease. The white pulp contains a proliferation of plasma cells, macrophages, lymphocytes, and eosinophils.

in association with plasma cell leukemia.[42] Clinically significant splenomegaly is uncommon in patients treated with chemotherapy. Kyle,[43] in a review of 869 cases, reported mild splenomegaly in 5 percent. Pasmantier and Azar[44] reported extraosseous involvement at postmortem examination in 70 percent of cases of multiple myeloma. The spleen was the most common site of either gross or microscopic extraosseous involvement in their series, followed by the liver, lymph nodes, and kidneys. Splenomegaly in multiple myeloma may also result from amyloid deposition.[45] In rare cases, light chain deposition only and not amyloid has been described in myeloma patients.[46] This may be accompanied by a foreign body type of giant cell reaction.[46]

Myeloma cells usually infiltrate the splenic red pulp diffusely, but less commonly may form grossly apparent nodules.[45] The white pulp is often obliterated. The structure of the cellular infiltrate is variable. Mature-appearing plasma cells are noted in some cases, whereas the cells in more poorly differentiated cases may appear large lymphoid or blastic (plasmablastic myeloma) (Fig. 9–5). The plasma cell origin of these more immature cells can usually be recognized by the abundant cytoplasm, eccentrically located nuclei, and occasional characteristic bi- or multinucleation. In some cases, in the absence of clinical data, it may be difficult to distinguish blastic myeloma/plasmacytoma from immunoblastic lymphoma of B-cell type. Immunohistochemistry may be helpful by showing cytoplasmic IgM staining as well as cell expression of B-cell

antigens in immunoblastic lymphoma cases. If the tumor cells contain IgG or IgA and do not react with B-cell markers, the most likely diagnosis is myeloma. Pasmantier and Azar[44] found that the degree of differentiation in multiple myeloma correlated with the stage of disease. Poorly differentiated tumors were more commonly associated with higher stages and greater likelihood of extraosseous involvement.

An osteosclerotic variant of myeloma occurs in the POEMS syndrome, which is the acronym for a clinical presentation of sensory **p**olyneuropathy, **o**rganomegaly, **e**ndocrinopathy, the presence of a **m**onoclonal paraprotein, usually of light λ chain type, and hyperpigmentation of the **s**kin.[47–50] The endocrinopathy is variable, including cases of diabetes mellitus, hypothyroidism, hypoadrenalism, and amenorrhea in females and gynecomastia in males.[49–51] Hepatosplenomegaly and lymphadenopathy are common features, in contrast to multiple myeloma, in which organomegaly is usually minimal. Recent evidence has suggested that increased production of interleukin-1 beta in affected lymph nodes of patients with POEMS[52] as well as increased circulating levels of proinflammatory cytokines (IL-beta, IL-6, and tumor necrosis factor-alpha)[53, 54] may mediate the systemic manifestations of the disease. The structure of the spleen in this syndrome has not been characterized.

PLASMA CELL LEUKEMIA

Plasma cell leukemia may arise either as a de novo acute leukemia or as a terminal mani-

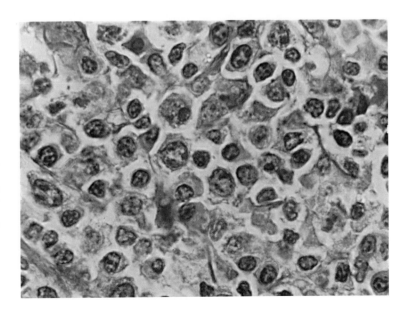

Figure 9–5. Multiple myeloma involving the spleen. In this case, some of the tumor cells appear blastic, with only the eccentric nuclei and prominent cytoplasm revealing a plasma cell origin. In the rare cases in which myeloma involves the spleen and forms tumor nodules with a morphologic picture such as this, it may be impossible to distinguish myeloma from immunoblastic sarcoma on morphologic grounds alone.

festation in the course of established multiple myeloma.[55-58] Occasional circulating immature plasma cells may be seen in 15 to 20 percent of patients with myeloma, and they are rarely abundant. Patients with plasma cell leukemia have more than 20 percent plasma cells in the peripheral blood and an absolute plasma cell count of at least $2.0 \times 10^9/L$. The peripheral blood in the leukemic phase may also show leukoerythroblastosis, reflecting extensive marrow involvement by tumor. The circulating plasma cells often appear immature, with nuclear/cytoplasmic dyssynchrony and prominent nucleoli.[59, 60] Compared with patients who

have the secondary form, those with primary plasma cell leukemia are younger and have a greater incidence of hepatosplenomegaly and lymphadenopathy, a higher platelet count, fewer lytic bone legions, a smaller M-protein component, and a longer survival.[61] The pathologic features of plasma cell leukemia resemble those of acute leukemias, with diffuse organomegaly and less bone disease than multiple myeloma.[62-64] Hepatosplenomegaly is much more common in plasma cell leukemia, particularly in de novo cases, than in multiple myeloma.[55] Splenomegaly is usually mild to moderate and may result in cytopenias second-

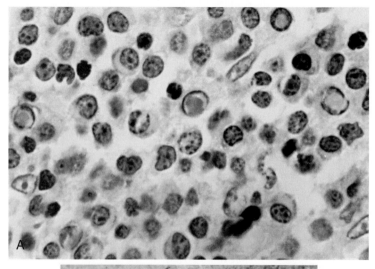

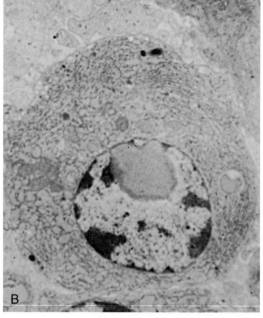

Figure 9–6. (A) Waldenström macroglobulinemia. The infiltrate is composed of lymphocytes, plasma cells, and plasmacytoid lymphocytes. Intranuclear inclusions of immunoglobulin, referred to as Dutcher bodies, may be seen. (B) A plasma cell with a Dutcher body from a case of Waldenström macroglobulinemia. Note that the so-called intranuclear inclusion is, in fact, an invagination of the perinuclear cisterna.

ary to hypersplenism.[58] The pattern of splenic involvement is similar to that of acute leukemias. Splenic rupture has been a reported complication of plasma cell leukemia.[64]

WALDENSTRÖM MACROGLOBULINEMIA

This disorder, first described by Waldenström,[65] is a clinicopathologic syndrome associated with a monoclonal IgM paraprotein, although we have seen rare cases of this syndrome associated with IgG paraprotein. The syndrome includes hepatosplenomegaly and lymphadenopathy, anemia, and often a bleeding diathesis.[66] Occasional cases occur in patients with a presentation similar to chronic lymphocytic leukemia. Although lytic bone lesions are rarely encountered in patients with Waldenström macroglobulinemia, they have been reported in cases with a predominant plasmacytic marrow morphology.[67] The hyperviscosity syndrome, seen in approximately 40 percent of patients with Waldenström macroglobulinemia, results from a clogging of small blood vessels by the high molecular weight IgM, often exceeding 10 g/dL.[68] Splenic involvement may be extensive in Waldenström macroglobulinemia and may sometimes be associated with hypersplenism.[69] The histologic features in spleens of patients with Waldenström macroglobulinemia are consistent with the morphologic appearance of lymphoplasmacytic lymphoma or immunocytoma (Fig. 9–6) (see Chapter 8).

REFERENCES

1. Craig EL, McClure JS, Brunning RD: Blood and bone marrow, in Damjanov I, Linder J (eds): Anderson's Pathology, 10th ed, p 1063. St. Louis, Mosby, 1996.
2. Kim H, Heller P, Rappaport H: Monoclonal gammopathies associated with lymphoproliferative disorders: A morphologic study. Am J Clin Pathol 1973; 59:282.
3. Azar HA, Hill WT, Osserman EF: Malignant lymphoma and lymphatic leukemia associated with myeloma-type serum proteins. Am J Med 1957; 23:239.
4. Michaux JL, Heremans JF: Thirty cases of monoclonal immunoglobulin disorders other than myeloma or macroglobulinemia. Am J Med 1969; 46:562.
5. Wolf BC, Kumar A, Vera JC, et al: Bone marrow morphology and immunology in systemic amyloidosis. Am J Clin Pathol 1986; 86:84.
6. Wu BD, Brady K, Anderson JJ, et al: The predictive value of bone marrow morphology and immunostaining in primary (AL) amyloidosis. Am J Clin Pathol 1991; 96:95.
7. Glenner GG: Amyloid deposits and amyloidosis: The beta-fibrilloses. N Engl J Med 1980; 302:1283.
8. Kyle RA: Amyloidosis: Introduction and overview. J Int Med 1992; 232:507.
9. Kyle RA: Primary systemic amyloidosis. J Int Med 1992; 232:523.
10. Kyle RA, Greipp PR: Amyloidosis (AL): Clinical and laboratory features in 229 cases. Mayo Clin Proc 1983; 58:665.
11. Pruzanski W, Katz A: Clinical and laboratory findings in primary generalized and multiple myeloma-related amyloidosis. Can Med Assoc J 1976; 114:906.
12. Glenner GG, Terry W, Harada M, et al: Amyloid fibril proteins: Proof of homology with immunoglobulin light chains by sequence analyses. Science 1971; 172:1150.
13. Solomon A, Frangione B, Franklin EC: Bence Jones proteins and light chain immunoglobulins: Preferential association of the lambda VI subgroup of human light chains with amyloidosis AL (lambda). J Clin Invest 1982; 70:453.
14. Cohen AS, Rubinow A, Goldberg DL: Amyloidosis. Rhode Island Med J 1976; 59:447.
15. Neiman, RS, Orazi A: Spleen, in Damjanov I, Linder J (eds): Anderson's Pathology, 10th ed, p 1201, St. Louis, Mosby, 1996.
16. Boyko WJ, Pratt R, Wass H: Functional hyposplenism—a diagnostic clue in amyloidosis: Report of six cases. Am J Clin Pathol 1982; 7:745.
17. Gertz MA, Kyle RA, Greipp PR: Hyposplenism in primary systemic amyloidosis, Ann Intern Med 1983; 98:475.
18. Frank JM, Palomino NJ: Primary amyloidosis with diffuse splenic infiltration presenting as fulminant pneumococcal sepsis. Am J Clin Pathol 1987; 87:405.
19. Shirahama T, Cohen AS, Skinner M: Immunohistochemistry of amyloid, in DeLellis RA (ed): Advances in Immunohistochemistry, p 277. New York, Masson Publishing, 1984.
20. Fujihara S, Balow JE, Costa JC, et al: Identification and classification of amyloid in formalin-fixed, paraffin-embedded tissue sections by the unlabeled immunoperoxidase method. Lab Invest 1980; 43:358.
21. Shirahama T, Skinner M, Cohen AS, et al: Histochemical and immunohistochemical characterization of amyloid associated with chronic hemodialysis as B$_2$-microglobulin. Lab Invest 1985; 53:705.
22. Chen KTK, Flam MS, Workman RD: Amyloid tumor of the spleen. Am J Surg Pathol 1987; 11:723.
23. Franklin EC, Lowenstein J, Bigelow B, et al: Heavy chain disease: A new disorder of serum gamma globulins. Am J Med 1964; 37:332.
24. Seligmann M, Mihaesco E, Preud'homme J, et al: Heavy chain diseases: Current findings and concepts. Immun Rev 1979; 48:155.
25. Bakhshi A, Guglielmi P, Coligan JE: A pre-translational defect in a case of human mu heavy chain disease. Mol Immunol 1986; 23:725.
26. Bakhshi A, Guglielmi P, Siebenlist U, et al: A DNA insertion/deletion necessitates an aberrant RNA splice accounting for a mu heavy chain disease protein. Proc Natl Acad Sci U S A 1986; 83:2689.
27. Levo Y, Recht B, Michaelsen T, et al: The interaction of immunoglobulin heavy and light chains in the absence of the V$_H$ domain. J Immunol 1977; 119:635.
28. Franklin EC, Lowenstein J, Bigelow B, et al: Heavy chain disease—a new disorder of serum gamma-globulins: Report of the first case. Am J Med 1964; 37:332.

29. Seligmann M: Immunochemical, clinical, and pathological features of alpha-heavy chain disease. Arch Intern Med 1975; 135:78.

30. Galian A, Lecestre MJ, Scotto J, et al: Pathological study of alpha-chain disease, with special emphasis on evolution. Cancer 1977; 39:2981.

31. Fermand JP, Brouet JC, Danon F, et al: Gamma heavy chain "disease"—heterogeneity of the clinicopathologic features: Report of 16 cases and review of the literature. Medicine 1989; 68:321.

32. Frangione B, Franklin EC: Heavy chain diseases: Clinical features and molecular significance of the disordered immunoglobulin structure. Semin Hematol 1973; 10:53.

33. Kyle RA, Greipp PR, Banks PM: The diverse picture of gamma heavy-chain diseases: Report of seven cases and review of the literature. Mayo Clin Proc 1981; 56:439.

34. Osserman EF, Takatsuki K: Clinical and immunochemical studies of four cases of heavy (H gamma 2) chain disease. Am J Med 1964; 37:351.

35. Seligmann M, Mihaesco E, Preud'homme JL, et al: Heavy chain disease: Current findings and concepts. Immunol Rev 1979; 48:145.

36. Li CY: The histopathology of heavy chain disease. Am J Clin Pathol 1982; 78:427.

37. Bonhomme J, Seligmann M, Mihaesco C, et al: Mu chain disease in an African patient. Blood 1974; 43:485.

38. Forte FA, Prelli F, Yount WJ, et al: Heavy chain disease of the mu (gamma M) type: Report of the first case. Blood 1970; 36:137.

39. Franklin EC: Mu chain disease. Arch Intern Med 1975; 135:71.

40. Johnsson V, Videbaek A, Axelsen NH, et al: Mu chain disease in a case of chronic lymphocytic leukaemia and malignant histiocytoma. I. Clinical aspects. Scand J Haematol 1976; 16:209.

41. Kyle RA, Greipp PR: Heavy chain diseases. III. Myeloma and related disorders, in Wiernik PH, Canellos GP, Kyle RA, et al (eds): Neoplastic Diseases of the Blood, 2nd ed, p 153. New York, Churchill Livingstone, 1991.

42. Azar HA: Plasma cell myelomatosis and other monoclonal gammopathies. Pathol Ann 1971; 7:1.

43. Kyle RA: Multiple myeloma: Review of 869 cases. Mayo Clin Proc 1975; 50:29.

44. Pasmantier MW, Azar HA: Extraskeletal spread in multiple plasma cell myeloma: A review of 57 autopsied cases. Cancer 1969; 23:167.

45. Rappaport H: Tumors of the hematopoietic system, in Atlas of Tumor Pathology, section 3, fascicle 8, p 207. Washington DC, Armed Forces Institute of Pathology, 1966.

46. Kirkpatrick CJ, Curry A, Galle J, et al: Systemic kappa light chain deposition and amyloidosis in multiple myeloma: Novel morphologic observations. Histopathology 1986; 10:1065.

47. Bardwick PA, Zvaifler NG, Gill GN, et al: Plasma cell dyscrasia with polyneuropathy, organomegaly, endocrinopathy, M protein, and skin changes: The POEMS syndrome. Medicine 1980; 59:311.

48. Kobayashi H, Ii K, Sano T, et al: Plasma-cell dyscrasia with polyneuropathy and endocrine disorders associated with dysfunction of salivary glands. Am J Surg Pathol 1985; 9:759.

49. Takatsuki K, Sanada I: Plasma cell dyscrasia with polyneuropathy and endocrine disorders (clinical aspects). Pathol Clin Med 1983; 12:1663.

50. Takatsuki K, Yodoi J, Uchiyama T, et al: Plasma cell dyscrasia with polyneuropathy and endocrine disorders: Review of 36 cases. Neurol Med 1977; 7:483.

51. Yodoi J, Takatsuki K, Wakisaka K: Association of atypical myeloma, polyneuropathy, pigmentation, and gynecomastia. A possible new syndrome. Acta Haematol Jpn 1973; 36:363.

52. Gherardi RK, Belec L, Fromont G, et al: Elevated levels of interleukin-1 beta (IL-1 beta) and IL-6 in serum and increased production of IL-1 beta mRNA in lymph nodes of patients with polyneuropathy, organomegaly, endocrinopathy, M protein, and skin changes (POEMS) syndrome. Blood 1994; 83:2587.

53. Rose C, Zandecki M, Copin MC, et al: POEMS syndrome: Report on six patients with unusual clinical signs, elevated levels of cytokines, macrophage involvement and chromosomal aberrations of bone marrow plasma cells. Leukemia 1997; 11:1318.

54. Gherardi RK, Belec L, Soubrier M, et al: Overproduction of proinflammatory cytokines imbalanced by their antagonists in POEMS syndrome. Blood 1996; 84:1458.

55. Kyle RA, Maldonado JE, Bayrd ED: Plasma cell leukemia: Report on 17 cases. Arch Intern Med 1974; 133:813.

56. Pedraza MA: Plasma-cell leukemia with unusual immunoglobulin abnormalities. Am J Clin Pathol 1975; 64:410.

57. Pruzanski W, Platts ME, Ogrylzo MA: Leukemic form of immunocyte dyscrasia (plasma cell leukemia). Am J Med 1969; 47:60.

58. Shaw MT, Twele TW, Nordquist RE: Plasma cell leukemia: Detailed studies and response to therapy. Cancer 1974; 33:619.

59. Woodruff RK, Malpas JS, Paxton AM, et al: Plasma cell leukemia (PCL): A report on 15 patients. Blood 1978; 52:839.

60. Andaloro VA, Babott D: Testicular involvement in plasma cell leukemia. Urology 1974; 3:636.

61. Noel P, Kyle RA: Plasma cell leukemia: An evaluation of response to therapy. Am J Med 1987; 83:1062.

62. Polliack A, Rachmilewitz D, Zlotnick A: Plasma cell leukemia. Arch Intern Med 1974; 34:131.

63. Thorling EB: Leukaemic myelomatosis (plasma cell leukaemia). Acta Haematol 1962; 28:222.

64. Stephens PJT, Hudson P: Spontaneous rupture of the spleen in plasma cell leukemia. Can Med Assoc J 1969; 100:31.

65. Waldenström J: Incipient myelomatosis or "essential" hyperglobulinemia with fibrinogenopenia: A new syndrome? Acta Med Scand 1944; 117:216.

66. MacKenzie MR, Fudenberg HH: Macroglobulinemia: An analysis of forty patients. Blood 1972; 39:874.

67. Berman HH. Waldenström's macroglobulinemia with lytic osseous lesions and plasma-cell morphology: Report of a case. Am J Clin Pathol 1975; 63:397.

68. McGrath MA, Penny R: Paraproteinemia: Blood hyperviscosity and clinical manifestations. J Clin Invest 1976; 58:1155.

69. Cohen RJ, Bohannon RA, Wallerstein RO: Waldenström's macroglobulinemia: A study of ten cases. Am J Med 1966; 41:274.

III

Disorders of the Red Pulp

10

NON-NEOPLASTIC DISORDERS OF ERYTHROCYTES, GRANULOCYTES, AND PLATELETS

The structure of the splenic red pulp provides a unique mechanism for monitoring the structural and functional status of the cellular elements of the blood. Circulating hematopoietic cells are continuously percolating through the cords of Billroth, where they are subject to constant scrutiny. These cells are preferentially sequestered in the cords of Billroth when they lack the plasticity necessary to traverse the walls of the splenic sinuses. The lack of plasticity may result from structural abnormalities of the cells themselves, from the attachment of antibodies to the cell surfaces, or from intracellular inclusions. The abnormal cells are removed from the blood by the spleen as part of its normal filtration function. Their entrapment in the cords of Billroth exposes them to an acidotic, hypoxic environment, facilitating cell lysis as well as phagocytosis by cordal macrophages.

Abnormal erythrocytes are sequestered in the spleen in a variety of congenital and acquired conditions. Three types of congenital disorders are associated with decreased erythrocyte deformability: (1) disorders of the red cell membrane, (2) hemoglobinopathies, and (3) erythrocyte enzyme deficiencies. The acquired disorders include a variety of hemolytic anemias and certain protozoal infections.

CONGENITAL DISORDERS OF ERYTHROCYTES

Disorders of the Erythrocyte Cell Membrane

The biconcave shape of the normal red cell results from a high surface-area-to-volume ratio.[1, 2] Erythrocytes with decreased surface area assume a spherocytic shape and are less deformable, resulting in their being trapped in the splenic cords.[3–9] Aging erythrocytes in normal individuals tend to become smaller, and therefore more spherocytic, resulting in their preferential sequestration in the spleen.[10–12] Spherocytes may also occur in the peripheral blood in a variety of pathologic conditions, both congenital and acquired.[13] In all of these conditions, the erythrocytes have a decreased survival time owing to splenic sequestration. Among the acquired hemolytic anemias, spherocytes may be associated with autoimmune hemolytic anemia, acute hemolytic transfusion reactions, and some Heinz body anemias.[14, 15] They may occasionally be formed as a result of direct physical or chemical injury, as in some patients with massive thermal burns, or due to toxins.[13] In all of these conditions the erythrocytes are either physically

147

damaged or coated with antibody. In cases in which the red cells are damaged, they lose surface membrane material, resulting in progressive spherocytosis. In cases in which red cells are coated with antibody, the antibody is recognized by the Fc receptors on the splenic macrophages, which remove the antibody and portions of the cell membrane as well, also resulting in spherocytosis.[16, 17]

Hereditary spherocytosis (HS) is the prototype of congenital disorders of the erythrocyte cell membrane. This condition is inherited as an autosomal-dominant trait with a variable degree of penetrance.[18] The majority of erythrocytes in the peripheral blood of patients with HS are spherocytic. They are smaller and thicker than normal erythrocytes and lack their central pallor. They have an increased mean corpuscular hemoglobin concentration.[19, 20] The accelerated red cell destruction in HS is now recognized to be a multistep process resulting from a deficiency or dysfunction of one of the proteins of the erythrocyte membrane. The ensuing destabilization of the normal lipid bilayer causes a release of lipids from the membrane,[21, 22] leading to surface-area deficiency and formation of spherocytes. The molecular basis of this membrane protein abnormality is heterogeneous. Based on the findings by polyacrylamide gel electrophoresis, HS can be divided into four principal subtypes: (1) isolated partial deficiency of spectrin, (2) combined partial deficiency of spectrin and ankyrin, (3) partial deficiency of band-3 protein, and (4) deficiency of protein 4.2.[18, 23] It has been postulated that spherocytosis may be the common morphologic result of all these different membrane defects of the red cell, all being associated with an increased permeability to sodium.[8, 24–27] Spherocytes are more susceptible to swelling and lysis in hypotonic solutions in vitro,[4] which forms the basis of the osmotic fragility test, and also have an increased rate of autohemolysis, which may be corrected by incubation with glucose.[21, 28]

Splenomegaly, usually of a moderate degree, is the rule in patients with HS[29, 30] (Color Plate 12). The spleen appears markedly congested, and the white pulp often appears atrophic (Fig. 10–1). The cords are packed with spherocytes,[29–32] and the sinuses appear empty and may be compressed (Fig. 10–2), although electron microscopic studies have shown that the sinuses contain red cell ghosts that have lost hemoglobin (laked cells).[31–33] Cordal macrophages are markedly increased, and the sinus lining cells are hypertrophied.[34] Hemosiderin deposition is usually minimal, except in cases in which transfusions or oral iron are administered.[30] Paradoxically, erythrophagocytosis by cordal macrophages is difficult to demonstrate by light microscopy, either in tissue sections or touch imprints. However, Molnar and Rappaport[33] demonstrated phagocytized red cells in their electron microscopic study of the spleen in HS; and Ferreira et al[31] demonstrated erythrophagocytosis by sinus lining cells as well. In contrast to most other examples of hemolytic conditions, extramedullary erythropoiesis or hematopoiesis is usually not noted.

The majority of patients with HS have a benign course, with hemolysis compensated by erythroid hyperplasia of the bone marrow, although there may be acute aplastic crises, usually associated with infection by parvovirus B19,[21, 35–38] which acts by selectively inhibiting erythropoiesis.[38] There may be a mild to moderate thrombocytopenia.[39] In common with all patients with chronic hemolysis, patients with HS are vulnerable to cholelithiasis composed of stones containing bilirubin.[40] Because the spleen plays a central role in the erythrocyte destruction in this disorder, splenectomy is almost invariably clinically curative, although the inherent membrane abnormality remains.[41–43] Splenectomy is usually performed once the diagnosis is established, although in cases manifested early in life splenectomy may be delayed beyond infancy.[43]

Hereditary elliptocytosis (ovalocytosis) is an uncommon disorder that is usually not associated with clinically significant hemolysis.[43, 44] Most cases are due to mutations of α- or β-spectrin, affecting the self-association of spectrin dimmers into tetrameres.[18] The peripheral blood shows ovalocytic and spherocytic microcytes that have an increased osmotic and mechanical fragility.[45] Occasionally, patients may have significant hemolysis with splenomegaly and pigmented gallstones, both of which are alleviated by splenectomy.[46–51] The pathologic features in the spleen are essentially the same as those in HS.

Hemoglobinopathies

The most common of the hemoglobinopathies is sickle cell disease, an inherited multisystem disorder characterized by the substitution of valine for glutamic acid at the sixth position of the hemoglobin β chain, producing hemo-

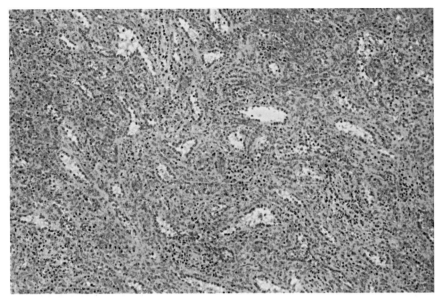

Figure 10–1. Hereditary spherocytosis. The cords are packed with erythrocytes, compressing the white pulp and producing atrophy of the lymphoid tissue. The sinuses appear relatively empty.

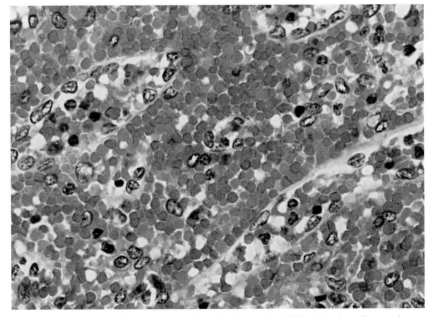

Figure 10–2. Spherocytic erythrocytes accumulate in the cords of Billroth in hereditary spherocytosis.

globin S.[52, 53] Hemoglobin-S molecules undergo polymerization on deoxygenation, resulting in the characteristic sickled shape of the erythrocyte.[54] Sickling is initially a reversible phenomenon, but with repeated episodes, membrane damage results in irreversibly sickled cells.[55–57] Patients homozygous for hemoglobin S are subject to a chronic hemolytic anemia. Occlusion of small blood vessels by sickled cells occurs in sites with reduced oxygen tension, including the spleen and renal medulla, resulting in chronic hypoxic organ damage.[54, 58–62] Sickling may also occur in heterozygous patients with sickle cell/hemoglobin C disease and sickle cell/β-thalassemia, but these diseases tend to be somewhat milder.[52]

Premature destruction of sickled erythrocytes occurs both extravascularly and intravascularly.[63] Extravascular hemolysis results from abnormalities of the sickle cells that permit their recognition by macrophages[64] and from impaired deformability of the cells, which causes their physical entrapment.[65]

The hypoxic environment of the cords of Billroth promotes deoxygenation and resultant sickling of erythrocytes in homozygous sickle cell patients. Sickle cells are rigid, lacking the plasticity to penetrate the splenic sinuses. Splenomegaly is prominent in early childhood, owing to the sequestration of sickled erythrocytes.[29] Although the spleen is enlarged, its function is usually impaired, and Howell-Jolly bodies may occur in the peripheral blood.[66–68] Painful splenic infarcts result from the stasis of sickled cells in small blood vessels. Infants and young children with homozygous sickle cell disease have a 30 percent incidence of sequestration crises due to sudden massive pooling of erythrocytes in the spleen, resulting in rapid enlargement of the organ associated with acute exacerbation of anemia, persistent reticulocytosis, and hypovolemic shock.[69, 70] Because splenic sequestration recurs in 50 percent of cases, splenectomy is recommended after the acute event remits.[71–75] Acute splenic sequestration has also been reported to occur in sickle cell/hemoglobin C disease, in sickle cell thalassemia, and in sickle cell trait associated with hereditary spherocytosis.[76, 77] Splenectomy is therefore indicated in these conditions as well.

Histologic examination of spleens in patients with sickle cell disease shows marked erythrostasis and sickling[69, 70] (Fig. 10–3). The marked stasis of sickled red cells results in localized hypoxia and pressure atrophy of underlying splenic tissue, with resultant focal hemorrhagic necrosis (Figs. 10–4, 10–5). In many cases the red cells seem to be preferentially sequestered in the marginal zone of the white pulp, with resultant atrophy of that region (Fig. 10–6). This phenomenon may play a role in increased susceptibility to infection in patients with sickle cell disease, even in the early splenomegalic phase. Aplastic crises and hemolytic crises, often associated with infec-

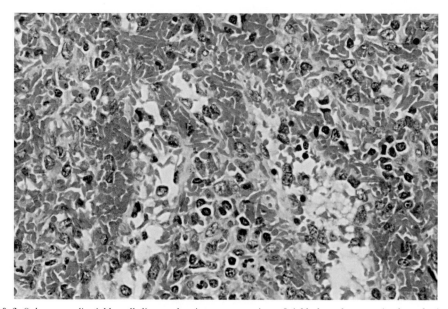

Figure 10–3. Splenomegalic sickle cell disease showing sequestration of sickled erythrocytes in the splenic red pulp.

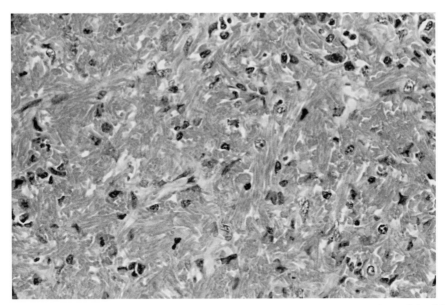

Figure 10–4. Marked stasis of sickled red cells in the red pulp producing pressure atrophy and focal hemorrhagic necrosis.

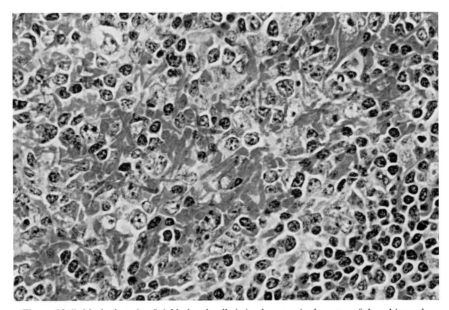

Figure 10–5. Marked stasis of sickled red cells is in the germinal center of the white pulp.

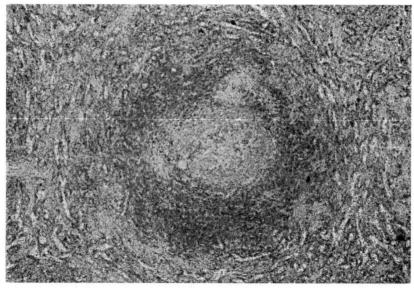

Figure 10–6. Marked sickling with resulting stasis in the marginal zone of the white pulp. Sickling in the early stages of sickle cell disease appears to occur preferentially in this region.

tion, particularly viral infection with parvovirus B19,[38] are other complications.

Splenomegaly is rare in adults with sickle cell disease, owing to progressive atrophy from repeated infarctions resulting in splenic fibrosis. Fibrotic nodules become encrusted with iron and calcium and may contain foreign body giant cells. These nodules are called Gamna-Gandy bodies (Fig. 10–7). In advanced stages the spleen becomes small and fibrotic,

resulting in functional autosplenectomy (Fig. 10–8; see also Color plate 4).[78] However, reversal of the progressive decrease in spleen size and function has been reported following transfusion,[79–81] bone marrow transplantation,[82] and hydroxyurea administration.[83, 84] Patients with sickle cell disease have increased blood viscosity that is thought to result in a shunting of splenic blood flow that decreases splenic filtration. All three therapeutic regi-

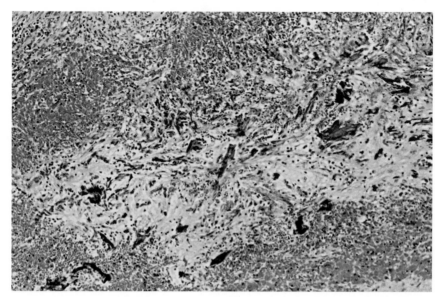

Figure 10–7. A Gamna-Gandy body in the spleen of a patient with long-standing sickle cell disease. Infarcts result in fibrotic nodules, which become encrusted with iron and calcium.

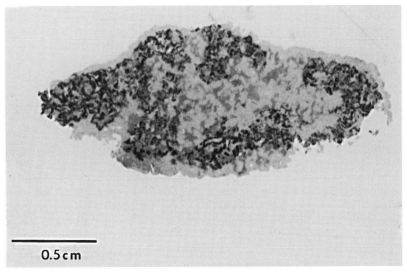

0.5 cm

Figure 10–8. Whole mount of cross section of the entire spleen in a patient with long-standing sickle cell disease. The organ was 3.5 cm in greatest diameter and weighed 11 g. The blackened areas represent deposits of calcium and iron, and the lighter gray areas represent areas of dense fibrosis. The only viable splenic tissue remaining is that of the darker gray areas.

mens just mentioned decrease blood viscosity in patients with sickle cell disease. The first two act by dilution or replacement of sickle cells. Hydroxyurea also functions to prevent sickling by increasing hemoglobin F synthesis.[84–86] This effect is potentiated by the additional administration of recombinant human erythropoietin.[87] The increase in both splenic size and function in the patients treated with these regimens may also be associated with nodular regeneration of splenic tissue in a manner analogous to the growth of splenotic implants.[81]

In some of the other diseases associated with sickling, such as sickle cell/hemoglobin C disease and sickle cell/thalassemia, splenomegaly may persist into adult life.[52, 88] Splenic infarction and other thromboembolic complications have been reported..[88–90] Splenomegaly is also common in homozygous hemoglobin C disease, in which erythrocytes are more rigid than normal and are fragmented in the circulation, producing microspherocytes.[52, 91–93]

The hemoglobinopathies associated with unstable hemoglobins result from the production of structurally abnormal globin chains. There are many examples of unstable hemoglobins, with a broad spectrum of clinical severity. Almost all are associated with splenomegaly, which is the result of increased sequestration of red cells in the red pulp. The unstable hemoglobins denature and precipitate as

Heinz bodies.[94, 95] These rigid inclusions are pitted out of the erythrocyte by the normal spleen and rarely occur in the peripheral blood unless the patient has been splenectomized.[94] However, episodes of infection and treatment with oxidant drugs may precipitate hemolytic crises.[96] Because of the pitting of portions of the erythrocyte, the surface area decreases, producing more spherocytic erythrocytes that are sequestered in the spleen, resulting in splenomegaly. Splenectomy has been useful in some patients with splenomegaly and severe hemolysis in these conditions.[97]

The thalassemia syndromes are a heterogenous group of disorders characterized by the diminished production of structurally normal globin chains, resulting in an excess of one type of chain.[98–100] β-Thalassemia is characterized by deficient synthesis of the β chain, whereas α-thalassemia results from deficient synthesis of the α chain. The excess chains precipitate to form inclusion bodies.[101] However, some rare forms of thalassemia are characterized by the production of structurally abnormal globin chains in reduced amounts. These thalassemic hemoglobinopathies share features of both thalassemia and structural hemoglobinopathies.[102] Two factors contribute to the anemia that may occur in these disorders. Erythroid precursors within the bone marrow may be destroyed before release into the peripheral circulation owing to membrane damage resulting from the precipitated globin chains (intramedullary hemolysis or ineffective erythropoiesis). In addition, erythrocytes containing these Heinz bodies are trapped and destroyed in the spleen. Homozygous β-thalassemia may be associated with mild to marked splenomegaly,[29, 103] which may result in cytopenias if the bone marrow is unable to compensate for the peripheral destruction.[104] Microscopically, the spleen shows prominent red cell sequestration in the red pulp. It has been stated that extramedullary hematopoiesis is common,[29] but in our experience the hematopoiesis is primarily or exclusively erythroid (extramedullary erythropoiesis). Foam cells resembling Gaucher cells have been described in the spleen in thalassemia.[105] Hemosiderosis may be prominent, particularly when many transfusions have been given, and fibrosis may occur in advanced disease.[29] Splenectomy may be indicated if rapidly progressive cytopenias or hypersplenism occurs, although the risk of postsplenectomy infection is enhanced in young children. To minimize this risk, partial splenic embolization has been advocated in thalassemic patients with hypersplenism.[106]

Erythrocyte Enzyme Deficiencies

Splenomegaly may be a feature of a variety of conditions associated with deficiency of an enzyme of either the Embden-Meyerhof glycolytic pathway or of the hexose monophosphate shunt. The most common of the glycolytic enzyme deficiencies is pyruvate kinase deficiency, which is associated with a form of hereditary nonspherocytic hemolytic anemia that is inherited as an autosomal-recessive trait.[107, 108] The enzyme deficiency affects only the erythroid cell line. Patients may have splenomegaly with anemia and jaundice.[107] The peripheral blood shows macrocytosis and reticulocytosis. Splenectomy is indicated to alleviate severe cytopenias.[107] Histologic findings in the spleen are not specific and resemble those of other hemolytic anemias. Hyperplasia of cordal macrophages with variable degrees of erythrophagocytosis and increased amounts of hemosiderin may be observed.[109, 110] Extramedullary hematopoiesis is usually not noted, although isolated normoblasts may occur.[108] Extensive erythrophagocytosis and prominent extramedullary hematopoiesis were recently described by Sandoval et al[111] in a spleen removed from a patient with pyruvate kinase

deficiency anemia who had failed to respond to partial splenectomy. Similar findings are associated with hexokinase deficiency and with deficiencies of other enzymes of the glycolytic pathway.

Glucose-6-phosphate dehydrogenase (G-6-PD) deficiency, an X-linked disorder, is the most common abnormality of the hexose monophosphate shunt.[112, 113] This path of carbohydrate metabolism is important because it results in the production of NADPH, which is needed as a cofactor for the red cell enzyme glutathione reductase to maintain glutathione in the reduced state. Reduced glutathione is necessary for the detoxification of oxidizing agents and for the maintenance of sulfhydryl groups in the cell membrane. G-6-PD deficiency is common in American black people and in Mediterranean populations.[113] Affected persons usually have a mild anemia. However, exposure to oxidizing agents, such as antimalarial drugs and sulfanilamides, causes Heinz body formation, facilitating increased erythrocyte destruction by the spleen, and a severe anemia may result.[103, 114–117] Splenectomy is only rarely helpful.

ACQUIRED DISORDERS OF ERYTHROCYTES

Autoimmune Hemolytic Anemia

Autoimmune hemolytic anemia (AIHA) is a term that refers to a group of disorders in which autoantibodies against antigens on the red blood cell (RBC) membrane cause a shortened RBC life span.[118] The autoantibodies involved in the diseases fall into three categories, each of which has distinct serologic properties: (1) IgG warm antibodies (warm autoimmune hemolytic anemia) bind to erythrocytes at 37° C but fail to agglutinate the cells; (2) cold agglutinins (cold autoimmune hemolytic anemia), almost always IgM type, agglutinate RBCs at cold temperatures; and (3) IgG Donath-Landsteiner antibodies (paroxysmal cold hemoglobinuria) fix to RBC membranes in the cold and activate the hemolytic complement cascade when the cells are warmed to 37° C. AIHA may occur as a primary disorder; may coexist with another disease, such as systemic lupus erythematosus, malignant lymphomas, chronic lymphocytic leukemia, certain nonhematopoietic tumors such as ovarian dermoid cysts and renal cell carcinoma; or may occur as a complication of the ingestion of certain drugs.[118-121] In these types of hemolytic disorders, the antibody acts as an opsonin, facilitating splenic destruction of the antibody-coated red cells.[122] The presence of antibody on the red cell surface may also render the cells less deformable, impeding passage into the splenic sinuses. The spleen is important both in the production of the autoantibody and as the site of erythrocyte destruction. In contrast, cold-acting antibodies, which react with erythrocytes best at 4° C, are usually complete agglutinins, inducing intravascular complement-mediated hemolysis without significant splenic sequestration.[122-124]

Moderate splenomegaly is usually present in patients with AIHA, but weights of more than 1 kg have been reported, even in the absence of coexisting lymphoma.[125] Infarcts are not uncommon. Microscopically, the white pulp in spleens of untreated patients with AIHA shows evidence of an evolving immune reaction, with reactive follicular hyperplasia showing partially or fully formed tripartite germinal centers. The marginal zone may also appear hyperplastic and widely expanded, especially in more chronic cases. However, we have observed that steroid therapy alters the splenic morphology. The white pulp of patients treated with corticosteroids before splenectomy usually does not show germinal center formation and resembles the early activated pattern of reactive lymphoid hyperplasia.[30] The red pulp may re-

veal sequestration of erythrocytes in the cords, and the sinuses may appear empty, resembling hereditary spherocytosis,[29, 30, 31] but usually there is less sequestration and more evidence of erythrophagocytosis by cordal macrophages, which can be demonstrated in touch imprints and in sections in both treated and untreated cases.[30] Hemosiderin deposition may be prominent, and a slight increase in reticulin fibrosis may occur in some cases.[29, 30, 125] Plasmacytosis is usually prominent in the red pulp in treated and untreated patients, and clusters of normoblasts may be frequent (Fig. 10–9). Although the white pulp changes in these disorders typically involve all of the organ to a similar degree, a peculiar type of localized lymphoid hyperplasia simulating malignant lymphoma was observed by Burke and Osborne[126] in a spleen from a patient with AIHA. The spleen was enlarged (268 g) and contained a solitary nodule of 1 cm in diameter. Microscopically, the lesion was characterized by a localized proliferation of lymphocytes, plasma cells, and immunoblasts associated with areas of sclerosis. We also have seen this process in a few cases.

The majority of cases of AIHA, particularly idiopathic and drug-induced cases, undergo spontaneous remission. In some cases, however, anemia may necessitate splenectomy.[127-130] The response to splenectomy is often favorable. Schwartz and coworkers[43] reported an excellent response in three of seven

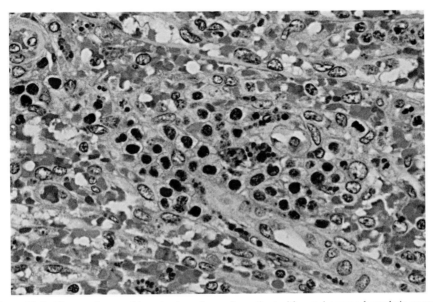

Figure 10–9. Cluster of normoblasts in the spleen of a patient with autoimmune hemolytic anemia.

cases, and Christensen and associates[129] reported significant improvement in five of six cases. Although some patients may achieve a permanent remission, the relapse rate is high, and some patients require continuing steroid therapy.[129, 130]

PROTOZOAL INFECTIONS

Malaria

Splenomegaly is characteristic in patients with malaria (see Chapter 11) and may reach gigantic proportions. It is more pronounced in acute infection with *Plasmodium vivax* than in infection with other malarial species.[131] Erythrocytes containing plasmodia are less pliable than are normal red cells, resulting in trapping of the parasitized cells in the red pulp, where they are phagocytized by cordal macrophages.[132, 133] Ultrastructural studies have demonstrated that parasites may be removed from infected erythrocytes by cordal macrophages by the process of pitting, resulting in an intact red cell that has lost some of its surface membrane. The once parasitized cell becomes more spherocytic and, therefore, more susceptible to destruction by cordal macrophages.[134] It has been shown that increased splenic size in malaria, in common with other disorders associated with splenomegaly, is associated with an enhanced clearance of labeled erythrocytes.[135] Splenectomy has been shown to increase susceptibility to malarial infection in experimental animals, and splenectomy prior to the resolution of an acute attack may result in a fulminant course.[136, 137]

On gross examination, spleens in patients with acute malaria are dark red due to congestion, hyperemia, and deposition of malarial pigment (hemozoin). Microscopically, the spleen shows a proliferation of cordal macrophages and desquamated sinus lining cells containing phagocytized erythrocytes in the splenic sinuses and pulp cords (Fig. 10–10) (see Chapter 11).[133, 138] Parasites may occur also in sinus lining cells. Macrophages and sinus lining cells may also contain hemozoin, imparting a black color to the organ.[29] Clumps of parasites may occlude arterioles, resulting in thrombosis with focal necrosis that can lead to infarction and, occasionally, splenic rupture.[138–142] The spleens in patients with chronic infection are usually markedly enlarged, are gray-black, and may show areas of fibrosis and scarring.[138, 142] Eventually the malarial pigment may disappear, leaving an enlarged fibrotic spleen without evidence of the underlying cause.

Worldwide, malaria is estimated to be the primary cause of spontaneous splenic rupture.[139, 140] There is general agreement that the rate of splenic rupture in induced (e.g., sharing of needles, laboratory accidents) malaria is higher than in naturally occurring infections.[138] Despite often massive splenic size in chronic malaria, spontaneous rupture occurs

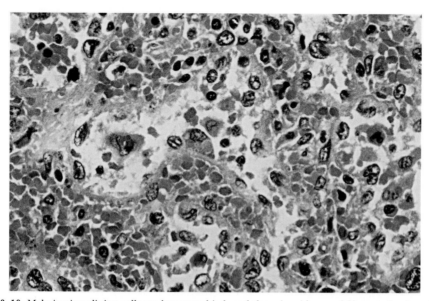

Figure 10–10. Malaria: sinus lining cells are hypertrophied, and there is evidence of fibercytosis of erythrocytes.

almost exclusively during acute infection, usually during the primary attack.[139, 142] This is thought to be a consequence of rapid stretching of the splenic parenchyma and capsule due to rapid splenic enlargement, high incidence of infarctions and hemorrhages, and an increased risk of splenic trauma (e.g., from vomiting). Conversely, the presence of fibrosis and capsular thickening found in chronic malarial spleens is thought to protect the organ from spontaneous rupture.[139] The malarial species most commonly reported in patients with splenic rupture is *P. vivax*,[139, 140] which, as previously mentioned, usually causes a more pronounced degree of splenic enlargement than other types.[132] However, cases of rupture have been observed in association with all plasmodial species.[139]

Immunity to malaria is both humoral and cell-mediated.[143, 144] Gamma/delta T cells,[145–148] a cell subset preferentially localized in the splenic red pulp, have been recently shown to have an important role in clearing parasitized erythrocytes from the blood and suppressing the disease in animal models.[148] By applying a double immunoenzymatic staining technique, Bordessoule et al[145] have demonstrated a greatly increased proportion of gamma/delta T cells within the pulp cords in a spleen obtained from a patient with malaria. It is postulated that the splenic gamma/delta T cell response in collaboration with macrophages and alpha/beta T cells is largely responsible for the self-limited course that occurs in most malaria patients.[144, 147, 148]

Whereas splenic rupture is the most serious splenic complication in malaria, idiopathic tropical splenomegaly (hyperreactive malarial splenomegaly) is a far more common complication in most endemic areas.[139] This splenomegalic syndrome develops when a chronic malarial challenge triggers an abnormal immune response, including decreased suppressor T cells, high titers of total serum IgM and malarial antibodies, and cryoglobulins and immune complexes.[139, 149] The patients show clinical and serologic response to antimalarial treatment. Genetic factors probably play an important role because idiopathic tropical splenomegaly is linked to particular HLA antigens, and cases cluster in families and tribes.[150, 151] Examination of the liver and the spleen in these cases reveals sinusoidal and reticuloendothelial hyperplasia, infiltration of hepatic sinuses by T cells, and intense splenic sequestration and phagocytosis of erythro-

cytes.[138] Prolonged antimalarial treatment results in complete resolution in most cases. Other unusual splenic complications reported in malaria include hypersplenism, torsion of a chronic malarial splenomegalic ectopic spleen, and the formation of splenic pseudocyst.[139] The latter may arise from a traumatic splenic hematoma or hemorrhagic infarct with subsequent encapsulation and cystic degeneration.

Babesiosis

Babesiosis is a tick-borne intraerythrocytic protozoal infection caused by organisms of the genus *Babesia*, which usually affects a variety of wild and domesticated animals. Humans are occasionally affected.[152, 153] The clinical features are an acute febrile illness with myalgia, fatigue, hemolytic anemia, and hemoglobinuria. Splenomegaly may be a feature of the disease. The parasites, which can be seen in Romanovsky-stained blood smears, cause similar physiologic changes in RBCs as do malarial parasites. The result is increased sequestration and destruction of parasitized erythrocytes in the spleen. The infection may be more common and more severe in patients who have undergone splenectomy.[154, 155]

DISORDERS OF PLATELETS

Idiopathic (immune) thrombocytopenic purpura (ITP) is a relatively common disorder in which antibody-coated platelets are sequestered and destroyed in the spleen in a manner analogous to erythrocyte sequestration in AIHA.[156–158] ITP may occur as an acute or chronic disorder.[158–160] The acute form, seen most commonly in children in association with viral infections, is usually self-limited.[159, 161, 162] Chronic ITP may occur as an isolated condition, most commonly in adult women,[163–167] or less frequently in association with other disorders,[168] including chronic lymphocytic leukemia,[168] AIHA ("Evans syndrome"),[169] or autoimmune disorders such as systemic lupus erythematosus,[170] in which it may be the presenting manifestation.[171] The spleen is a major site of production of the autoantibody as well as the site of platelet destruction.[157, 172–181] Platelet phagocytosis is facilitated by the binding of antiplatelet IgG to platelet-associated antigen, with or without complement fixation.[157, 177, 182, 183]

As in other types of autoimmune disorders (e.g., Sjögren syndrome),[184] oligoclonal B-cell proliferations are frequently detected in patients with ITP.[185] The nature of these clonal populations is, however, unknown. Although it might be postulated that these clones produce antiplatelet antibodies, such a direct involvement remains doubtful. It seems more likely that both the presence of B-cell clones and the production of antiplatelet antibodies in ITP may be the result of B-cell dysfunction present in this disorder.[185] A weak association with B-cell lymphomas, however, exists, particularly in patients with chronic ITP.[186, 187]

Therapeutic splenectomy is frequently performed in patients with chronic ITP. The spleen is usually only mildly enlarged and frequently weighs no more than 200 g.[29, 188] The morphologic features of the spleen in untreated ITP display both the evolving immune reaction, reflecting IgG production, and increased platelet destruction.[188–191] The white pulp shows well-developed germinal centers that are accompanied by plasmacytosis in the red pulp and marginal zones.[191] The presence of platelets in varying stages of degeneration imparts a "dirty" appearance to the cords of Billroth, with granular, acidophilic material within cordal macrophages and extracellularly (Fig. 10–11).[172, 180, 192–196] Platelet sequestration and phagocytosis can be more clearly demonstrated using touch imprints (Fig. 10–12) and electron microscopy.[180, 197] Lipid-laden macrophages may be seen in the red pulp,[197–202] sometimes showing the staining characteristics of ceroid (see Chapter 11). The red pulp also contains an increased number of neutrophilic granulocytes[196, 203] and granulocytic precursors.[196, 202, 204] Erythroblasts and megakaryocytes occur less frequently.[204] The presence of concentric periarterial fibrosis, similar to the vascular "onion skinning" that commonly occurs in the spleens of patients with systemic lupus erythematosus, has also been reported.[205] The splenic morphology is altered by steroid therapy, which suppresses the immune response.[192] The white pulp in steroid-treated cases shows little or no immunologic activation or may resemble the early immune reaction, consisting of lymphocytes, immunoblasts, and tingible body macrophages in the white pulp without germinal center formation. Platelet phagocytosis, however, can still be demonstrated, as can foamy macrophages in some cases.[192] It has been postulated that in those cases in which steroid therapy is ineffective, antibody production is curtailed, but platelet phagocytosis persists, necessitating splenectomy.[192]

Immune thrombocytopenia with both increased antiplatelet antibodies and circulating immune complexes may be observed in HIV-

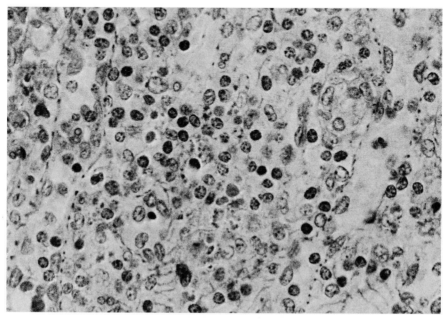

Figure 10–11. Chronic idiopathic thrombocytopenic purpura (ITP). The presence of numerous platelets trapped in the cords of Billroth results in a granular, "dirty" appearance.

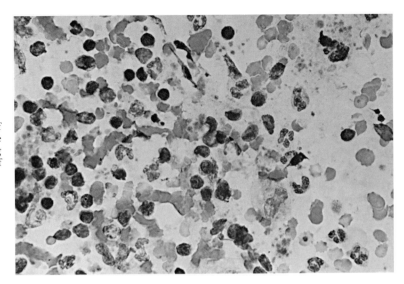

Figure 10–12. Touch imprints of the spleen in ITP reveal large numbers of platelets, both lying free and within the cytoplasm of macrophages.

positive patients, especially in intravenous drug abusers.[206–209] Histologic findings in the spleen in these patients are similar to those of ITP. Marti et al[196] compared several morphometric and morphologic features of the spleen in HIV-positive drug abusers with thrombocytopenia refractory to steroid therapy to those of spleens of ITP patients. Although several similarities were present in the two groups, the spleen from drug-abuser patients showed increased weights, larger lymphoid follicles, and more abundant granulopoietic cells, with fewer macrophages and ceroid histiocytes than spleens from ITP patients.[196]

The course of chronic ITP is often characterized by multiple relapses. JiJi and co-workers[210] reported a 70 percent complete remission rate following splenectomy in a series of 52 patients in whom steroid therapy had failed, and other investigators have reported similar success.[42, 157, 211–215] In the majority of cases the antiplatelet antibody titer level falls following splenectomy. In some cases, however, the antibody persists, and the patient may relapse, suggesting that other lymphoid organs are also involved in the pathogenesis of the disorder.[214] Our morphologic observations provide some support for this suggestion. We have noted that splenic hilar lymph nodes from splenectomized patients with ITP usually demonstrate prominent follicular hyperplasia. Karpatkin and associates[170] reported that patients who failed to respond to splenectomy had a higher antibody titer level, suggesting that the higher level of antibody might result in the more highly sensitized platelets being

destroyed by the liver. Presently, it is impossible to accurately predict the long-term therapeutic effect of splenectomy in a given patient. However, some investigators have suggested a correlation between splenic lymphoid follicle size in the excised spleen and long-term response to splenectomy.[216] Occasionally, accessory splenic tissue, either previously present or accidentally implanted at the time of splenectomy, may assume enough function to cause clinical relapse in ITP.[213, 217] We have had the opportunity to study several spleniculi removed in patients with relapsed ITP after initial splenectomy. In these cases, ceroidlike histiocytes filled with platelets virtually filled the organs.

DISORDERS OF GRANULOCYTES

Selective splenic sequestration of granulocytes is uncommon. The majority of cases occur in patients with chronic rheumatoid arthritis (Felty syndrome).[218–221] Felty syndrome consists of the triad of rheumatoid arthritis, splenomegaly, and neutropenia.[222, 223] The syndrome usually develops in less than 1 percent of patients with rheumatoid arthritis; these patients frequently have a high titer of rheumatoid factor and extra-articular manifestations, including refractory leg ulcers and an increased susceptibility to bacterial infection.[224] Splenomegaly may also result in mild anemia and/or thrombocytopenia and, occasionally, lymphopenia. However, the granulocytopenia is out of proportion to the other cytopenias.

Some patients also have hepatomegaly and lymphadenopathy, which correlate with a more severe degree of neutropenia.

Several mechanisms are known to play a role in the pathogenesis of granulocytopenia in Felty syndrome. Decreased neutrophil production has been reported in some cases.[225] Increased suppressor T-cell activity has also been implicated as a mechanism of the neutropenia.[226, 227] However, in the majority of cases, the granulocytopenia is due to a shift of granulocytes from the circulating to the marginating pool.[225, 228, 229] Previous studies have shown that in Felty syndrome the interaction of immune complexes with granulocytes leads to peripheral sequestration of granulocytes.[230, 231] Van Krieken et al[229] suggested on the basis of detailed morphologic, morphometric, and immunohistologic analysis of spleens from patients with Felty syndrome that the spleen is the principal site of interaction between immune complexes and granulocytes. Because the level of immune complexes is not decreased after splenectomy in patients with Felty syndrome, it is unlikely that the splenic lymphoid tissue plays a significant role in formation of immune complexes.[229] Nonetheless, the fact that the spleen plays a crucial role in the cytopenias observed in Felty syndrome is also suggested by the clinical observation that corticosteroid therapy is rarely effective, but splenectomy often corrects the cytopenias.[232–234] Granulocytes are found in T-cell areas (periarterial lymphoid sheaths), even in patients with severe granulocytopenia. Spleens in Felty syndrome may be markedly enlarged. The red pulp shows expansion of the perifollicular zones as well as sinusoidal dilatation and an increased number of macrophages. The number of red pulp plasma cells is usually not increased, and perivascular fibrosis is absent.[229] The spleens may be markedly enlarged, with morphologic evidence of an evolving immune reaction.[233–234] Splenectomy results in an improvement in the number of granulocytes in 60 to 70 percent of patients.[233, 235, 236] Perhaps paradoxically, a decreased incidence of infection has been reported in 73 percent of patients following splenectomy.[233, 236] Although some investigators recommend splenectomy at the time of diagnosis,[237] surgical intervention is usually reserved for cases with severe neutropenia and infections.[238] Oral methotrexate has also been found to be an effective long-term therapy in selected patients with Felty syndrome.[239]

Selective neutropenia may also occur in association with other disorders, including other forms of arthritis, hemolytic anemia, sarcoidosis, and cirrhosis.[240] Certain drugs may also produce neutropenia.[241, 242] Isolated neutropenia associated with splenomegaly has also been reported in the absence of an underlying disorder.[243] Splenectomy has been occasionally successfully used to increase neutrophil counts in patients with chronic idiopathic neutropenia.[244]

REFERENCES

1. LaCelle PL: Alterations of membrane deformability in hemolytic anemias. Semin Hematol 1970; 7:355.
2. Weed RI: The importance of erythrocyte deformability. Am J Med 1970; 49:147.
3. Crosby WH: The pathogenesis of spherocytes and leptocytes (target cells). Blood 1952; 7:261.
4. Jacob HS: The defective red blood cell in hereditary spherocytosis. Ann Rev Med 1969; 20:41.
5. Jandl JH, Simmons RL, Castle WB: Red cell filtration and the pathogenesis of certain hemolytic anemias. Blood 1961; 18:133.
6. Lux SE, Glader BE: Disorders of the red cell membrane, in Nathan DG, Oski FA (eds): Hematology of Infancy and Childhood, p 456. Philadelphia, WB Saunders, 1981.
7. Mohandas N, Phillips WM, Bessis M: Red blood cell deformability and hemolytic anemias. Semin Hematol 1979; 16:95.
8. Weisman R Jr, Hurley TH, Harris JW, et al: Studies of the function of the spleen in the hemolysis of red cells in hereditary spherocytosis and sickle cell disorders. J Lab Clin Med 1953; 42:965.
9. Young LE, Platzer RF, Ervin DM, et al: Hereditary spherocytosis. II. Observations on the role of the spleen. Blood 1951; 6:1099.
10. Danon D, Marikowsky Y: Determination of density distribution of red cell population. J Lab Clin Med 1964; 64:668.
11. Ganzoni AM, Oakes R, Hellman RS: Red cell aging in vivo. J Clin Invest 1971; 50:1373.
12. Piomelli S, Lurinsky Y, Wasserman LR: The mechanism of red cell aging. I. Relationship between cell age and specific gravity evaluated by ultra configuration in a discontinuous density gradient. J Lab Clin Med 1967; 69:659.
13. Scamurra D, Davey FR: Anemias associated with spherocytic erythrocytes. Lab Med 1985; 16:83.
14. Petz LD, Garraty G: Acquired Immune Hemolytic Anemias. New York, Churchill Livingstone, 1980.
15. Weed RI: Membrane structure and its relation to hemolysis. Clin Haematol 1975; 4:3.
16. Brown DL, Nelson DA: Surface microfragmentation of red cells as a mechanism for complement-mediated immune spherocytosis. Br J Haematol 1973; 24:301.
17. LoBuglio AF, Cotran RS, Jandl JH: Red cells coated with immunoglobulin G₁ binding and sphering by mononuclear cells in man. Science 1967; 158:1582.
18. Palek J, Jarolim P: Red cell membrane disorders, in Hoffman et al: Hematology: Basic Principles and

Practice, p 667. New York, Churchill Livingstone, 1995.

19. Erslev AJ, Atwater J: Effect of mean corpuscular hemoglobin concentration on viscosity. J Lab Clin Med 1963; 62:401.

20. Valentine WN: Hereditary spherocytosis revisited. West J Med 1978; 128:35.

21. Cooper RA, Jandl JH: The selective and conjoint loss of red cell lipids. J Clin Invest 1969; 48:906.

22. Reed CF, Swisher SN: Erythrocyte lipid loss in the pathogenesis of hereditary spherocytosis. J Clin Invest 1966; 45:777.

23. Gallagher PG, Ferriera JD: Molecular basis of erythrocyte membrane disorders. Curr Opin Hematol 1997; 4:128.

24. Bertles JF: Sodium transport across the surface membrane of red blood cells in hereditary spherocytosis. J Clin Invest 1957; 36:816.

25. Jacob HS: Hereditary spherocytosis: A disease of the red cell membrane. Semin Hematol 1965; 2:139.

26. Jacob HS, Jandl JH: Increased cell membrane permeability in the pathogenesis of hereditary spherocytosis. J Clin Invest 1964; 43:1704.

27. Jacob HS, Ruby A, Overland ES, et al: Abnormal membrane protein of red blood cells in hereditary spherocytosis. J Clin Invest 1971; 50:1800.

28. Simon ER: Expanded autohemolysis as an investigative and diagnostic tool in hemolytic disorders. Clin Res 1963; 11:200.

29. Jensen OM, Kristensen J: Red pulp of the spleen in autoimmune haemolytic anaemia and hereditary spherocytosis: Morphometric light and electron microscopy studies. Scand J Haematol 1986; 36:263.

30. Chang C, Li C, Liang Y, et al: Clinical features and splenic pathologic changes in patients with autoimmune hemolytic anemia and congenital hemolytic anemia. Mayo Clin Proc 1993; 68:757.

31. Ferreira JA, Feliu E, Rozman C, et al: Morphologic and morphometric light and electron microscopic PIC studies of the spleen in patients with hereditary spherocytosis and autoimmune haemolytic anaemia. Br J Haematol 1989; 72:146.

32. Matsumoto N, Ishihara I, Shibata M, et al: Electron microscopic studies of the spleen and liver in hereditary spherocytosis. Acta Pathol Jpn 1973; 23:507.

33. Molnar Z, Rappaport H: Fine structure of the spleen in hereditary spherocytosis. Blood 1972; 39:81.

34. Rappaport H: The pathologic anatomy of the splenic red pulp, in Lennert K, Harms D (eds): Die Milz, p 24. Berlin, Springer-Verlag, 1970.

35. Kelleher JF, Luban NLC, Mortimer PP, et al: Human serum "parvovirus:" A specific cause of aplastic crisis in children with hereditary spherocytosis. J Pediatr 1983; 102:720.

36. Saarinen UM, Chorba TL, Tattersall P, et al: Human parvovirus B19–induced epidemic acute red cell aplasia in patients with hereditary hemolytic anemia. Blood 1986; 67:1411.

37. Young N: Hematologic and hematopoietic consequences of B19 parvovirus infection. Semin Hematol 1988; 25:159.

38. Mortimer PP, Humphries RK, Moore JG, et al: A human parvovirus-like virus inhibits haematopoietic colony formation in vitro. Nature 1983; 302:426.

39. Krueger HC, Burgert EO: Hereditary spherocytosis in 100 children. Mayo Clin Proc 1966; 41:281.

40. Gairdner D: The association of gallstones with acholuric jaundice in children. Arch Dis Child 1963; 14:109.

41. Chapman RG, McDonald LL: Red cell life-span after splenectomy in hereditary spherocytosis. J Clin Invest 1968; 47:2263.

42. Crosby WH: Splenectomy in hematologic disorders. N Engl J Med 1972; 286:1252.

43. Schwartz SI, Bernard RP, Adams JT, et al: Splenectomy for hematologic disorders. Arch Surg 1970; 101:338.

44. Cooper RA: Hereditary elliptocytosis and related disorders, in Williams WJ, Beutler, E, Erslev AJ, et al (eds): Hematology, 3rd ed, p 553. New York, McGraw-Hill, 1983.

45. Geerdink RA, Helleman PW, Verloop MC: Hereditary elliptocytosis and hyperhaemolysis: A comparative study of six families with 145 patients. Acta Med Scand 1966; 179:715.

46. Cutting HO, McHugh WJ, Conrad FG, et al: Autosomal dominant hemolytic anemia characterized by ovalocytosis: A family study of seven involved members. Am J Med 1965; 39:21.

47. Blackburn EK, Jordan A, Lytle WJ, et al: Hereditary elliptocytic haemolytic anaemia. J Clin Pathol 1958; 11:316.

48. Lipton EL: Elliptocytosis with hemolytic anemia: The effect of splenectomy. Pediatrics 1955; 15:67.

49. Lux SE, Wolfe LC: Inherited disorders of the red cell membrane skeleton. Pediatr Clin North Am 1980; 27:436.

50. Wilson HE, Long MH: Hereditary ovalocytosis (elliptocytosis) with hypersplenism. Arch Intern Med 1955; 95:438.

51. Wilson HE: Long MH: Ovalocytosis with hypersplenism: Report of two cases and observations on the pathogenesis of the hypersplenism. Am J Med 1953; 14:534.

52. Beutler E: The sickle cell diseases and related disorders, in Williams WJ, Beutler E, Erslev AJ, et al (eds): Hematology, 3rd ed, p 583. New York, McGraw-Hill, 1983.

53. Ingram VM: Gene mutations in human hemoglobin: The chemical difference between normal and sickle cell hemoglobin. Nature 1957; 180:326.

54. Dean J, Schechter AN: Sickle-cell anemia: Molecular and cellular bases of therapeutic approaches. N Engl J Med 1978; 299:752.

55. Bertles JF, Milner PFA: Irreversibly sickled erythrocytes: A consequence of the heterogeneous distribution of hemoglobin types in sickle-cell anemia. J Clin Invest 1968; 47:1731.

56. Eaton JW, Hebbel RP: Pathogenesis of sickle cell disease. Pathobiol Ann 1981; 11:31.

57. McCurdy PR, Sherman AS: Irreversibly sickled cells and red cell survival in sickle cell anemia: A study with both DF^{32}P and ^{51}Cr. Am J Med 1978; 64:253.

58. Diggs LW: Sickle cell crises. Am J Clin Pathol 1965; 44:1.

59. Dintenfass L: Rheology of packed red blood cells containing hemoglobin A-A, S-A, S-S. J Lab Clin Med 1964; 64:594.

60. Finch CA: Pathophysiologic aspects of sickle cell anemia. Am J Med 1972; 53:1.

61. Jensen M, Shoket SB, Nathan DG: The role of red cell energy metabolism in the generation of irreversibly sickled cells in vitro. Blood 1973; 42:835.

62. Walters JH: Vascular occlusion in sickle-cell disease. Proc R Soc Med 1958; 51:646.

63. Crosby WH: The metabolism of hemoglobin and bile pigment in hemolytic disease. Am J Med 1995; 18:112.

64. Hebbel RP, Miller WJ: Phagocytosis of sickle erythrocytes: Immunologic oxidative determinants of hemolytic anemia. Blood 1984; 64:733.

65. Kaul DK, Fabry ME, Nagel RL: Vaso-occlusion by sickle cells: Evidence for selective trapping of dense cells. Blood 1986; 68:1162.

66. Pearson HA, McIntosh S, Ritchey AK, et al: Developmental aspects of splenic function in sickle cell diseases. Blood 1979; 53:358.

67. Pearson HA, Spencer RP, Cornelius EA: Functional asplenia in sickle-cell anemia. N Engl J Med 1969; 281:923.

68. Schwartz AD: The splenic platelet reservoir in sickle cell anemia. Blood 1972; 40:678.

69. Yang YM, Donnell C, Wilborn W, et al: Splenic sequestration associated with sickle cell trait and hereditary spherocytosis. Am J Hematol 1992; 40:110.

70. Pekrun A, Linne S, Schroter W: Fatal course of a sequestration crisis in hemoglobin SC disease. Monatsschr Kinderheilk 1993; 141:573.

71. Egdahl RH, Marin WW, Hilkovitz G: Splenectomy for hypersplenism in sickle cell anemia. JAMA 1963; 186:745.

72. Jenkins ME, Scott RB, Baird RL: Studies in sickle cell anemia. XVI. Sudden death during sickle cell anemia crises in young children. J Pediatr 1960; 56:30.

73. Pearson HA, Diamond LK: The critically ill child. XXI. Sickle cell disease. Pediatrics 1971; 48:629.

74. Rossi EC, Westring DW, Santos AS, et al: Splenectomy for hypersplenism in sickle cell anemia. Arch Intern Med 1964; 114:408.

75. Solanki DL, Kletter GG, Castro O: Acute splenic sequestration crises in adults with sickle cell disease. Am J Med 1986; 80:985.

76. Yang YM, Donnell C, Wilborn W, et al: Splenic sequestration associated with sickle cell trait and hereditary spherocytosis. Am J Hematol 1992; 40:110.

77. Seeler RA, Shwiaki MZ: Acute splenic sequestration crises (ASSC) in young children with sickle-cell anemia. Clin Pediatr 1972; 1:701.

78. Diggs LW: Siderofibrosis of the spleen in sickle cell anemia. JAMA 1935; 104:538.

79. Buchanan GR, McKie V, Jackson EA, et al: Splenic phagocytic function in children with sickle cell anemia receiving long-term hypertransfusion. J Pediatr 1989; 115:568.

80. Wethers DL, Grover R: Reversibility of splenic function by transfusion in two young adults with sickle cell anemia. Am J Pediatr Hematol Oncol 1987; 9:209.

81. Pearson HA, Cornelius EA, Schwartz AD, et al: Transfusion-reversible functional asplenia in young children with sickle-cell anemia. N Engl J Med 1970; 83:334.

82. Ferster A, Bryan W, Corazza F, et al: Bone marrow transplantation corrects the splenic reticuloendothelial dysfunction in sickle cell anemia. Blood 1993; 81: 1102.

83. Claster S, Vichinsky E: First report of reversal of organ dysfunction in sickle cell anemia by the use of hydroxyurea: Splenic regeneration. Blood 1996; 88:1951.

84. Charache S, Dover GJ, Moyer MA, et al: Hydroxyurea-induced augmentation of fetal hemoglobin production in patients with sickle cell anemia. Blood 1987; 69:109.

85. Charache S, Dover GJ, Moore RD, et al: Hydroxyurea: Effects on hemoglobin F production in patients with sickle cell anemia. Blood 1992; 79:2555.

86. Goldberg MA, Brugnara C, Dover GJ, et al: Treatment of sickle cell anemia with hydroxyurea and erythropoietin. N Engl J Med 1990; 323:366.

87. Rodgers GP, Dover GJ, Vyesaka N, et al: Augmentation by erythropoietin of the fetal-hemoglobin response to hydroxyuria in sickle cell disease. N Engl J Med 1993; 328:73.

88. Smith EW, Conley CL: Clinical features of the genetic variants of sickle disease. Bull Johns Hopkins Hosp 1954; 94:289.

89. Fishbone G, Nunez D Jr, Leon R, et al: Massive splenic infarction in sickle cell–hemoglobin C disease: Angiographic findings. Am J Roentgenol 1977; 129:927.

90. Geola F, Kukreja SC, Schade SG: Splenic sequestration with sickle cell-C disease. Arch Intern Med 1978; 138:307.

91. Ballas SK, Lewis CN, Noone AM, et al: Clinical, hematological, and biochemical features of Hb SC disease. Am J Hematol 1982; 13:37.

92. Charache S, Conley CL, Waugh DF, et al: Pathogenesis of hemolytic anemia in homozygous hemoglobin-C disease. J Clin Invest 1967; 46:1795.

93. Thomas ED, Motulsky AG, Walters DH: Homozygous hemoglobin C disease. Am J Med 1955; 18:832.

94. Beutler E: Hemoglobinopathies associated with unstable hemoglobin, in Williams WJ, Beutler E, Erslev AJ, et al (eds): Hematology, 3rd ed, p 609. New York, McGraw-Hill, 1983.

95. Rifkind RA: Heinz body anemia: An ultrastructural study. II. Red cell sequestration and destruction. Blood 1965; 26:433.

96. Jandl JH, Engle LK, Allen DW: Oxidative hemolysis and precipitation of hemoglobin. I. Heinz body anemias as an acceleration of aging. J Clin Invest 1960; 39:1818.

97. Vichinsky EP, Lubin BH: Unstable hemoglobins, hemoglobins with altered oxygen affinity, and M-hemoglobins. Pediatr Clin North Am 1980; 27:421.

98. Benz EJ, Forget BG: Pathogenesis of the thalassemia syndromes. Pathobiol Ann 1980; 10:1.

99. Benz EJ, Forget BG: The thalassemia syndromes: Models for molecular analysis of human disease. Ann Rev Med 1982; 33:363.

100. Weatherall DJ, Clegg JB: The Thalassemia Syndromes, 3rd ed. Oxford, Blackwell Scientific, 1981.

101. Fessas P: Inclusions of hemoglobin in erythroblasts and erythrocytes of thalassemia. Blood 1963; 21:21.

102. Adams JG III, Coleman MB: Structural hemoglobin variants that produce the phenotype of thalassemia. Semin Hematol 1990; 27:229.

103. Videbaek AA, Christensen BE, Jonsson V: The Spleen in Health and Disease, p 164. Chicago, Year Book Medical Publishers, 1982.

104. Weatherall DJ: The thalassemias, in Williams WJ, Beutler E, Erslev AJ, et al (eds): Hematology, 3rd ed. p 493. New York, McGraw-Hill, 1983.

105. Sen Gupta PC, Chatterjea JB, Mukherjee AM, et al: Observations on the foam cell in thalassemia. Blood 1960; 16:1039.

106. Stanley P, Shen JC: Partial embolization of the spleen in patients with thalassemia. J Vasc Intervent Radiol 1955; 6:137.

107. Beutler E: Hereditary nonspherocytic hemolytic anemia-pyruvate kinase deficiency and other abnormalities, in Williams WJ, Beutler E, Erslev AJ, et al (eds): Hematology, 3rd ed, p 574. New York, McGraw-Hill, 1983.

108. Miwa S, Kanno H, Fujii H: Concise review: Pyruvate kinase deficiency—historical perspective and recent progress of molecular genetics. Am J Hematol 1993; 42:31.

109. Bowman HS, Oski FA: Splenic macrophage interaction with red cells in pyruvate kinase deficiency and hereditary spherocytosis. Vox Sang 1970; 19:168.

110. Tanaka KR, Paglia DE: Pyruvate kinase deficiency. Sem Hematol 1971; 8:367.

111. Sandoval C, Stringel G, Weisberger J, et al: Failure of partial splenectomy to ameliorate the anemia of pyruvate kinase deficiency. J Ped Surg 1997; 132:641.

112. Beutler E: Glucose-6-phosphate dehydrogenase deficiency, in Stanbury JB, Wyngaarden JB, Fredrickson DS, et al (eds): Metabolic Basis of Inherited Disease, 5th ed, p 1629. New York, McGraw-Hill, 1983.

113. Marks PA, Gross RT: Erythrocyte glucose-6-phosphate dehydrogenase deficiency: Evidence of differences between Negroes and Caucasians with respect to this genetically determined trait. J Clin Invest 1959; 38:2253.

114. Allen DW, Jandl JH: Oxidative hemolysis and precipitation of hemoglobin. II. J Clin Invest 1961; 40:454.

115. Beutler E, Dern RJ, Alving AS: The hemolytic effect of primaquine. VI. An in vitro test for sensitivity of erythrocytes to primaquine. J Lab Clin Med 1955; 45:40.

116. Fertman MH, Fertman MD: Toxic anemias and Heinz bodies. Medicine 1955; 34:131.

117. Harley JD, Mauer AM: Studies on the formation of Heinz bodies. I. Methemoglobin production and oxyhemoglobin destruction. Blood 1960; 16:1722.

118. Axelson JA, LoBuglio AF: Immune hemolytic anemia. Med Clin North Am 1980; 64:597.

119. DeGruchy GC: Drug-Induced Blood Disorders, p 169. Oxford, Blackwell Scientific, 1975.

120. Petz LD: Drug-induced immune hemolytic anemia. Clin Haematol 1980; 9:455.

121. Bowdler AJ: The role of the spleen and splenectomy in autoimmune hemolytic disease. Semin Hematol 1976; 13:335.

122. Abramson N, LoBuglio AF, Jandl JH, et al: The interaction between human monocytes and red cells. J Exp Med 1970; 132:1191.

123. Hughes-Jones NC: Red-cell antigens, antibodies and their interaction. Clin Haematol 1975; 4:29.

124. Matsumoto N, Ishihara T: Electron microscopic studies on the process of intrasplenic hemolysis in autoimmune hemolytic anemia. Jpn J Clin Hematol 1983; 24:1192.

125. Rappaport H, Crosby WH: Auto-immune hemolytic anemia. II. Morphologic observations and clinicopathologic correlations. Am J Pathol 1957; 33:429.

126. Burke JS, Osborne BM: Localized reactive lymphoid hyperplasia of the spleen simulating malignant lymphoma. Am J Surg Pathol 1983; 7:373.

127. Allgood JW, Chaplin H Jr: Idiopathic acquired autoimmune hemolytic anemia: A review of forty-seven cases treated from 1955 through 1965. Am J Med 1967; 43:254.

128. Goldberg A, Hutchinson HE, MacDonald E: Radiochromium in the selection of patients with haemolytic anaemia for splenectomy. Lancet 1966; 1:109.

129. Christensen BE, Hansen LK, Kristensen JK, et al: Splenectomy in haematology: Indications, results and complications in 41 cases. Scand J Haematol 1970; 7:249.

130. Ikkala E, Kivilaakso E, Hästbacka J: Splenectomy in blood diseases: A report of 80 cases. Ann Clin Res 1974; 6:290.

131. Russell PF, West LS, Manwell RD, et al: Practical Malariology, 2nd ed, pp 371–373, 429, 480–485; London, Oxford University Press, 1963.

132. Cranston HA, Boylan CW, Carroll GL, et al: *Plasmodium falciparum* maturation abolishes physiologic red cell deformability. Science 1984; 223:400.

133. Schnitzer B, Sodeman TM, Mead ML, et al: An ultrastructural study of the red pulp of the spleen in malaria. Blood 1973; 41:207.

134. Schnitzer B, Sodeman TM, Mead ML, et al: Pitting function of the spleen in malaria: Ultrastructural observations. Science 1972; 177:175.

135. Looareesuwan S, Ho M, Wattanagoon Y, et al: Dynamic alteration in splenic function during acute falciparum malaria. N Engl J Med 1987; 317:675.

136. Wyler DJ: Splenic functions in malaria. Lymphology 1983; 16:121.

137. Wyler DJ, Oster CN, Quinn TC: The role of the spleen in malaria infections. In UNDP/World Bank/WHO Special Programme for Research and Training in Tropical Diseases—role of the spleen in the immunology of parasitic diseases: Proceedings of the Meeting held in Geneva 12–14 June 1978, p 183. Basel, Schwabe, 1970.

138. Zingman BS, Viner BL: Splenic complications in malaria: Case report and review. Clin Infect Dis 1993; 16:223.

139. Lubitz JM: Pathology of the ruptured spleen in acute vivax malaria. Blood 1949; 4:1168.

140. Schwartz SI: Spleen, in Schwartz SI, Shires GT, Spencer FC, et al (eds): Principles of Surgery, 5th ed, p 1445. New York: McGraw-Hill, 1989.

141. Covell G: Spontaneous rupture of the spleen. Trop Dis Bull 1955; 52:705.

142. Edington GM: Pathology of malaria in West Africa. Br Med J 1967; 1:715.

143. Kabilan L: T-cell immunity in malaria. Indian J Med Res 1997; 106:130.

144. Good MF, Currier J: The importance of T-cell homing and the spleen in reaching a balance between malaria immunity and immunopathology: The molding of immunity by early exposure to cross-reactive organisms. Immunol Cell Biol 1992; 70:405.

145. Bordessoule D, Gaulard P, Mason DY: Preferential localization of human lymphocytes bearing gamma delta T-cell receptors to the red pulp of the spleen. J Clin Pathol 1990; 43:461.

146. Behr C: Immunopathology of malaria: Emergence of a new T-lymphocyte reactivity. C R Seances Soc Biol Fil 1996; 190:357.

147. Rzepczyk CM, Anderson K, Stamatiou S, et al: Gamma delta T cells: Their immunobiology and role in malaria infections. Intern J Parasitol 1997; 27:191.

148. Nakazawa S, Brown AE, Maeno Y, et al: Malaria-induced increase of splenic gamma delta T cells in humans, monkeys, and mice. Exp Parasitol 1994; 79:391.

149. Ackerman L: Hyperreactive malarial syndrome. J Am Board Fam Pract 1996; 9:356.

150. Ziegler JL, Stuiver PC: Tropical splenomegaly syndrome in Rwandan kindred in Uganda. Br Med J 1972; 3:79.

151. Riley EM: The role of MCH- and non-MCH–associated genes in determining the human immune response to malaria antigens. Parasitol 1996; 111:S39.

152. Dammin GJ: Babesiosis, in Weinstein L, Fields B

(eds): Seminars in Infectious Disease, p 169. New York, Stratton Intercontinental Medical Book Corp., 1978.

153. Dammin GJ, Spielman A, Benach JL, et al: The rising incidence of clinical *Babesia microti* infection. Hum Pathol 1981; 12:398.

154. Rosner F, Zarrabi MH, Benach JL, et al: Babesiosis in splenectomized adults: Review of 22 reported cases. Am J Med 1984; 76:696.

155. Ruebush TK, Cassaday PB, Marsh HL, et al: Human babesiosis on Nantucket Island: Clinical features. Ann Intern Med 1977; 86:6.

156. Karpatkin S: Autoimmune thrombocytopenic purpura. Blood 1980; 56:329.

157. Kelton JG, Gibbons S: Autoimmune platelet destruction: Idiopathic thrombocytopenic purpura. Semin Thromb Hemost 1982; 8:83.

158. Bussel J, Cines D: Immune thrombocytopenic purpura, neonatal alloimmune thrombocytopenia, and post-transfusion purpura, in Hoffman R, Benz S Jr, Shattil S, et al (eds): Hematopathology: Basic Principles and Practice, 2nd ed, p 1849. New York, Churchill Livingstone, 1995.

159. Mueller-Eckhardt C: Idiopathic thrombocytopenic purpura (ITP): Clinical and immunologic considerations. Semin Thromb Hemost 1977; 3:125.

160. Hirsh EO, Dameshek W: Idiopathic thrombocytopenia: Review of 89 cases with particular reference to the differentiation and treatment of acute (self-limited) and chronic types. Arch Intern Med 1951; 88:701.

161. Laros RK Jr, Penner JA: "Refractory" thrombocytopenic purpura treated successfully with cyclophosphamide. JAMA 1971; 215:445.

162. Cines DB, Schreiber AD: Immune thrombocytopenia: Use of Coombs antiglobulin test to detect IgG and C₃ on platelets. N Engl J Med 1979; 300:106.

163. Dixon R, Rosse W, Ebbert L: Quantitative determination of antibody in idiopathic thrombocytopenic purpura. N Engl J Med 1975; 292:230.

164. Hymes K, Shulman S, Karpatkin S: A solid-phase radioimmunoassay for bound anti-platelet antibody: Studies on 45 patients with autoimmune platelet disorders. J Lab Clin Med 1979; 94:639.

165. Van Boxtel CJ, Oosterhof F, Engelfriet CP: Immunofluorescence microphotometry for the detection of platelet antibodies. III. Demonstration of autoantibodies against platelets. Scand J Immunol 1975; 4:657.

166. DiFino SM, Lachant NA, Kirshner JJ, et al: Adult idiopathic thrombocytopenic purpura: Clinical findings and response to therapy. Am J Med 1980; 69:430.

167. Doan CA, Bouroncle BA, Wiseman BK: Idiopathic and secondary thrombocytopenic purpura: Clinical study and evaluation of 381 cases over a period of 28 years. Ann Intern Med 1960; 53:861.

168. Ebbe S, Wittels B, Dameshek W: Autoimmune thrombocytopenic purpura ("ITP" type) with chronic lymphocytic leukemia. Blood 1962; 19:23.

169. Evans RS, Takahashi K, Duane RT, et al: Primary thrombocytopenic purpura and acquired hemolytic anemia: Evidence for a common etiology. Arch Intern Med 1951; 87:48.

170. Karpatkin S, Siskind GW: In vitro detection of platelet antibody in patients with idiopathic thrombocytopenic purpura and systemic lupus erythematosus. Blood 1969; 33:795.

171. Karpatkin S, Strick N, Karpatkin M, et al: Cumulative experience in the detection of antiplatelet antibody in 234 patients with idiopathic thrombocytopenic purpura, systemic lupus erythematosus and other clinical disorders. Am J Med 1976; 52:776.

172. Aster RH, Keene WR: Sites of platelet destruction in idiopathic thrombocytopenic purpura. Br J Haematol 1969; 16:61.

173. Gugliotta L, Isacchi G, Guarini A, et al: Chronic idiopathic thrombocytopenic purpura (ITP): Site of platelet sequestration and results of splenectomy—a study of 197 patients. Scand J Haematol 1981; 26:407.

174. Karpatkin S, Strick N, Siskind GW: Detection of splenic anti-platelet antibody synthesis in idiopathic autoimmune thrombocytopenic purpura (ATP). Br J Haematol 1972; 23:167.

175. McMillan R: Chronic idiopathic thrombocytopenic purpura. N Engl J Med 1981; 304:1135.

176. McMillan R, Longmire RL, Tavassoli M, et al: In vitro platelet phagocytosis by splenic leukocytes in idiopathic thrombocytopenic purpura. N Engl J Med 1974; 290:249.

177. McMillan R, Longmire RL, Yelenosky R, et al: Quantitation of platelet binding IgG produced in vitro by spleens from patients with idiopathic thrombocytopenic purpura. N Engl J Med 1974; 291:812.

178. McMillan R, Longmire RL, Yelenosky R, et al: Immunoglobulin synthesis in vitro by splenic tissue in idiopathic thrombocytopenic purpura. N Engl J Med 1972; 286:681.

179. Najean Y, Ardaillou N: The sequestration site of platelets in idiopathic thrombocytopenic purpura: Its correlation with results of splenectomy. Br J Haematol 1971; 21:156.

180. Tavassoli M, McMillan R: Structure of the spleen in idiopathic thrombocytopenic purpura. Am J Clin Pathol 1975; 64:180.

181. Clancy RL, Trent RJ: Current concepts of pathogenesis and management of idiopathic thrombocytopenic purpura. Aust N Z J Med 1977; 7:312.

182. Lightsey AL Jr, McMillan R: The role of the spleen in autoimmune blood disorders. Am J Pediatr Hematol Oncol 1979; 1:331.

183. Moore SB: Immune thrombocytopenias and platelet antibodies. Mayo Clin Proc 1982; 57:778.

184. Fishleder A, Tubbs R, Hesse B, et al: Uniform detection of immunoglobulin-gene rearrangement in benign lymphoepithelial lesions. N Engl J Med 1987; 316:1118.

185. van der Harst D, de Jong D, Limpens J, et al: Clonal B-cell populations in patients with idiopathic thrombocytopenic purpura. Blood 1990; 76:2321.

186. Fink K, Al-Mondhiry H: Idiopathic thrombocytopenic purpura in lymphoma. Cancer 1976; 37:1999.

187. Kaden BR, Rosse WF, Hauch TW: Immune thrombocytopenia in lymphoproliferative diseases. Blood 1979; 53:545.

188. Nickerson DA, Sunderland DA: The histopathology of idiopathic thrombocytopenic purpura hemorrhagica. Am J Pathol 1937; 13:463.

189. Bowman HE, Pettit VD, Caldwell FT, et al: Morphology of the spleen in idiopathic thrombocytopenic purpura. Lab Invest 1955; 4:206.

190. Lasser A: Diffuse histiocytosis of the spleen and idiopathic thrombocytopenic purpura (ITP): Histochemical and ultrastructural studies. Am J Clin Pathol 1983; 80:529.

191. Kristensen J, Jensen OM: Splenic pulp, plasma cells and foamy histiocytes in immune thrombocytopenia:

Combined morphometric immunohistochemical and ultrastructural studies. Scand J Haematol 1985; 34:340.

192. Hassan NMR, Neiman RS: The pathology of the spleen in steroid-treated immune thrombocytopenic purpura. Am J Clin Pathol 1985; 84:433.

193. Luk SC, Musclow E, Simon GT: Platelet phagocytosis in the spleen of patients with idiopathic thrombocytopenic purpura (ITP). Histopathology 1980; 4:127.

194. Rubenstein JH, Sidhu GS, Schonetag R: Ultrastructural diagnosis of histologically atypical idiopathic thrombocytopenic purpura. Ultrastruct Pathol 1981; 2:269.

195. Chang C, Li C, Cha SS: Chronic idiopathic thrombocytopenic purpura: Splenic pathologic features and their clinical correlation. Arch Pathol Lab Med 1993; 117:981.

196. Marti M, Feliu E, Campo E, et al: Comparative study of spleen pathology in drug abusers with thrombocytopenia related to human immunodeficiency virus infection and in patients with idiopathic thrombocytopenic purpura: A morphometric, immunohistochemical, and ultrastructural study. Am J Clin Pathol 1993; 100:633.

197. Cohn J, Tygstrup J: Foamy histiocytosis of the spleen in patients with chronic thrombocytopenia. Scand J Haematol 1976; 16:33.

198. Czernobilsky B, Freedman HH, Frumin AM: Foamy histiocytes in spleens removed for chronic idiopathic thrombocytopenic purpura. Blood 1962; 19:99.

199. Firkin BG, Wright R, Miller S, et al: Splenic macrophages in thrombocytopenia. Blood 1969; 33:240.

200. Landing BH, Strauss L, Crocker AC, et al: Thrombocytopenic purpura with histiocytosis of the spleen. N Engl J Med 1961; 265:572.

201. Saltzstein SL: Phospholipid accumulation in histiocytes of splenic pulp associated with thrombocytopenic purpura. Blood 1961; 18:73.

202. Rywlin AM, Hernandez JA, Chastain DE, et al: Ceroid histiocytosis of spleen and bone marrow in idiopathic thrombocytopenic purpura (ITP): A contribution to the understanding of the sea-blue histiocyte. Blood 1971; 35:587.

203. Jakubovsky J, Zaviacic M, Schnorrer M, et al: The human spleen in idiopathic thrombocytopenic purpura. Bratisl Lek Listy 1994; 95:498.

204. Yam LT, McMillan R, Tavassoli M, et al: Splenic hemopoiesis in idiopathic thrombocytopenic purpura. Am J Clin Pathol 1974; 62:830.

205. Berendt HL, Mant MJ, Jewell LD: Periarterial fibrosis in the spleen in idiopathic thrombocytopenic purpura. Arch Pathol Lab Med 1986; 110:1152.

206. Karpatkin S: Immunologic thrombocytopenic purpura in HIV-seropositive homosexuals, narcotic addicts and hemophiliacs. Semin Hematol 1988; 25:219.

207. Savona S, Nardi M, Lennette E, et al: Thrombocytopenic purpura in narcotic addicts. Ann Intern Med 1985; 102:737.

208. Adams W, Rufo R, Talarico L, et al: Thrombocytopenia and intravenous heroin use. Ann Intern Med 1978; 89:207.

209. Rousselet MC, Andouin J, Le Tourneau A, et al: Idiopathic thrombocytopenic purpura in patients at risk for acquired immunodeficiency syndrome: Histopathologic study, immunohistochemistry, and ultrastructural study on six spleens. Arch Pathol Lab Med 1988; 112:1242.

210. JiJi RM, Firozvi T, Spurling CL: Chronic idiopathic thrombocytopenic purpura: Treatment with steroids and splenectomy. Arch Intern Med 1973; 132:380.

211. Choi SI, McClure PD: Idiopathic thrombocytopenic purpura in childhood. Can Med Assoc J 1967; 97:562.

212. Meyers MC: Results of treatment in 71 patients with idiopathic thrombocytopenic purpura. Am J Med Sci 1961; 242:295.

213. Mazur EM, Field WW, Cahow CE, et al: Idiopathic thrombocytopenic purpura occurring in a subject previously splenectomized for traumatic splenic rupture: Role of splenosis in the pathogenesis of thrombocytopenia. Am J Med 1978; 65:843.

214. Shulman NR, Weinrach RS, Libre EP, et al: The role of the reticuloendothelial system in the pathogenesis of idiopathic thrombocytopenic purpura. Trans Assoc Am Phys 1965; 78:374.

215. Bussel J, Cines D: Immune thrombocytopenic purpura, neonatal alloimmune thrombocytopenia, and post-transfusion purpura, in Hoffman R, et al: Hematology: Basic Principles and Practice, p 1489. New York, Churchill Livingstone, 1995.

216. Arendt T, Nizze H, Konrad H: Prognostic significance of splenic follicle size in splenectomized idiopathic thrombocytopenic purpura patients. Blut 1988; 57:347.

217. Facon T, Caulier MT, Fenaux P, et al: Accessory spleen in recurrent chronic immune thrombocytopenic purpura. Am J Hematol 1992; 41:184.

218. Cryer PE, Kissane JM: Rheumatoid arthritis with Felty's syndrome, hyperviscosity, and immunologic hyperactivity. Am J Med 1981; 70:89.

219. Price TH, Dale DC: The selective neutropenias. Clin Haematol 1978; 7:501.

220. Sienknecht CW, Urowitz MB, Pruzanski W, et al: Felty's syndrome: Clinical and serological analysis of 34 cases. Ann Rheum Dis 1977; 36:500.

221. Spivak JL: Felty's syndrome: An analytical review. Johns Hopkins Med J 1977; 141:156.

222. Barnes CG, Turnbull AL, Vernon-Roberts B: Felty's syndrome: A clinical and pathological survey of 21 patients and their response to treatment. Ann Rheum Dis 1971; 30:359.

223. Louie JS, Pearson CM: Felty's syndrome. Semin Hematol 1971; 8:216.

224. Franklin EC, Kunkel HG, Ward JR: Clinical studies of seven patients with rheumatoid arthritis and uniquely large amounts of rheumatoid factor. Arthritis Rheum 1958; 1:400.

225. Gupta RC, Robinson WAS, Albrecht D: Granulopoietic activity in Felty's syndrome. Ann Rheum Dis 1975; 34:156.

226. Abdou NI, Na Pombejara C, Belentine L, et al: Suppressor cell-mediated neutropenia in Felty's syndrome. J Clin Invest 1978; 61:738.

227. Bagby GC Jr: T lymphocytes involved in inhibition of granulopoiesis in two neutrophilic patients are of the cytotoxic/suppressor (T3+,T8+) subset. J Clin Invest 1981; 68:1597.

228. Vincent PC, Levi JA, MacQueen A: The mechanism of neutropenia in Felty's syndrome. Br J Haematol 1974; 27:463.

229. van Krieken JH, Breedveld FC, te Velde J: The spleen in Felty's syndrome: A histological, morphmetrical, and immunohistochemical study. Eur J Haematol 1988; 40:58.

230. Breedveld FC, Lefeber GJM, de Vries E, et al: Immune complexes and the pathogenesis of neutro-

penia in Felty's syndrome. Ann Rheum Dis 1986; 45:696.

231. Breedveld FC, Lafeber GJM, Doekes G, et al: Felty's syndrome: Autoimmune neutropenia or immune complex–mediated disease? Rheumatol Int 1985; 5:253.

232. Logue G: Felty's syndrome: Granulocyte-bound immunoglobulin G and splenectomy. Ann Intern Med 1976; 85:437.

233. Laszlo J, Jones R, Silberman HR, et al: Splenectomy for Felty's syndrome: Clinicopathologic study of 27 patients. Arch Intern Med 1978; 38:597.

234. Mason DT, Morris JJ: The variable features of Felty's syndrome. Am J Med 1964; 36:463.

235. Goldberg J, Pinals RS: Felty's syndrome. Semin Arthritis Rheum 1980; 10:52.

236. Moore RA, Brunner CM, Sandusky WR, et al: Felty's syndrome: Long-term follow-up after splenectomy. Ann Intern Med 1971; 75:381.

237. Riley SM, Aldrete JS: Role of splenectomy in Felty's syndrome. Am J Surg 1975; 130:51.

238. Crosby WH: What to treat in Felty's syndrome. JAMA 1973; 225:1114.

239. Gerster JC: Long-term effect of methotrexate in Felty's syndrome: A 12-year follow-up. J Rheumatol 1996; 23:200.

240. Welch CS, Dameshek W: Splenectomy in blood dyscrasias. N Engl J Med 1950; 242:601.

241. Pisciotta AV: Drug-induced agranulocytosis. Drugs 1978; 15:132.

242. Weitzmen SA, Stossel TP: Drug-induced immunological neutropenia. Lancet 1978; 1:1068.

243. Kyle RA, Linman JW: Chronic idiopathic neutropenia: A newly recognized entity? N Engl J Med 1968; 279:1015.

244. Dale D, Guerry D, Wewerka J, et al: Chronic neutropenia. Medicine 1979; 58:283.

11

DISORDERS OF THE MONOCYTE-MACROPHAGE SYSTEM

Disorders of the monocyte-macrophage system include a variety of etiologically unrelated conditions that may be either neoplastic or non-neoplastic (Table 11–1). The majority involving the spleen are characterized by a proliferation causing a widening of the cords of Billroth with resultant splenomegaly and hy-

Table 11–1. Disorders of the Monocyte-Macrophage System

I. Proliferations of Cordal Macrophages
  A. Non-neoplastic
    1. Status post blood transfusion
    2. Nonspherocytic hemolytic anemias
    3. Parasitic infections
      a. Malaria
      b. Kala-azar
    4. Storage diseases
      a. Lipidoses
      b. Mucopolysaccharidoses
      c. Glycogenoses
      d. Gangliosidoses
    5. Hemophagocytic syndromes
      a. Familial
      b. Viral (infection)-associated
  B. Neoplastic
    1. Malignant histiocytosis
    2. Malignant histiocytosis/secondary to mediastinal germ cell tumors
    3. True histiocytic lymphoma
II. Proliferations of Langerhans cells
  A. Probably neoplastic (clonal) in most cases
    1. Langerhans cell histiocytosis
    2. "Malignant histiocytosis X"
III. Other Proliferations
  A. Neoplastic
    1. Follicular dendritic cell tumor
    2. Malignant fibrous histiocytoma

persplenism. These disorders are almost always systemic, although splenic involvement may be the predominant manifestation in some cases. Hypersplenism results specifically from the increased number of proliferating cells, which widen the cords of Billroth, and from a variable degree of increased hemophagocytosis. Blood cytopenias may also result from the decreased hematopoiesis caused by proliferation of macrophages in the bone marrow.

NON-NEOPLASTIC PROLIFERATIONS OF SPLENIC MACROPHAGES

The cordal macrophages of the spleen are efficient phagocytic cells that may proliferate in a variety of unrelated conditions that include immune-mediated hemolytic anemias; status post blood transfusion; parasitic infections; hemophagocytic syndromes; and storage diseases. Such conditions as nonspherocytic hemolytic anemias, idiopathic thrombocytopenic purpura, and other disorders associated with abnormalities of the formed elements of the blood are discussed in greater detail in Chapter 10. In many of these conditions, there is morphologic evidence of proliferation of sinus lining cells of the splenic red pulp, which frequently display clear-cut evidence of phagocytosis. As was discussed in Chapter 1, these cells display both vascular endothelial and monocyte-macrophage antigens, so it is not surprising that they may, under certain circumstances, demonstrate a phagocytic function.

Probably the most frequent cause of proliferation of splenic macrophages with evidence of phagocytosis is blood transfusion. The majority of these cases, of course, go undetected; however, in a number of cases, we have had the opportunity to study spleens removed for other reasons from patients after the patients have had multiple blood transfusions. Spleens in these conditions reveal a varying degree of proliferation of cordal macrophages as well as sinus lining cells, with prominent erythrophagocytosis and hemosiderosis, even in cases in which the transfusions were compatible by conventional crossmatching techniques (Fig. 11–1).

PARASITIC INFECTIONS

Although numerous infectious agents may involve the spleen, there are two intracellular parasites in particular that invade the cells of the lymphoreticular system and cause massive splenomegaly by virtue of proliferation of cordal macrophages. These are visceral leishmaniasis and malaria.[1] Visceral leishmaniasis, also known as kala-azar, is caused by the intracellular protozoan *Leishmania donovani*. This infection is endemic in many tropical and subtropical regions of the world. It is characterized by hepatosplenomegaly with pancytopenia, lymphadenopathy, fever, and weight loss. Massive splenomegaly is common and is caused by the ingestion of the parasites by the macrophages of the cords of Billroth (Fig. 11–2).

Plasmacytosis is also frequent, and a polymorphonuclear leukocytic infiltrate may be present as well. There is atrophy of the splenic white pulp because of proliferation of the macrophages, and focal necrosis and fibrosis of the white pulp may occur.[2] Fatal hemorrhage may result from thrombocytopenia and hemorrhagic necrosis of the spleen.

A similar picture is seen in patients with malaria. Splenomegaly is so characteristic in this group of diseases that gross evaluation of splenic involvement by evaluation of clinical splenomegaly has been used for the assessment of the prevalence of malaria in endemic areas; the incidence of splenomegaly has been referred to as the spleen rate. The spleen in malaria is hyperemic, and numerous macrophages occur in the red pulp. The macrophages contain numerous parasites, red blood cells, and a large amount of characteristic pigment referred to as hemozoin. Fibrosis and atrophy of the white pulp is also present, and hemorrhagic infarcts may occur as well as focal areas of extramedullary erythropoiesis.[1, 3]

STORAGE DISEASES

The spleen is involved in many of the lysosomal storage diseases, including the lipidoses, mucopolysaccharidoses, and glycogenoses. However, only those disorders in which splenic involvement is a predominant feature are discussed here in detail.

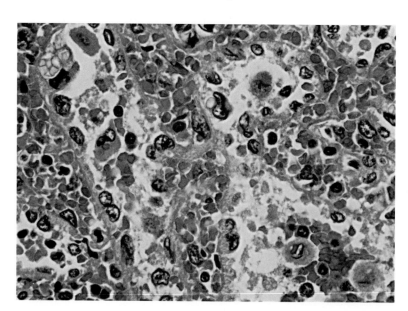

Figure 11–1. Status post blood transfusion. There is a proliferation of cordal macrophages as well as hyperplasia of sinus lining cells with erythrophagocytosis.

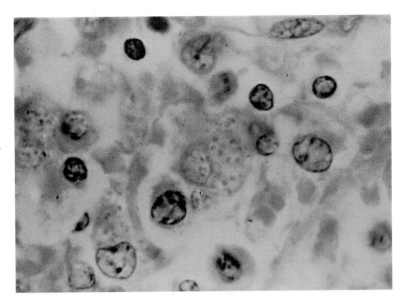

Figure 11–2. Visceral leishmaniasis. The organisms can be seen within cordal macrophages.

Lipidoses

Gaucher Disease

The lipid storage disorders, the majority of which are inherited as autosomal-recessive traits, may result in significant splenomegaly and hypersplenism.[4] Gaucher disease is characterized by the accumulation of glucocerebroside due to the deficiency of the enzyme glucocerebrosidase A.[5-7] The enzyme deficit is caused by mutations at the glucocerebrosidase locus on chromosome 1q21.[8] The disorder has several clinical variants. The adult form of Gaucher disease (type 1) is usually progressive but compatible with long life, in contrast to the acute infantile neuronopathic variety (type 2), which is rapidly fatal.[9] A third type, intermediate in severity, also involves the central nervous system but affects young adults rather than infants. The adult form is usually a chronic disorder limited to the lymphoreticular and skeletal systems, whereas the clinical picture in the infantile form is usually dominated by involvement of the central nervous system. The disease varies in severity. Anemia is almost always present in affected adults and may have multiple causes. The proliferating Gaucher cells in the marrow may result in depressed erythropoiesis; the enlargement of the spleen may produce increased red cell sequestration with resultant shortening of red cell survival; and the marked expansion of the patient's macrophage pool with concomitant shifting of the body's iron stores may cause relative iron deficiency.

Although the spleen is enlarged in all three subtypes of Gaucher disease, neurologic impairment is usually the dominant manifestation of types 2 and 3. Splenomegaly is a presenting feature only in type 1 Gaucher disease, and massively enlarged spleens are recorded. Lymphadenopathy is usually mild. Pancytopenia may be a dominant clinical feature; it may result from both hypersplenism and replacement of normal hematopoietic marrow by proliferating Gaucher cells.[6, 10]

The cut surface of the spleen in Gaucher disease is usually uniformly pale, dry, and firm owing to the diffuse proliferation of histiocytes; however, it may occasionally be mottled because of focal accumulations of these cells (Color Plate 13).[6] Rarely, fibrous scars may result in a truly nodular appearance. Microscopically, the red pulp is expanded because of the accumulation of numerous histiocytes in the cords of Billroth (Fig. 11–3). Characteristic Gaucher cells range in size from 20 to 100 μm in diameter and have fibrillar cytoplasm that appears brownish in hematoxylin-and-eosin and Romanovsky-stained preparations (Fig. 11–4).[11] Multinucleated cells may occur. The cytoplasm is intensely periodic acid–Schiff (PAS)-positive, and the PAS positivity is resistant to diastase digestion.[6] The glucocerebroside in Gaucher cells is autofluorescent. Because Gaucher cells are macrophages and ingest red blood cells, they may frequently stain positively for iron.[12, 13] Lipid stains are only weakly positive. Ultrastructural studies reveal numerous lysosomes containing lipid bi-

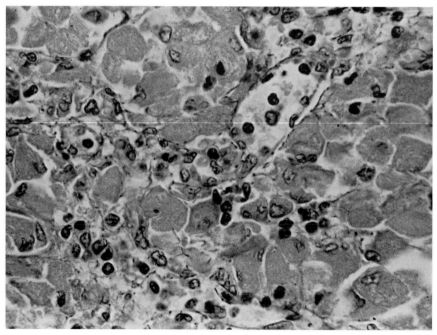

Figure 11–3. Gaucher cells in the red pulp of the spleen. Note that the cells occupy principally the cords, whereas the sinuses and sinus lining cells appear uninvolved. This is because cordal macrophages have a greater ability to ingest lipid than sinus lining cells.

layers 6 nanometers in diameter with a right-handed twist.[6, 14–16] Iron is seen as individual micelles of ferritin, mainly within vacuoles.[17] Extramedullary hematopoiesis often occurs in the spleen and is thought to be caused by the disruption of the marrow architecture by proliferating macrophages.[6] Gaucher cells also occur in other lymphoid organs, the liver, and occasionally the lung and may produce tumorous masses involving the skeletal system.[11]

Although splenectomy has been utilized as a therapeutic measure to combat hyperple-

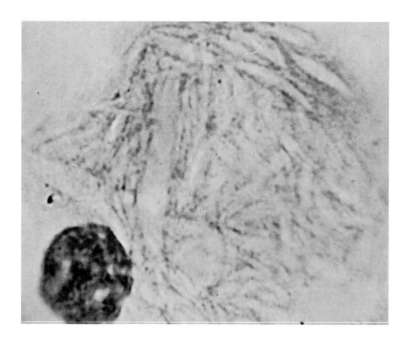

Figure 11–4. Gaucher cells in imprint preparations reveal characteristic fibrillar cytoplasm.

nism in Gaucher disease,[18] it is largely palliative and not without adverse effects. It has been reported to hasten the development of destructive bone changes[19] and also to accelerate central nervous system deterioration.[20] In addition, it places young splenectomized patients in danger of postsplenectomy sepsis. Partial splenectomy[21] and splenic embolization[22] have been attempted to alleviate hypersplenism while preserving splenic function in these patients. However, these techniques have been of questionable added benefit. Bone marrow transplantation, using cells from an HLA-compatible donor, has also been used as a treatment approach.[23] Results have been ameliorated by pretreatment splenectomy.[24] The most recent therapeutic approach to the disease, and the one with the most promise, is the administration to the patient of glucocerebrosidase.[25] However, a suboptimal response to an adequate trial of this enzyme replacement therapy may occur, and splenectomy may then be necessary.[26]

Niemann-Pick Disease

Splenomegaly is a frequent finding in all types of Niemann-Pick disease. Niemann-Pick disease is a group of autosomal-recessive disorders that are clinically, biochemically, and genetically heterogenous.[27, 28] Of the five types (A, B, C, D, E), two (A and B) are the consequence of a deficiency of sphingomyelinase.[29–33] Type C is characterized by accumulation of tissue cholesterol and sphingomyelin.[34–37] Types D and E have been shown to have normal levels of sphingomyelinase. In patients with types D and E, defects in intracellular cholesterol homeostasis have been suggested.[38] The D variant has been reported only in descendants of an Acadian couple who lived in Nova Scotia in the early 18th century.[39] The metabolic abnormalities in all forms of Niemann-Pick disease result in the accumulation of either sphingomyelin or cholesterol in cells of the lymphoreticular and neural system. Type A, the infantile neurologic form, accounts for approximately three quarters of all cases and is usually clinically evident by 6 months of age. Central nervous system involvement is characteristic and is associated with prominent hepatosplenomegaly, mental retardation, generalized lymphadenopathy, and skin xanthomas.[29, 40] Type B has a more variable clinical picture and is characterized by hepatosplenomegaly without neurologic involvement. Other rare variants with late onset and atypical features have also been described.[27, 41, 42] Adults with type B Niemann-Pick disease usually have massive splenomegaly and clinically significant hypersplenism. Type C Niemann-Pick disease affects older individuals. Patients usually have neurologic symptoms and hepatosplenomegaly.[34] Types D and E diseases are clinically similar to one another as both types feature moderate degrees of hepatosplenomegaly. They differ in that neurologic involvement is present only in type D.[38]

Affected spleens are usually pale and homogenous on cut section. The Niemann-Pick cells proliferate in the cords of Billroth (Fig. 11–5). They are large, ranging from 20 to 100 micrometers in diameter, and appear foamy or bubbly owing to numerous small vacuoles (Fig. 11–6). They are clearer than Gaucher cells and usually stain only faintly with the PAS stain but contain neutral fat as demonstrated by Sudan black B and oil red O stains. The lipid deposits are birefringent and, under ultraviolet light, display yellow-green fluorescence. Electron microscopy reveals lamellated structures resembling myelin figures within lysosomes.[42] The membranous cytoplasmic bodies may take the form of parallel lamellae, termed "zebra bodies." Qualitatively different inclusions are found by ultrastructural analysis in type C disease.[43] The lipid-laden macrophages may also occur in other lymphoid organs as well as in the liver, gastrointestinal tract, and lung. Hepatic parenchymal cells may also be affected. Sphingomyelin accumulates in neurons as well as in Schwann cells of the peripheral nerves in the neuronopathic forms.[40] Foam cells resembling sea-blue histiocytes may occur in these organs, particularly in type C Niemann-Pick disease, and it has been postulated that this type of Niemann-Pick disease may be related to the ceroid histiocytoses.[44, 45] Splenectomy is rarely performed in Niemann-Pick disease because death usually occurs from other complications before significant hypersplenism develops.

CEROID HISTIOCYTOSIS

Ceroid, a product of the oxidation and polymerization of unsaturated lipids, may accumulate in the lymphoreticular system either secondarily in a number of seemingly unrelated disorders or primarily in the so-called syndrome of the sea-blue histiocyte.[46, 47] Ceroid

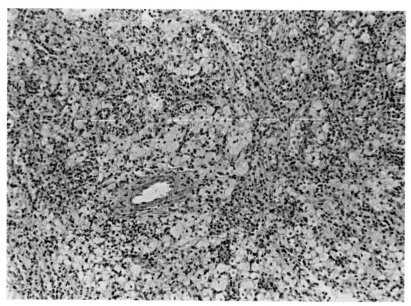

Figure 11–5. Niemann-Pick disease. Foamy cells proliferate within the cords of Billroth.

histiocytosis is characterized by prominent splenomegaly and often hepatomegaly. Lymphadenopathy is usually not prominent.[48] Cytopenias, particularly thrombocytopenia, may be clinically significant, but the course of the disease is usually mild.[47, 49] Occasionally, however, the disorder may lead to cirrhosis and liver failure.[46, 50] Other uncommon manifestations include a white foveal ring in the ocular fundus, abnormal skin pigmentation, central nervous system involvement with mental and motor retardation, and pulmonary involvement.[51] Affected patients often have increased mucopolysaccharides in the urine.[46, 50] The sea-blue histiocyte syndrome may be familial, probably with an autosomal-recessive inheritance pattern.[49]

Ceroid-containing histiocytes may also occur in many tissues as part of the familial Hermansky-Pudlak syndrome, a rare, often fatal, autosomal-recessive disorder caused by mutations at the HPS gene located in chromosome 10q23.[52] The Hermansky-Pudlak syndrome also includes tyrosinase-positive oculocutaneous albinism and platelet defects, consisting of storage-pool deficiency resulting in defective platelet aggregation. CD63, a protein that is present in platelet-dense granules, lysosomes, and melanocytes, was found to be defective in a patient with this syndrome.[53, 54] This disorder is particularly frequent in Puerto Rico and in an isolated village in the Swiss Alps.[54, 56] The melanocytes of affected patients show decreased numbers of melanosomes, which are often incomplete. Occasionally patients have pulmonary fibrosis or Crohn disease.[57, 58]

The spleen in ceroid histiocytosis is usually moderately enlarged and firm. Ceroid-containing histiocytes accumulate in the cords of Billroth and in the splenic sinuses (Fig. 11–7).[51] Ceroid-containing histiocytes measure up to 20 micrometers and contain cytoplasmic granules that measure 3 to 4 micrometers. The histiocytes show a variable degree of granulation (Fig. 11–8). Foamy histiocytes with smaller, darker granules may occur.[49] Ceroid is composed of phospholipids and glycosphingolipids and is similar to lipofuscin in its physical and chemical properties.[59, 60] Histiocytes containing ceroid appear faintly yellow-brown in hematoxylin-and-eosin–stained sections, but blue-green with Romanovsky stains, resulting in the term "sea-blue histiocyte." Ceroid is PAS-positive and resistant to diastase digestion and stains positively with lipid stains. It shows a strong affinity for basic dyes such as fuchsin and methylene blue. Ceroid is acid-fast and becomes autofluorescent with aging of the pigment.[61] Ultrastructural studies reveal inclusions of lamellated membranous material with 4.5 to 5 nanometers periodicity. Extramedullary hematopoiesis may occur in the spleen secondary to bone marrow replacement by ceroid-containing histiocytes. Silverstein and Ellefson[51] also described blood lakes partially lined by histiocytes. These histiocytes occur

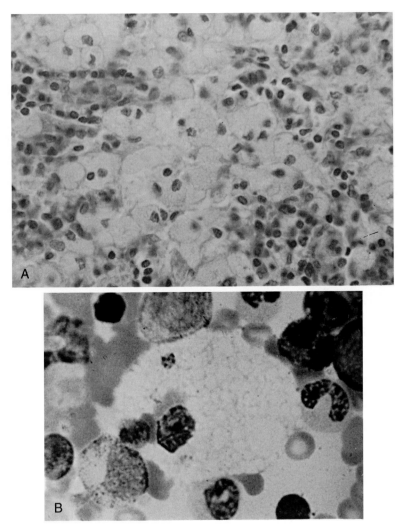

Figure 11–6. (A) Niemann-Pick cells appear pale and foamy in tissue sections. (B) In touch imprints, they display multiple small vacuoles.

also in the sinuses of lymph nodes and in the periportal regions of the liver.

Ceroid-containing histiocytes may occur also in the spleen and bone marrow of patients with a variety of disorders, including other lipidoses,[62–64] chronic myelogenous leukemia,[65, 66] immune thrombocytopenic purpura,[67–71] chronic granulomatous disease of childhood,[72] and sickle cell anemia.[72] Several investigators have reported ceroid-containing histiocytes in the spleen and occasionally in other organs in association with certain types of hyperlipidemia.[64, 73–75] Long and colleagues[45] described sea-blue histiocytes in a number of organs in adults with Niemann-Pick disease and postulated that in its adult form this disease is actually a form of ceroid histiocytosis.

In all of these conditions, the ceroid-containing histiocytes are much less numerous than in the idiopathic form and are usually restricted to the bone marrow and/or spleen. Occasionally, scattered ceroid-containing histiocytes may occur in the spleen as an isolated finding.

GANGLIOSIDOSES

GM_2 gangliosidoses are a group of three lysosomal diseases caused by an inability to catabolize GM_2 gangliosides. Degradation of GM_2 gangliosides requires three polypeptides encoded by three separate loci. Splenomegaly may be a feature of the gangliosidoses.[76] The

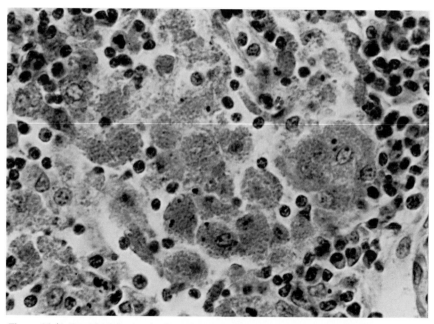

Figure 11–7. Ceroid histiocytes in the spleen of a patient with Hermansky-Pudlak syndrome.

most common of these disorders is Tay-Sachs disease, in which a sphingolipid termed "GM$_2$ ganglioside" accumulates caused by a deficiency of the enzyme hexosaminidase A, resulting from a mutation of the alpha-subunit locus on chromosome 15.[76–79] The lymphoreticular system and the parenchymal cells of some viscera, including the heart, may be involved. However, the involvement of the central and peripheral nervous systems usually dominates the clinical picture. Affected cells appear ballooned with fine cytoplasmic vacuoles due to lysosomes distended with the sphingolipid. The sphingolipid stains moderately with Sudan black B and faintly with stains for triglycerides. Electron microscopic studies of glial cells and neurons have revealed several types of cytoplasmic inclusion bodies.[80] The most common type consists of prominent lysosomes containing concentrically arranged membranes surrounding an inner zone that is homogeneous or finely granular. The clinical features of the two other forms of GM$_2$ gangliosidoses, Sandhoff disease and GM$_2$-activator deficiencies, are similar to those of Tay-Sachs disease.

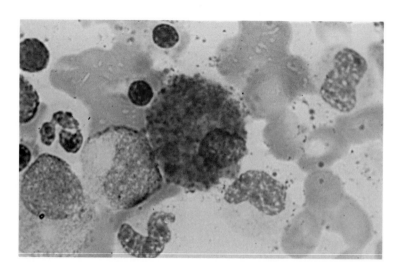

Figure 11–8. Ceroid histiocytes in bone marrow aspirates or touch imprints with Romanovsky stains appear blue; hence the term "sea-blue histiocyte."

Fabry disease, an X-linked lysosomal storage disease caused by α-galactosidase deficiency, is characterized by the accumulation of glycosphingolipid ceramide trihexoside in lymphoreticular and epithelial cells.[81, 82] Affected cells appear foamy and, by electron microscopy, have been shown to contain lamellated membranous structures.[82] Symptoms relating to renal and cardiac involvement usually dominate the clinical picture, and cutaneous angiokeratomas are characteristic. The lymphoreticular system is involved, although to a lesser degree,[83] and splenomegaly is usually not a prominent finding. In Wolman disease, foamy histiocytes—some resembling ceroid cells—accumulate in many organs, including the liver, spleen, and lymph nodes, owing to the accumulation of triglyceride and cholesterol esters.[84–86] Wolman disease results from a deficiency of the enzyme acid esterase and is similar to Niemann-Pick disease in its clinical course. Hepatosplenomegaly may be prominent (Fig. 11–9). In Tangier disease, histiocytes containing cholesterol esters also accumulate in the spleen, liver, lymph nodes, thymus, and bone marrow. This disease is caused by a deficiency of one of the high-density lipoproteins.[87–89] Splenomegaly with hypersplenism and lymphadenopathy may also be features. In von Gierke disease (type 1 glycogen-storage disease),[90] foam cells may also accumulate in the lymphoreticular system. Clusters of foamy histiocytes have also been described in the spleens of patients with tuberous sclerosis (Fig. 11–10).[91]

Mucopolysaccharidoses

The mucopolysaccharidoses (MPS) are a group of closely related lysosomal storage disorders that result from genetically determined deficiencies of specific enzymes involved in the degeneration of mucopolysaccharides.

Hepatosplenomegaly may be a feature of the mucopolysaccharidoses, in which the glycosaminoglycamines dermatan sulfate, heparan sulfate, keratin sulfate, and chondroitin sulfate accumulate in many organs.[92] The best known of these disorders are Hurler (MPS-IH) and Hunter (MPS-II) syndromes, in which, respectively, a deficiency of the enzymes α-L-iduronidase and α-L-iduronosulfate sulfatase results in an accumulation of heparan sulfate and dermatan sulfate. These metabolites occur in lymphoreticular cells, in intimal smooth muscle and endothelial cells, and in fibroblasts. Common sites of involvement, therefore, are the liver, spleen, and lymph nodes as well as the heart and blood vessels, leading to hepatosplenomegaly, cardiac valve lesions, and skeletal deformities. Affected cells, termed "balloon cells," appear clear because of minute cytoplasmic vacuoles.[93] The cytoplasm appears finely granular with the PAS stain. Ultrastructural studies have demonstrated that the

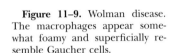

Figure 11–9. Wolman disease. The macrophages appear somewhat foamy and superficially resemble Gaucher cells.

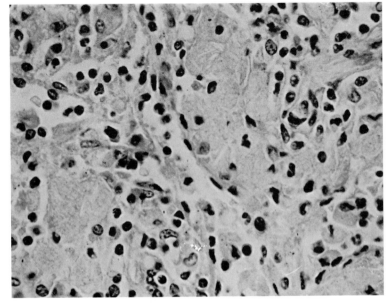

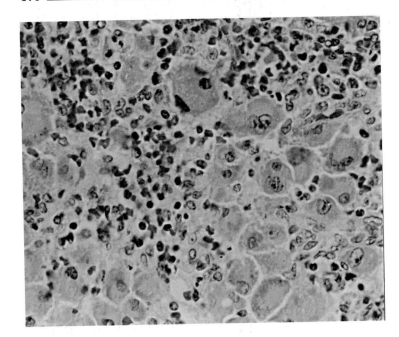

Figure 11–10. Tuberous sclerosis. Cordal macrophages proliferate in clusters.

intracellular inclusions can be visualized as swollen lysosomes filled with mucopolysaccharidoses. Zebra bodies within neurons similar to those seen in Niemann-Pick disease may also occur.

HEMOPHAGOCYTIC SYNDROMES

The hemophagocytic syndromes are a group of disorders characterized by the proliferation of cordal macrophages associated with prominent phagocytosis of hematopoietic elements. These syndromes have no immediately apparent cause and are usually acute in their clinical course.[94] Because of the acute clinical course (with death in many cases), no obvious cause, systemic distribution, and striking proliferation of cells in all lymphoreticular organs, these cases were usually considered in the past to represent malignant histiocytosis. The distinction of these disorders from true malignant histiocytosis was complicated by the fact that no reliable criteria for identifying clonality in histiocytes were available. Chandra et al[95] were the first to recognize that the hemophagocytic syndrome may be a benign process. However, Risdall et al[96] were the first to describe the disorder in detail. Their cases were both adult and pediatric patients who demonstrated a distinct clinical syndrome characterized by a proliferation of benign histiocytes demonstrating prominent hematophagocytosis

and a fulminant clinical course characterized by fever and varying cytopenias in a clinical context of underlying immunosuppression in most cases. In all their cases, a viral origin was implicated. As a result, they termed the disorder "viral-associated hematophagocytic syndrome." A later publication from the same group[97] reported a bacterial association with this syndrome, and numerous subsequent studies have revealed that a large number of organisms—bacterial,[98–103] microbacterial,[104–106] fungal,[107] rickettsial,[108] and parasitic[109, 110] as well as viral[96, 111–116]—may be associated with hematophagocytic syndrome. In addition, hematophagocytosis may occur in association with a variety of neoplastic disorders, in particular T-cell lymphomas.[117–125] The clinical course of infection-associated hemophagocytic syndrome is variable. Most cases present with a fulminant clinical course with overwhelming infections and significant evidence of immunosuppression. However, hematophagocytic syndromes have more recently been described in patients who were previously healthy.[126, 127]

The mechanism of hematophagocytosis, regardless of whether it is associated with an infectious agent or a neoplastic process, is thought to be mediated by abnormalities in the immunoregulatory system that cause an overproduction of cytokines.[128, 129] A number of these agents, including interleukin-1 (IL-1),[130] IL-2,[131, 132] interferon-γ,[131, 133, 134] tumor necrosis factor-α,[130] and macrophage colony-stimulating factor,[133–135] have been associated with hematophagocytic syndromes.

The spleen is invariably involved in cases of hematophagocytic syndrome but is rarely the first organ studied. Bone marrow aspiration and biopsy are usually studied first. In some cases, the phagocytic activity is marked. However, the marrow may show little, if any, evidence of hematophagocytosis, particularly in the early phases of the disease. Splenectomy may therefore be performed as a diagnostic procedure, although in the majority of cases it is performed as a therapeutic maneuver to alleviate the cytopenias that are characteristic of this syndrome. Spleens are usually moderately enlarged, although significant enlargement of more than 1 kg does occur. Infarcts of the organ are common. Histologically, the red pulp displays a proliferation of macrophages as well as prominent hematophagocytosis, most characteristically of erythrocytes, but also of granulocytes, lymphocytes, and platelets (Fig. 11–11). Occasionally, ingestion of nucleated red blood cells may occur in cases associated with the normoblastemia associated with hemolysis. Fibrosis, focal infarctions, and gradual obliteration of the white pulp may occur. Hemosiderin deposition may be prominent, both because of the hemolytic component and because of blood transfusions that may have been given because of the anemia.[136] The phagocytic histiocytes may be accompa-

nied by more primitive cells of similar lineage, but these cells do not display cytologic evidence of malignancy. Variations in the extent of the disease in the spleen appear related to the severity of the individual case and do not appear to be related to the particular type of infectious agent. Hematophagocytic syndromes associated with malignancies of the hematopoietic system differ morphologically and contain a component of malignant cells. This is particularly true in cases associated with T-cell lymphoma. In cases in which the neoplastic T cells infiltrate the splenic red pulp diffusely, the resemblance to malignant histiocytosis may be considerable. The diagnosis of T-cell lymphoma in these cases can be confirmed by demonstration of a rearranged configuration of the T-cell receptor genes.

Familial Hemophagocytosis

A familial variant of hemophagocytic syndrome was first described in 1952 by Farquhar and Claireau,[137] who termed the disorder "familial hemophagocytic reticulosis." Although it has been described using a variety of names such as generalized lymphohistiocytic infiltration,[138] familial reticuloendotheliosis,[139] familial histiocytic reticulosis,[140] and familial erythrophagocytic lymphohistocytosis,[141–143] the current accepted term is familial hemophago-

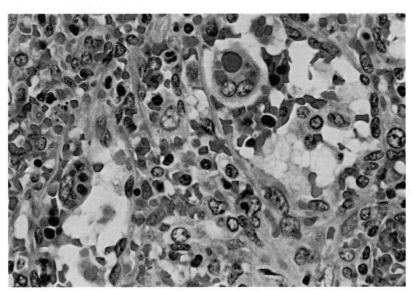

Figure 11–11. Viral (infection)-associated hemophagocytic syndrome. Macrophages proliferate in the cords of Billroth. Sinus lining cells frequently demonstrating erythrophagocytosis and lymphophagocytosis desquamate into the lumen of the red pulp sinuses.

cytic lymphohistiocytosis (FHL).[144] The disease affects infants and young children, with over three quarters of the cases presenting in patients younger than two years of age.[145] FHL is characterized by fever, irritability, nausea and vomiting, progressive pancytopenia, and hepatosplenomegaly. Neurologic symptoms are common.[146, 147] Laboratory findings include anemia, usually associated with leukopenia and thrombocytopenia. In addition, jaundice and hypofibrinogenemia, as well as hyperlipidemia with elevated triglycerides in the absence of hypercholesterolemia, are common.[145] The disease is fulminant and leads to death in the majority of cases in a matter of weeks. It has been suggested on the basis of genetic studies that there is an autosomal-recessive manner of inheritance.[148] Evidence has been presented that FHL may result from immunodeficiency.[149, 150] Abnormalities in both cellular and humoral immune systems have been described.[151, 152]

The morphology of the spleen in these disorders is essentially indistinguishable from those in virus-associated hemophagocytic syndrome. There may be focal necrosis within the red pulp as well as proliferation of histiocytes.[153] However, recent immunohistologic studies have shown phenotypic differences between these two conditions. Specifically, histiocytes in the FHL cases express CD35, CD21, and CD11b, the monocyte antigen CD36, and the activation markers CD25 and CD30, whereas the histiocytes in infection-associated hemophagocytic syndrome do not.[154]

Studies[155–158] have shown that in a significant percentage of cases of presumable FHL, Epstein-Barr virus, cytomegalovirus, and parvovirus can be implicated in the origin of the disease. It is frequently impossible to determine in a given case whether a young child has the familial form of histiocytosis or histiocytosis in association with an infection.[158] Because the genetic analysis suggests an autosomal-recessive manner of inheritance, many patients with the familial disease may not have parents or siblings who are affected. Similarly, several patients with FHL in the same family may be infected with the same virus. It has been suggested that viral infections may trigger FHL in genetically predisposed individuals.[155] However, because of the great similarity, both morphologically and clinically, between the familial and nonfamilial varieties of hemophagocytosis, it has been suggested that FHL and infection-associated hemophagocytic syndrome not be considered separate disorders.[143, 145]

LANGERHANS CELL HISTIOCYTOSIS

In 1953, Liechtenstein[159] proposed the term histiocytosis X to encompass the three clinical syndromes Hand-Schüller-Christian disease, eosinophilic granuloma of bone, and Letterer-Siwe syndrome. He based this proposal on his own and previous studies demonstrating an overlap in the clinical and pathologic features of these disorders.[159, 160] Recognizing that these three names defined different clinical syndromes of unifocal, multifocal, and disseminated disease, respectively, Rappaport[161] proposed the term "progressive histiocytoses" for this group of diseases and divided them into chronic differentiated histiocytosis, which refers to Hand-Schüller-Christian syndrome and eosinophilic granuloma of bone, and acute differentiated histiocytosis, which refers to Letterer-Siwe disease. Although dissenting opinions have been expressed,[162] it is now generally accepted that these three syndromes represent varying manifestations of the same disorder. The publication of Nezelof et al,[163] demonstrating that the cells of histiocytosis X contain Birbeck granules,[164] was the first to suggest the relationship between the proliferating cell of this disorder and the Langerhans cell of the skin. Subsequent studies[165, 166] have confirmed the Langerhans cell origin of this disorder and have provided the unified term Langerhans cell histiocytosis (LCH) for these proliferations.[167] The Langerhans cell is derived from the bone marrow and is normally distributed in skin, lymph nodes, bronchial mucosa, and thymus.[168] It is one of the most effective antigen-presenting cells and provides immune surveillance in detecting foreign antigen entering the body through the skin.[169] The LCH cell appears to have the antigenic phenotype of an early stage of Langerhans cell activation.[170] It is defective in its ability to present antigen, and its distribution in disseminated LCH is different from the normal distribution of the Langerhans cell; it commonly involves bone marrow, lymph nodes, lung, spleen, liver, and the central nervous system.[169]

There has been historical controversy regarding the etiology of LCH, particularly in the case of Letterer-Siwe syndrome. Despite the aggressive clinical course of the latter disorder, the morphologic appearance of the proliferating cell appears bland. A syndrome closely resembling Letterer-Siwe disease has been described in neonates with severe immunodeficiency,[171] and some investigators have suggested that, at least in some cases, disseminated histiocytosis may be a manifestation of an immunodeficiency syndrome.[172] Several studies have documented defective T-cell function in LCH,[173–175] and thymic extract or hormone has been successfully used to treat the disorder.[173, 175] There is little evidence to suggest an infectious cause of LCH. There is no evidence of a bacterial cause, and although one study demonstrated evidence of herpesvirus type 6 in lesions of LCH,[176] others have failed to demonstrate evidence of viruses in an extensive study.[177] However, molecular studies using X-linked DNA probes that can detect clonal or polyclonal X-chromosome inactivation patterns in female tissues have demonstrated that LCH in all its clinical subtypes is a proliferation of CD1a-positive, clonal histiocytes.[178, 179]

LCH has multiple clinical presentations, ranging from an isolated lytic lesion of bone to a fulminating, disseminated disorder mimicking leukemia. This latter disorder is most common in children and is the form of the disease in which splenic involvement occurs. Children with Letterer-Siwe disease usually present with fever and skin lesions.[180] Hepatosplenomegaly is common, and splenomegaly is a poor prognostic factor.[181–184] Cytopenias result from hypersplenism and from infiltration of the bone marrow. The spleen may be massive and often shows areas of hemorrhage, necrosis, and infarction (Color Plate 14). On rare occasions, the infiltrate in the spleen may be so extensive as to cause pathologic rupture of that organ.[185] Involvement occurs in the red pulp and may be in the form of a diffuse infiltrate, ill-defined tumor aggregates resembling loosely formed granulomas, or on rare occasions single tumor masses.[186] The characteristic cell of this disorder is large with abundant pale and sometimes vacuolated cytoplasm.[187] Erythrophagocytosis may be noted in some cells, especially in touch imprints. Nuclei are frequently deeply indented or grooved, with regular chromatin and one or two small nucleoli (Fig. 11–12). Although scattered eosinophils and multinucleated giant cells may be seen, they are much less numerous in Letterer-Siwe syndrome than in localized eosinophilic granuloma.[188]

Electron microscopy usually reveals characteristic structures, termed Birbeck or Langerhans granules, within the cytoplasm of the cells.[189–192] These structures are rod-shaped with rounded ends and are usually curved. They are composed of two electron-dense outer lines with a central less dense line, resulting in an external diameter of approximately 40 nanometers (Fig. 11–13). Although these structures may vary significantly in incidence from case to case, they are usually identifiable in every specimen if sought carefully. LCH cells are typically S-100-positive and

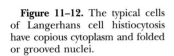

Figure 11–12. The typical cells of Langerhans cell histiocytosis have copious cytoplasm and folded or grooved nuclei.

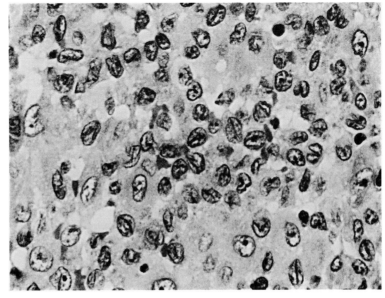

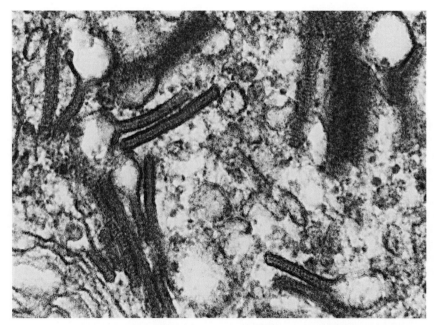

Figure 11–13. Birbeck or Langerhans granules in a Langerhans cell in Langerhans cell histiocytosis.

CD1a-positive and also express *HLA-DR (LN2), CD74 (LN3)*, vimentin, *CD68 (KP-1)*, and peanut agglutinin[169, 193–199] in most cases. Some cells may demonstrate α_1-antichymotrypsin and lysozyme.[197, 198, 200] CD1a is also characteristically positive.[146, 176]

The Histiocyte Society has adopted diagnostic criteria for LCH.[201] It has suggested that a definitive diagnosis cannot be made on morphologic grounds alone but must be accompanied by the presence of ultrastructural confirmation of Birbeck granules or the presence of CD1a by immunohistochemistry. We agree with Warnke et al[202] that these criteria are unnecessarily strict and believe that a definitive diagnosis can be made in many cases by examination of carefully prepared histologic sections.

Rare cases of so-called malignant LCH have been reported.[203, 204] These patients have a male predominance, an older age, disseminated involvement with frequent splenic distribution, and cytologically malignant-appearing cells. However, not all cases in which cytologic atypia occur are necessarily associated with a malignant clinical course.[204]

MALIGNANT HISTIOCYTOSIS

The existence of a clinically malignant disseminated proliferation of histiocytes was first noted by Scott and Robb-Smith in 1939.[205] Because the proliferating histiocytes occurred in the medullary sinuses of lymph nodes, the lesion was termed "histiocytic medullary reticulosis." It is now recognized that this disorder is heterogeneous, being composed of a variety of neoplastic and non-neoplastic proliferations.[206, 207] Rappaport[208] originated the term "malignant histiocytosis" for "a systemic, progressive invasive proliferation of morphologically atypical histiocytes and their precursors." Numerous subsequent studies defined malignant histiocytosis as a disease occurring at any age and characterized by systemic symptoms; fever; hepatosplenomegaly; lymphadenopathy, particularly in children[209, 210]; and frequent preterminal jaundice. Common laboratory findings include varying degrees of peripheral blood cytopenias, attributed to phagocytosis by tumor cells[211, 212]; hyperbilirubinemia; multiple liver enzyme abnormalities; and a rapidly progressive clinical course that is usually fatal.[208, 213–217] However, the disease may present as isolated splenomegaly. Vardiman et al[218] described four patients who presented with massive splenomegaly in the absence of systemic symptoms and who had a more protracted course. Once the systemic symptoms appeared, however, the course was rapidly progressive.

The morphologic features of the spleen in malignant histiocytosis resemble those of acute

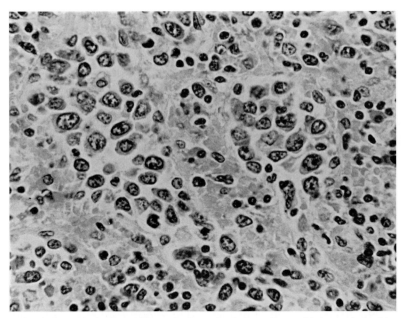

Figure 11–14. Cytologically atypical cells proliferate in the red pulp in malignant histiocytosis. In this case, immunologic studies revealed that the tumor cells were B lymphocytes.

leukemia, with diffuse infiltration of the red pulp (Fig. 11–14) sometimes obliterating the white pulp.[213, 214] Necrosis may be prominent. The infiltrate is pleomorphic, with the proliferating cells showing a variable degree of differentiation and cytologic atypia.[219] The nuclei are often bean-shaped and eccentric. The majority of cases show highly atypical bizarre cells with irregularly clumped chromatin, prominent nucleoli, and numerous mitoses (Fig. 11–15).[213, 214] Multinucleated giant cells, some re-

sembling Reed-Sternberg cells, may occur; and an admixture of eosinophils and plasma cells may result in a resemblance to Hodgkin's disease. Abnormal histiocytes and monocytoid cells often occur in the peripheral blood.[219, 220] Warnke and colleagues[214] reported that the degree of cytoplasmic atypia of the histiocytes increases with the course of the disease. Erythrophagocytosis by malignant cells is usually difficult to demonstrate, and most phagocytic cells are benign-appearing histiocytes. Ultra-

Figure 11–15. Malignant histiocytosis. Cellular atypia and mitotic activity are usually frequent. Erythrophagocytosis occurs in reactive macrophages (lower right).

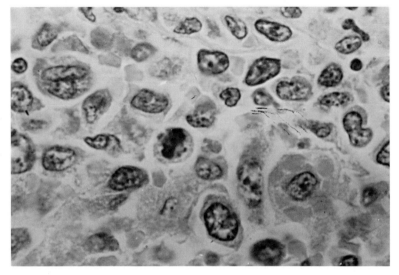

structural studies show numerous phagolyso-somes, residual bodies, and short strands of rough endoplasmic reticulum. Birbeck granules are not found.[217, 221] Malignant histiocytosis is usually rapidly fatal. Rarely, patients have experienced prolonged survival following splenectomy.[222]

With the advent of more sophisticated immunologic and molecular techniques, the disorder termed malignant histiocytosis has been reappraised.[223] A large number of the cases reported in the literature were based only on morphologic evidence of histiocytic lineage, such as the presence of phagocytosis by the proliferating cells. Confirmation of the true nature of the malignant-appearing cells was hampered by the fact that in the majority of cases hemophagocytosis could be demonstrated only in morphologically normal-appearing, mature histiocytes.[208, 213, 220] In addition, evidence of the histiocytic nature of the proliferating cells provided by cytochemical studies such as acid phosphatase and nonspecific esterase and by immunohistologic staining for such enzymes as lysozyme, α_1-antitrypsin, and α_1-antichymotrypsin are not reliable because these stains are now known to be not specific.[224–226]

Recent development of more sophisticated immunophenotypic studies has indicated that many diseases once termed malignant histiocytosis are in fact malignant lymphomas,[223, 219–230] including but not limited to the subtypes anaplastic large cell lymphoma[231, 232]; erythrophagocytic T-gamma lymphoma,[233] and Epstein-Barr virus–related[234, 235] and non-Epstein-Barr virus–related T-cell lymphomas.[236] The proliferation of histiocytes is presumably related to the elaboration by tumor cells of cytokines, such as tumor necrosis factor-α or macrophage colony-stimulating factor, that induce macrophage proliferation. In addition, the hemophagocytic syndromes are believed to have been mistakenly diagnosed as malignant histiocytosis in many cases.[94, 237–239]

Although few would disagree that the majority of cases of so-called malignant histiocytosis published in the literature represent either reactive hemophagocytic processes or malignancies of lymphocytes, it is clear that true malignant histiocytosis does exist but that the term should be restricted to those cases that demonstrate convincing evidence of histiocytic lineage, as evidenced by the absence of T-cell or B-cell immunophenotype or gene rearrangements, and by the demonstration of such markers as CD68, CD11c, CD14, Mac-387, and lysozyme.

"Malignant Histiocytosis" Associated with Mediastinal Germ Cell Tumor

An unusual association occurs between mediastinal nonseminomatous germ cell tumors (MNSGCT) and hematologic malignancies.[240, 241] Approximately one half of the hematologic malignancies have been characterized in the literature as malignant histiocytosis.[241–247] We have reported one case in which the histiocytic nature has been confirmed.[244] More recently, we have studied two more such cases. Proliferations of histiocytes in this condition may occur either diffusely or in the form of ill-defined nodules of CD68-positive cells within the red pulp of the spleen (Fig. 11–16). These proliferations are thought to represent an unusual form of metastasis from hematologic elements originating within the MNSGCT through aberrant hematologic differentiation of malignant germ cells.[244, 247] However, there is the possibility that the histiocytes are reactive because it has not been shown by cytogenetic or other means that they are clonal as are the other hematologic proliferations in this syndrome.

TRUE HISTIOCYTIC LYMPHOMA (HISTIOCYTIC SARCOMA)

The term "true histiocytic lymphoma" is used to define malignant tumors of the lymphoreticular system that are composed of cells that demonstrate monocyte-macrophage lineage, in contrast to the tumors previously called histiocytic lymphoma, which are now recognized to be malignancies of large lymphoid cells in virtually all cases.[248–252] For a tumor to be considered a true histiocytic lymphoma, it must demonstrate immunologic and/or molecular confirmation of monocyte-macrophage lineage. As such, the distinction from tumors of lymphocytic origin must be as rigorous as it is in cases of true malignant histiocytosis.

The distinction between true malignant histiocytosis and true histiocytic lymphoma may be somewhat arbitrary.[250] By our criteria, true histiocytic lymphoma of the spleen must be a tumor mass, as opposed to a disseminated infiltration of the red pulp, which better de-

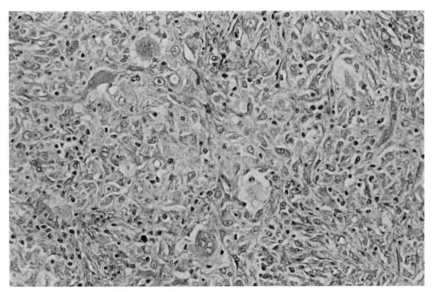

Figure 11–16. Malignant histiocytosis in the spleen of a patient with mediastinal germ cell tumor. These cells may proliferate either as tumor masses or diffusely within the red pulp of the spleen. Although immunologic studies confirm the monocyte-macrophage nature of these cells, it is not known whether they are truly neoplastic.

fines malignant histiocytosis. True histiocytic lymphomas are extremely uncommon and have been estimated to represent significantly less than 1 percent of all non-Hodgkin's lymphomas. Almost all cases involve lymph nodes, skin, and the mediastinum,[250–252] and confirmed cases involving the spleen are quite rare. Most of the few cases we have been able to find in the literature describe diffuse infiltration of the red pulp by tumor cells, which we believe are more appropriately classified as malignant histiocytosis. Franchino et al[253] reported a case of a splenic malignancy that presented as discrete tumor nodules, which we believe fulfills the criteria for true histiocytic lymphoma. The cells expressed a histiocytic immunophenotype and lacked both immunoglobulin and T-cell receptor β chain gene rearrangements. In spite of its localized presentation, the tumor disseminated and eventually killed the patient.

OTHER TUMORS

Follicular dendritic cell sarcoma, or follicular dendritic cell tumor, is a rare neoplasm derived from the follicular dendritic cell of the germinal center.[254–258] The cells are typically CD21-positive, CD35-positive, *HLA-DR*-positive, CD11a-positive, and CD18-positive. They may be negative for CD45RB; CD1a is

not expressed, and S-100 is variably positive. Almost all of these tumors arise in lymph nodes; however, rare examples have been described in the spleen. In the case reported by Perez-Ordonez et al,[256] the tumor was massive and solitary. Microscopically, these tumors resemble soft-tissue sarcomas with oval or spindle cells usually growing in bundles and whorls. Nuclei are bland in appearance and have a low mitotic rate (Fig. 11–17). Electron microscopy demonstrates elongated cells with long, slender processes connected to each other through numerous desmosomes.[258] The clinical behavior of these tumors appears to be more aggressive than the relatively bland cytology would suggest.

Interdigitating dendritic cell sarcoma is a rare neoplasm that shows differentiation similar to that of normal lymph node interdigitating dendritic cells.[258–261] The disease usually presents in a lymph node, although extranodal presentation may occur. In a variable proportion of cases the disease is disseminated, with involvement of spleen, bone marrow, skin, liver, kidney, and lung.[258, 261] The histologic features of interdigitating dendritic cell sarcoma are similar to those described for follicular dendritic cell sarcoma. In paraffin sections, the cells are positive for S-100 and CD68 and lack CD1a, B-cell, T-cell, and specific follicular dendritic cell antigen expression. On ultrastructural examination, the tumor is seen to

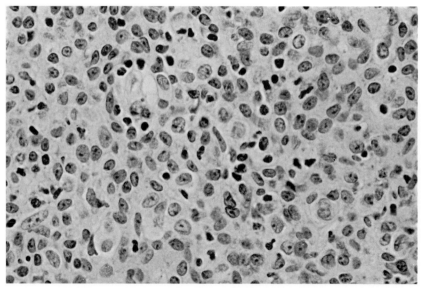

Figure 11–17. Follicular dendritic cell tumor. Tumor cells appear bland and demonstrate an oval or spindle-shaped appearance.

lack desmosomes. These rare tumors must be distinguished from rare cases of primary malignant fibrous histiocytoma of the spleen.[262]

SINUS HISTIOCYTOSIS WITH MASSIVE LYMPHADENOPATHY

Sinus histiocytosis with massive lymphadenopathy (SHML), or Rosai-Dorfman disease,[263] is an uncommon non-neoplastic proliferation of macrophages that typically express S-100, CD14, and CD68 but do not express CD1a. SHML most typically presents with massive cervical adenopathy, but it may involve most organs of the body. The proliferating histiocytes demonstrate characteristic phagocytosis of lymphocytes, but phagocytosis of other hematopoietic cells may also be noted. Although the cause of the disease is unknown, antibodies to human herpesvirus type 6 and Epstein-Barr virus have been described in some patients. Laboratory findings in SHML include anemia that may be either normocytic/normochromic or hemolytic in type. Patients frequently have polyclonal hyperglobulinemia, and some may show abnormalities in CD4/CD8 ratios in the peripheral blood. Patients may undergo spontaneous remission or develop recurrent disease. Other patients may have progressive disease and die of disseminated involvement. Despite the aggressive clinical course, there is no molecular evidence confirming that these lesions are clonal. Splenomegaly is an uncommon finding in SHML.[263] There is a single case report of splenic involvement[264] in SHML. Rosai and Dorfman[263] mention this case report in their review of SHML but comment that they themselves have not seen a case.

REFERENCES

1. Gutierrez Y: Diagnostic Pathology of Parasitic Infections with Clinical Correlations, p 140. Philadelphia, Lea & Febiger, 1990.
2. Veress B, Omer A, Satir AA, et al: Morphology of the spleen and lymph node in fatal visceral leishmaniasis. Immunology 1977; 33:605.
3. Schnitzer B, Sodeman TM, Mead ML, et al: An ultrastructural study of the red pulp of the spleen in malaria. Blood 1973; 41:207.
4. Reidbord HR, Horvat BL, Fisher ER: Splenic lipodoses: Histochemical and ultrastructural differentiation with special reference to the syndrome of the sea-blue histiocyte. Arch Pathol 1972; 93:518.
5. Beutler E, Grabowski GA: Gaucher disease, in Scriver CR, Beaudet AL, Sly WS, et al (eds): The Metabolic and Molecular Bases of Inherited Disease, p 2641. New York, McGraw-Hill, 1995.
6. Lee RE, Peters SP, Glew RH: Gaucher's disease: Clinical, morphologic and pathogenetic considerations. Pathol Ann 1977; 2:309.
7. Beutler E: Gaucher's disease. N Engl J Med 1991; 325:1354.
8. Mistry PK, Smith SJ, Ali M, et al: Genetic diagnosis of Gaucher's disease. Lancet 1992; 339:889.
9. Glew RH, Basu A, Prence EM, et al: Lysozomal storage diseases. Lab Invest 1985; 53:250.
10. Groopman JE, Golde DW: The histiocytic disorders:

A pathophysiologic analysis. Ann Intern Med 1981; 94:95.

11. Kahn LB: Pathology of Gaucher's disease. S Afr Med J 1974; 48:1098.

12. Lorber M: Adult-type Gaucher's disease: A secondary disorder of iron metabolism. J Mt Sinai Hosp 1970; 37:404.

13. Lorber M, Nemes JL: Identification of ferritin within Gaucher cells: An electron microscopic and immunofluorescent study. Acta Haematol 1967; 37:189.

14. Fisher ER, Reidbord HE: Gaucher's disease: Pathogenetic considerations based on electron microscopic and histochemical observations. Am J Pathol 1962; 41:679.

15. Lee RE: The fine structure of cerebroside occurring in Gaucher's disease. Proc Natl Acad Sci U S A 1968; 61:484.

16. Lee RE, Worthington CR, Glew RH: The bilayer nature of deposits occurring in Gaucher's disease. Arch Biochem Biophys 1973; 159:259.

17. Lee RE, Balcerzak SP, Westerman MP: Gaucher's disease: A morphologic study and measurements of iron metabolism. Am J Med 1967; 42:891.

18. Fleshner PR, Aufses AH Jr, Grabowsky GA, et al: A 27-year experience with splenectomy for Gaucher's Disease. Am J Surg 1991; 161:69.

19. Ashkenazi A, Zaizov R, Matoth Y: Effect of splenectomy on destructive bone changes in children with chronic (type I) Gaucher Disease. Eur J Pediatr 1986; 145:138.

20. Ross JS, Grabowski GA, Barnett SH, et al: Accelerated skeletal deterioration after splenectomy in Gaucher type I disease. Am J Roentgenol 1982; 139:1202.

21. Rodgers BM, Tribble C, Joob A: Partial splenectomy for Gaucher's disease. Ann Surg 1987; 205:693.

22. Thanopoulos BD, Frimas CA, Mantagos SP, et al: Gaucher disease: Treatment of hypersplenism with splenic embolization. Acta Pediatr Scand 1987; 76:1003.

23. Hobbs JR: Bone marrow transplantation for genetic diseases. N Engl J Med 1985; 312:1260.

24. Hobbs JR, Shaw PJ, Jones KH, et al: Beneficial effect of pretransplant splenectomy on displacement bone marrow transplantation for Gaucher's syndrome. Lancet 1987; 1:1111.

25. Zimran A, Hadas-Halpern I, Abrahamov A: Enzyme replacement therapy for Gaucher's Disease. N Engl J Med 1991; 325:1810.

26. Kranewich D, Dietrich K, Bauer L, et al: Splenectomy in Gaucher disease: New management dilemmas. Blood 1998; 91:3085.

27. Elleder M: Niemann-Pick disease. Pathol Res Pract 1989; 185:293.

28. Weisz B, Spirer Z, Reif S: Niemann-Pick disease: Newer classification based on genetic mutations of the disease. Adv Pediatr 1994; 41:415.

29. Schuchman EH, Desnick RT: Niemann-Pick disease types A & B: Acid sphingomyelinase deficiencies, in Scriver CR, Beaudet AL, Sly WS, et al (eds): The Metabolic and Molecular Bases of Inherited Disease, p 2601. New York, McGraw-Hill, 1995.

30. Levran O, Desnick RJ, Schuchman EH: Niemann-Pick disease: A frequent missense mutation in the acid sphingomyelinase gene of Ashkenazi Jewish type A and B patients. Proc Natl Acad Sci U S A 1991; 88:3748.

31. Levran O, Desnick RJ, Schuchman EH: Niemann-Pick type B disease: Identification of a single codon deletion in the acid sphingomyelinase gene and genotype/phenotype correlations in type A and B patients. J Clin Invest 1991; 88:806.

32. Ida H, Rennert OM, Maekawa K, et al: Identification of the three novel mutations in the acid sphinogomyelinase gene of Japanese patients with Niemann-Pick disease type A and B. Hum Mutat 1996; 7:65.

33. Schuchman EH: Two new mutations in the acid sphingomyelinase gene causing type A Niemann-Pick disease: N389T and R441X. Hum Mutat 1995; 6:352.

34. Pentchev PG, Vanier MT, Suzuki K, et al: Niemann-Pick disease type C: A cellular cholesterol lipidosis, in Scriver CR, Beaudet AL, Sly WS, et al (eds): The Metabolic and Molecular Bases of Inherited Disease, p 2625. New York, McGraw-Hill, 1995.

35. Pentchev PG, Comly ME, Kruth SH, et al: A defect in cholesterol esterification in Niemann-Pick disease (type C) patients. Proc Natl Acad Sci U S A 1985; 82:8247.

36. Brady RO, Filling-Katz MR, Barton NW, et al: Niemann-Pick disease types C and D. Neurol Clin 1989; 7:75.

37. Carstea ED, Morris JA, Coleman KG, et al: Niemann-Pick C1 disease gene: homology to mediators of cholesterol hemostasis. Science 1997; 277:228.

38. Gilbert-Barness E, Barness LA, Rapola J, et al: Metabolic disorders, in Anderson's Pathology, 10th ed, p 283. St. Louis, Mosby, 1996.

39. Winsor EJT, Welch JP: Genetic and demographic aspects of Nova Scotia Niemann-Pick disease (type D). Am J Hum Genet 1978; 30:530.

40. Arey JB: The lipidoses: Morphologic changes in the nervous system in Gaucher's disease, GM$_2$ gangliosidoses and Niemann-Pick disease. J Clin Lab Sci 1975; 5:475.

41. McCusker JJ, Parsons DB: Niemann-Pick disease: Report of two cases in siblings including the necropsy and histochemical findings in one. Arch Pathol 1962; 74:127.

42. da Silva V, Vassella F, Bischoff A, et al: Niemann-Pick's disease: Clinical, biochemical, and ultrastructural findings in a case of infantile form. J Neurol 1975; 211:61.

43. Dumontel C, Girod C, Dijoud F, et al: Fetal Niemann-Pick disease type C: Ultrastructural and lipid findings in liver and spleen. Virchows Arch 1993; 422:253.

44. Dawson PJ, Dawson G: Adult Niemann-Pick disease with sea-blue histiocytes in the spleen. Hum Pathol 1982; 13:1115.

45. Long RG, Lake BD, Pettie JE, et al: Adult Niemann-Pick disease: Its relationship to the syndrome of the sea-blue histiocyte. Am J Med 1977; 62:627.

46. Silverstein MN, Young DG, ReMine WH, et al: Splenomegaly with rare morphologically distinct histiocytes: A syndrome. Arch Intern Med 1964; 114:251.

47. Silverstein MN, Ellefson RD, Ahern EJ: The syndrome of the sea-blue histiocyte. N Engl J Med 1970; 282:1.

48. Rosner F, Kagen MD, Dana M: The sea-blue histiocyte syndrome. N Engl J Med 1970; 282:1100.

49. Sawitsky A, Rosner F, Chodsky S: The sea-blue histiocyte syndrome—a review: Genetic and biochemical studies. Semin Hematol 1972; 9:285.

50. Karayalgin G, Rosner F, Sawitsky A: Sea-blue histiocyte syndrome in an octogenarian. Lancet 1971; 2:318.

51. Silverstein MN, Ellefson RD: The syndrome of the sea-blue histiocyte. Semin Hematol 1972; 9:299.

52. Oh J, Bailin T, Fukai K, et al: Positional cloning of a gene for Hermansky-Pudlak syndrome, a disorder of cytoplasmic organelles. Nat Genet 1996; 14:300.

53. Schinella RA, Greco MA, Garay SM, et al: Hermansky-Pudlak syndrome: A clinicopathologic study. Hum Pathol 1985; 16:366.

54. Nishibori M, Cham B, McNichol A, et al: The protein CD63 is in platelet-dense granules, is deficient in a patient with Hermansky-Pudlak syndrome, and appears identical to granulophysin. J Clin Invest 1993; 91:1775.

55. Wildenberg SC, Oetting WS, Almodovar C, et al: A gene causing Hermansky-Pudlak syndrome in a Puerto Rican population maps to chromosome 10q2. Am J Hum Genet 1995; 57:755.

56. Fukai K, Oh J, Frenk E, Almodovar C, et al: Linkage disequilibrium mapping of the gene for Hermansky-Pudlak syndrome to chromosome 10q23.1–q23.3. Hum Mol Genet 1995; 4:1665.

57. Garay SM, Gardella JE, Fazzini EP, et al: Hermansky-Pudlak syndrome: Pulmonary manifestations of a ceroid-storage disorder. Am J Med 1979; 66:737.

58. Schinella RA, Greco MA, Cobert BL, et al: Hermansky-Pudlak syndrome with granulomatous colitis. Ann Intern Med 1980; 92:20.

59. Hartroft WS, Porta EA: Ceroid. Am J Med Sci 1965; 250:324.

60. Porta EA, Hartroft WS: Lipid pigments in relation to aging and dietary factors (lipofuscins), in Wolman M (ed): Pigments in Pathology, p 191. New York, Academic Press, 1969.

61. Endicott KM, Lillie RD: Ceroid, the pigment of dietary cirrhosis of rats: Its characteristics and its differentiation from hemofuscin. Am J Pathol 1944; 20:149.

62. Kattlove HE, Gaynor E, Spivack M, et al: Sea-blue indigestion. N Engl J Med 1970; 282:630.

63. Jacobsen CD, Gjone E, Hovig T: Sea-blue histiocytes in familial lecithin: Cholesterol acyltransferase deficiency. Scand J Haematol 1972; 9:106.

64. Ferrans VJ, Buja LM, Roberts WC, et al: The spleen in type I hyperlipoproteinemia: Histochemical, biochemical, microfluorimetric and electron microscopic observations. Am J Pathol 1971; 64:67.

65. Dosik H, Rosner F, Sawitsky A: Acquired lipidosis: Gaucher-like cells and "blue cells" in chronic granulocytic leukemia. Semin Hematol 1972; 9:309.

66. Steinberg MH, Dreiling BJ: Chronic granulocytic leukemia: Prolonged survival, muscle infiltration and sea-blue histiocytosis. Am J Med 1973; 55:93.

67. Chandra P, Rosner F, Sawitsky A: Sea-blue histiocytes in thrombocytopenia purpura. Ann Intern Med 1973; 79:901.

68. Dollberg L, Casper J, Djaldetti M, et al: Lipid-laden histiocytes in the spleen in thrombocytopenic purpura. Am J Clin Pathol 1965; 43:16.

69. Firkin BG, Wright R, Miller S, et al: Splenic macrophages in thrombocytopenia. Blood 1963; 33:240.

70. Hill JM, Speer RJ, Gedikoglu H: Secondary lipidosis of spleen associated with thrombocytopenia and other blood dyscrasias treated with steroids. Am J Clin Pathol 1963; 39:607.

71. Rywlin AM, Hernandez JA, Chastain DE, et al: Ceroid histiocytosis of spleen and bone marrow in idiopathic thrombocytopenic purpura (ITP): A contribution to the understanding of the sea-blue histiocyte. Blood 1971; 37:587.

72. Bartman J, van de Velde RL, Friedman F: Pigmented lipid histiocytosis and susceptibility to infection: Ultrastructure of splenic histiocytes. Pediatrics 1967; 40:1000.

73. Parker AC, Bain AD, Brydon WG, et al: Sea-blue histiocytosis associated with hyperlipidemia. J Clin Pathol 1976; 29:634.

74. Roberts WC, Levy RI, Fredrickson DS: Hyperlipoproteinemia: A review of the five types with first report of necropsy findings in type 3. Arch Pathol 1970; 90:46.

75. Rywlin AM, Lopez-Gomez A, Tachmes P, et al: Ceroid histiocytosis of the spleen in hyperlipemia: Relationship to the syndrome of the sea-blue histiocyte. Am J Clin Pathol 1971; 56:572.

76. Sandhoff K, Conzelmann E, Neufeld EF, et al: The GM_2 gangliosidoses, in Scriver CR, Beaudet AL, Sly WS, et al (eds): The Metabolic and Molecular Bases of Inherited Disease, 6th ed, p 1807. New York, McGraw-Hill, 1989.

77. Sandhoff K, Harzer K, Wassle W, et al: Enzyme alterations and lipid storage in three variants of Tay-Sachs disease. J Neurochem 1971; 18:2469.

78. Tallman JF, Johnson WG, Brady RO: The metabolism of Tay-Sachs ganglioside: Catabolic studies with lysosomal enzymes from normal and Tay-Sachs brain tissue. J Clin Invest 1972; 51:2339.

79. Sandhoff K, Conzelmann E, Neufeld EF, et al: The GM_2 gangliosidoses, in Scriver CR, Beaudet AL, Sly WS, et al (eds): The Metabolic and Molecular Bases of Inherited Disease, 6th ed, p 1824. New York, McGraw-Hill, 1989.

80. Volk BW, Adachi M, Schneck L: The gangliosidoses. Hum Pathol 1975; 6:555.

81. Desnick RJ, Bishop DE: Fabry disease—alpha-galactosidase deficiency and Schindler disease: Alpha-N-acetylgalactosaminidase deficiency, in Scriver CR, Beaudet AL, Sly WS, et al (eds): The Metabolic and Molecular Bases of Inherited Disease, 6th ed, p 1751. New York, McGraw-Hill, 1989.

82. Beutler E, Kuhl W: Biochemical and electrophoretic studies of alpha-galactosidase in normal man, in patients with Fabry's disease, and in equidae. Am J Hum Genet 1972; 24:237.

83. Bagdade JD, Parker F, Ways PO, et al: Fabry's disease. A correlative clinical, morphological and biochemical study. Lab Invest 1968; 18:681.

84. Lough J, Fawcett L, Weigensberg B: Wolman's disease. Arch Pathol 1970; 89:103.

85. Ferrans VJ, Roberts WC, Levy RI, et al: Chylomicrons and the formation of foam cells in type I hyperlipoproteinemia: A morphologic study. Am J Pathol 1973; 70:253.

86. Wolman M, Sterk VV, Gatts FM: Primary familial xanthomatosis with involvement and calcification of the adrenals: Report on two more cases in siblings of a previously described infant. Pediatrics 1961; 28:742.

87. Ferrans VJ, Fredrickson DS: The pathology of Tangier disease: A light and electron microscopic study. Am J Pathol 1975; 78:101.

88. Herbert PN, Forte T, Heinen RJ, et al: Tangier disease: One explanation of lipid storage. N Engl J Med 1978; 299:519.

89. Hoffman HN, Fredrickson DS: Tangier disease (familial high density lipoprotein deficiency): Clinical and genetic features in two adults. Am J Med 1965; 39:582.

90. Chen Y-T: Glycogen storage disease, in Scriver CR, Beaudet AL, Sly WS, et al (eds): The Metabolic and Molecular Bases of Inherited Disease, 7th ed, p 935. New York, McGraw-Hill, 1995.

91. Bender BL, Yunis EJ: The pathology of tuberous sclerosis. Pathol Ann 1982; 17:369.

92. Neufeld EF, Muenzer J: The mucopolysaccharidoses, in Scriver CR, Beaudet AL, Sly WS, et al (eds): The Metabolic and Molecular Bases of Inherited Disease, 7th ed, p 2465. New York, McGraw-Hill, 1995.

93. Legum CP, Schor RS: The genetic mucopolysaccharidoses and mucolipidoses: Review and comment. Adv Pediatr 1976; 22:305.

94. Reiner AP, Spivak JL: Hematophagic histiocytosis: A report of 23 new patients and a review of the literature. Medicine 1988; 67:369.

95. Chandra P, Chaudhery SA, Rosner F, et al: Transient histiocytosis with striking phagocytosis of platelets, leukocytes, and erythrocytes. Arch Intern Med 1975; 135:989.

96. Risdall RJ, McKenna RW, Nesbit ME, et al: Virus-associated hemophagocytic syndrome: A benign histiocytic proliferation distinct from malignant histiocytosis. Cancer 1979; 44:993.

97. Risdall RJ, Brunning RD, Hernandez JI, et al: Bacteria-associated hemophagocytic syndrome. Cancer 1984; 54:2968.

98. Gill K, Marrie TJ: Hemophagocytosis secondary to mycoplasma pneumonia infection. Am J Med 1987; 82:668.

99. Kokkini G, Giotaki HG, Moutsopoulos HM: Transient hemophagocytosis in *Brucella melitensis* infection. Arch Pathol Lab Med 1984; 108:213.

100. Manoharan A, Painter D: Histiocytic medullary reticulosis. Lancet 1992; 2:881.

101. Martin-Moreno S, Soto-Guzman O, Bernaldo-de-Quiros J, et al: Pancytopenia due to hemophagocytosis in patients with brucellosis: A report of four cases. J Infect Dis 1983; 147:445.

102. Prokocimer M, Inbal A, Gelber M, et al: Hemophagocytosis simulating malignant histiocytosis: A terminal event of the myelodysplastic syndrome. Acta Haematol 1985; 74:164.

103. Udden MM, Banez E, Sears DA: Bone marrow histiocytic hyperplasia and hemophagocytosis with pancytopenia in typhoid fever. Am J Med Sci 1986; 291:396.

104. Barnes N, Bellamy D, Ireland R, et al: Pulmonary tuberculosis complicated by haemophagocytic syndrome and rifampicin-induced tubulointerstitial nephritis. Br J Dis Chest 1984; 78:395.

105. Campo E, Condom E, Miro J-J, et al: Tuberculosis-associated hemophagocytic syndrome. Cancer 1986; 58:2640.

106. Weintraub M, Siegman-Igra Y, Josiphov J, et al: Histiocytic hemophagocytosis in miliary tuberculosis. Arch Intern Med 1984; 114:2055.

107. Keller FG, Kurtzberg J: Disseminated histoplasmosis: A cause of infection-associated hemophagocytic syndrome. Am J Pediatr Hematol Oncol 1994; 16:368.

108. Estrov Z, Bruck R, Shtalrid M, et al: Histiocytic hemophagocytosis in Q fever. Arch Pathol Lab Med 1984; 108:7.

109. Broeckaert-von Orshoven A, Michielsen P, Vandepitte J: Fatal leishmaniasis in renal transplant patient. Lancet 1979; 2:740.

110. Matzner Y, Behar A, Berri E, et al: Systemic leishmaniasis mimicking malignant histiocytosis. Cancer 1979; 43:398.

111. Boruchoff SE, Woda BA, Pihan GA, et al: Parvovirus B-19–associated hemophagocytic syndrome. Arch Intern Med 1990; 150:897.

112. Muir K, Todd WTA, Watson WH, et al: Viral-associated haemophagocytosis with parvovirus-B19–related pancytopenia. Lancet 1992; 339:1139.

113. Reisman RP, Greco MA: Virus-associated hemophagocytic syndrome due to Epstein-Barr virus. Hum Pathol 1984; 15:290.

114. Danish EH, Dahms BB, Kumar ML: Cytomegalovirus-associated hemophagocytic syndrome. Pediatr 1985; 75:280.

115. Sugita K, Kurumada H, Eguchi M, et al: Human herpesvirus-6 infection associated with hemophagocytic syndrome. Acta Haematol 1995; 93:108.

116. Spivak JL, Bender BS, Quinn TC: Hematologic abnormalities in the acquired immune deficiency syndrome. Am J Med 1984; 77:224.

117. Ezdinli EZ, Kucuk O, Chedid A, et al: Hypogammaglobulinemia and hemophagocytic syndrome associated with lymphoproliferative disorders. Cancer 1986; 57:1024.

118. Jaffee E, Costa J, Fauci AS, et al: Malignant lymphoma and erythrophagocytosis simulating malignant histiocytosis. Am J Med 1983; 75:741.

119. Korman LY, Smith JR, Landaw SA, et al: Hodgkin's disease: Intramedullary phagocytosis with pancytopenia. Ann Intern Med 1979; 91:60.

120. Manoharan A, Catovsky D, Lampert IA, et al: Histiocytic medullary reticulosis complicating chronic lymphocytic leukemia: Malignant or reactive? Scand J Haematol 1981; 26:5.

121. Ng C-S, Chan JKC, Cheng PNM, et al: Nasal T-cell lymphoma associated with hemophagocytic syndrome. Cancer 1986; 58:67.

122. Rubin M, Rothenberg SP, Panchacharam P: A histiocytic medullary reticulosis-like syndrome as the terminal event in lymphocytic lymphoma. Am J Med Sci 1984; 287:62.

123. Theodorakis ME, Zamkoff KW, Davey FR, et al: Acute nonlymphocytic leukemia complicated by severe cytophagocytosis of formed blood elements by nonmalignant histiocytes: Cause of significant clinical morbidity. Med Pediatr Oncol 1983; 11:20.

124. James LP, Stass SA, Peterson V, et al: Abnormalities of bone marrow simulating histiocytic medullary reticulosis in a patient with gastric carcinoma. Am J Clin Pathol 1979; 7:600.

125. Dargent JL, Vermylen P, Abramowicz D, et al: Disseminated angiosarcoma presenting as a hemophagocytic syndrome in a renal allograft recipient. Transpl Int 1997; 10:61.

126. Shirono K, Tsuda H: Virus-associated haemophagocytic syndrome in previously healthy adults. Eur J Haematol 1995; 55:240.

127. Shirono K, Tsuda H: Parvovirus B19–associated haemophagocytic syndrome in healthy adults. Br J Haematol 1995; 89:923.

128. Imashuku S, Hibi S: Cytokines in haemophagocytic syndrome. Br J Haematol 1991; 77:438.

129. Fujiwara F, Hibi S, Imashuku S: Hypercytokinemia in hemophagocytic syndrome. Am J Pediatr Hematol Oncol 1993; 15:92.

130. Ishii E, Ohga S, Aoki T, et al: Prognosis of children with virus-associated hemophagocytic syndrome and malignant histiocytosis: Correlation with levels of serum interleukin-1 and tumor necrosis factor. Acta Hematol 1991; 85:93.

131. Komp DM, McNamara J, Buckley P: Elevated soluble interleukin-2 receptor in childhood hemophagocytic histiocytic syndromes. Blood 1989; 73:2128.

132. Imashuku S, Ikushima SA, Esumi N, et al: Serum

levels of interferon-gamma, cytotoxic factor and soluble interleukin-2 receptor in childhood hemophagocytic syndromes. Leuk lymph 1991; 3:287.

133. Akashi K, Hayashi S, Gondo H, et al: Involvement of interferon-gamma and macrophage colony-stimulating factor in pathogenesis of haemophagocytic lymphohistiocytosis in adults. Br J Haemathol 1994; 87:243.

134. Imashuku S, Hibi S, Fujiwara F, et al: Haemophagocytic lymphohistiocytosis, interferon-gamma-anemia and Epstein-Barr virus involvement. Br J Haemathol 1994; 88:656.

135. Tsuda H, Shirono K: Possible role of macrophage-colony stimulating factor in the development of hemophagocytic syndrome. Eur J Haematol 1995; 54:197.

136. Zoubek A, Haas OA, Ladenstein R, et al: Hemophagocytic syndrome with restricted organ involvement: Excessive hemosiderosis and fibrosis of the spleen. Pediatr Hematol Oncol 1986; 3:135.

137. Farquhar JW, Claireau AE: Familial hemophagocytic reticulosis. Arch Dis Child 1952; 27:519.

138. Nelson P, Santa Maria A, Olson RL, et al: Generalized lymphohistiocytic infiltration: A familial disease not previously described and different from Letterer-Siwe disease and Chediak-Higashi syndrome. Pediatrics 1961; 27:931.

139. Miller DR: Familial reticuloendothelioses: Concurrence of disease in five siblings. Pediatrics 1966; 38:986.

140. Marrian VJ, Sanekin NG: Familial histiocytic reticulosis (familial haemophagocytic reticulosis). J Clin Pathol 1963; 16:65.

141. O'Brien RT, Schwartz AD, Pearson HA, et al: Reticuloendothelial failure in familial erythrophagocytic lymphohistiocytosis. J Pediatr 1972; 81:543.

142. Perry MC, Harrison EG, Burgert EO, et al: Familial erythrophagocytic lymphohistiocytosis: Report of two cases and clinicopathologic review. Cancer 1976; 38:209.

143. Loy, TS, Diaz-Arias AA, Perry MC: Familial erythrophagocytic lymphohistiocytosis. Semin Oncol 1991; 18:34.

144. Janka G: Familial hemophagocytic lymphohistiocytosis. Eur J Pediatr 1983; 140:221.

145. Henter J-I, Elinder G, Ost A, et al: Diagnostic guidelines for hemophagocytic lymphohistiocytosis. Semin Oncol 1991; 18:29.

146. Henter J-I, Elinder G: Familial hemophagocytic lymphohistiocytosis: Clinical review based on the findings in seven children. Acta Paediatr Scand 1991; 80:269.

147. Henter J-I, Elinder G, Soder O, et al: Incidence and clinical features of familial hemophagocytic lymphohistiocytosis. Acta Paediatr Scand 1991; 80:428.

148. Gencik A, Signer E, Muller H: Genetic analysis of familial erythrophagocytic lymphohistiocytosis. Eur J Pediatr 1984; 142:248.

149. Barth RF, Vergara GG, Khurana SK, et al: Rapidly fatal familial histiocytosis associated with eosinophilia and primary immunological deficiency. Lancet 1972; 2:503.

150. Ladisch S, Poplack DG, Holiman B, et al: Immunodeficiency in familial erythrophagocytic lymphohistiocytosis. Lancet 1978; 1:581.

151. Henter J-I, Elinder G, Soder O, et al: Hypercytokinemia in familial hemophagocytic lymphohistiocytosis. Blood 1991; 78:2918.

152. Fullerton P, Ekert H, Hosking C, et al: Hemophagocytic reticulosis: A case report with investigations of immune and white cell function. Cancer 1975; 36:441.

153. Perry MC, Harrison EG Jr, Burgert EO, et al: Familial erythrophagocytic lymphohistiocytosis: Report of two cases and clinicopathologic review. Cancer 1976; 38:209.

154. Buckley PJ, O'Laughlin S, Komp DM: Histiocytes in familial and infection-induced/idiopathic hemophagocytic syndromes may exhibit phenotypic differences. Pediatr Pathol 1992; 12:51.

155. Henter J-I, Ehrnst A, Anderson J, et al: Familial hemophagocytic lymphohistiocytosis and viral infections. Acta Paediatr 1993; 82:369.

156. McClain K, Gehrz R, Grierson H, et al: Virus-associated histiocytic proliferations in children: Frequent association with Epstein-Barr virus and congenital and acquired immunodeficiencies. Am J Pediatr Hematol Oncol 1988; 10:196.

157. Janka-Schaub GE, Hansmann ML: Familial hemophagocytic lymphohistiocytosis terminating in fatal infectious mononucleosis. Med Pediatr Oncol 1989; 17:252.

158. The Writing Group of the Histiocyte Society: Histiocytosis syndromes in children. Lancet 1987; 1:208.

159. Liechtenstein L: Histiocytosis X: Integration of eosinophilic granuloma of bone, "Letterer-Siwe disease," and "Schuller-Christian disease" as related manifestations of a single nosologic entity. Arch Pathol 1956; 56:84.

160. Farber S: The nature of "solitary eosinophilic granuloma" of bone. Am J Pathol 1941; 17:625.

161. Rappaport H: Tumors of the hematopoietic system, in Atlas of Tumor Pathology, section III, fascicle 8, p 63. Washington, DC, Armed Forces Institute of Pathology, 1966.

162. Lieberman P, Jones C, Dargeon H, et al: A reappraisal of eosinophilic granuloma of bone, Hand-Schüller-Christian disease and Letterer-Siwe syndrome. Med 1969; 48:375.

163. Nezelof C, Basset F, Rousseau MF: Histiocytosis X: Histogenetic arguments for a Langerhans cell origin. Biomedicine 1973; 18:365.

164. Birbeck MS, Breathnach AS, Everall JD: An electron microscopic study of basal melanocytes and high-level clear cells (Langerhans cells) in vitiligo. J Invest Dermatol 1961; 37:51.

165. Nezelof C: Histiocytosis X: A histological and histogenetic study, In Rosenberg HS, Bolande RP (eds): Perspectives in Pediatric Pathology, vol V, p 153. New York, Masser, 1979.

166. Beckstead JH, Wood GS, Turner RR: Histiocytosis X cells and Langerhans cells: Enzyme histochemical and immunologic similarities. Hum Pathol 1984; 15:826.

167. Callihan TR: Langerhans cell histiocytosis (histiocytosis X), In Jaffe ES (ed): Surgical Pathology of the Lymph Nodes and Related Organs, p 534. Philadelphia, WB Saunders, 1995.

168. Favara BE: Langerhans cell histiocytosis: Pathology and pathogenesis. Semin Oncol 1991; 18:3.

169. Chu T, Jaffe R: The normal Langerhans cell and the LCH cell. Br J Cancer 1994; 70:S4.

170. Ruco LP, Remotti D, Monardo F, et al: Letterer-Siwe disease: Immunohistochemical evidence for a proliferative disorder involving immature cells of Langerhans lineage. Virchows Arch 1988; 413:239.

171. Cederbaum SD, Niwayama G, Stiehm ER, et al: Combined immunodeficiency presenting as the Letterer-Siwe syndrome. J Pediatr 1974; 85:466.

172. Favara BE, McCarthy RC, Mierau GW: Histiocytosis X. Hum Pathol 1983; 14:663.

173. Shannon, BT, Newton WA: Suppressor cell dysfunction in children with histiocytosis X. J Clin Immunol 1986; 6:510.

174. Kragballe K, Zachariae M, et al: Histiocytosis X: An immune deficiency disease? Studies on antibody-dependent monocyte-mediated cytotoxicity. Br J Dermatol 1981; 105:13.

175. Osband ME, Lipton JM, Lavin P, et al: Histiocytosis X. N Engl J Med 1981; 304:146.

176. Leahy MA, Knejei SM, Friedmanash M, et al: Human herpesvirus-6 is present in lesions of Langerhans cell histiocytosis. J Invest Dermatol 1993; 101:642.

177. McClain K, Jin H, Gresik V, et al: Langerhans cell histiocytosis: Lack of viral etiology. Am J Hematol 1994; 47:16.

178. Willman CL: Detection of clonal histiocytes in Langerhans cell histiocytosis: Biology and clinical significance. Br J Cancer 1994; 23:S29.

179. Willman CL, Busque L, Griffith BB, et al: Langerhans cell histiocytosis (histiocytosis X): A clonal proliferative disease. N Engl J Med 1994; 331:154.

180. The French Langerhans Cell Histiocytosis Study Group: A multicentre retrospective survey of Langerhans cell histiocytosis: 348 cases observed between 1983 and 1993. Arch Dis Child 1996; 75:17.

181. Komp DM: Langerhans cell histiocytosis. N Engl J Med 1987; 316:747.

182. Komp DM, Herson J, Starling KA, et al: A staging system for histiocytosis X: A Southwest Oncology Group study. Cancer 1981; 47:798.

183. Lahey ME: Prognostic factors in histiocytosis X. Am J Pediatr Hematol Oncol 1981; 3:57.

184. Nezelof C, Frileux-Herbert F, Cronier-Sachot J: Disseminated histiocytosis X: Analysis of prognostic factors based on a retrospective study of 50 cases. Cancer 1979; 44:1824.

185. Broadbent V, Williams M, Dosetor J: Ruptured spleen as a cause of death in an infant with Langerhans cell histiocytosis (histiocytosis X). Pediatr Hematol Oncol 1990; 7:297.

186. Lam KY, Chan AC, Wat MS: Langerhans cell histiocytosis forming an asymptomatic solitary nodule in the spleen. J Clin Pathol 1996; 49:262.

187. Jaffe R: Pathology of histiocytosis X. Perspect Pediatr Pathol 1987; 9:4.

188. Risdall RJ, Dehner LP, Duray P, et al: Histiocytosis X (Langerhans cell histiocytosis): Prognostic role of histopathology. Arch Pathol Lab Med 1983; 107:59.

189. Tarnowski WM, Hashimoto K: Langerhans cell granule in histiocytosis X: The epidermal Langerhans cell as a macrophage. Arch Dermatol 1967; 96:298.

190. Shamoto M: Langerhans cell granule in Letterer-Siwe disease: An electron microscopic study. Cancer 1970; 26:1102.

191. Basset F, Escaig J, LeCrom M: A cytoplasmic membranous complex in histiocytosis X. Cancer 1972; 29:1380.

192. Mierau GW, Favara BE, Brenman JM: Electron microscopy in histiocytosis X. Ultrastruct Pathol 1982; 3:137.

193. Mierau, GW, Favara BE: S-100 protein immunohistochemistry and electron microscopy in the diagnosis of Langerhans cell proliferative disorders: A comparative assessment. Ultrastruct Pathol 1986; 10:303.

194. Ree HJ, Kadin ME: Peanut agglutinin: A useful marker for histiocytosis X and interdigitating reticulum cells. Cancer 1986; 57:282.

195. Azumi N, Sheibani K, Swartz WG, et al: Antigenic phenotype of Langerhans cell histiocytosis: An immunohistochemical study demonstrating the value of LN-2, LN-3, and vimentin. Hum Pathol 1988; 19:1376.

196. Ornvold K, Ralfkiaer E, Carstensen H: Immunohistochemical study of the abnormal cells in Langerhans cell histiocytosis (histiocytosis X). Virchows Arch 1990; 416:403.

197. Hage C, Willman CL, Favara BE, et al: Langerhans cell histiocytosis (histiocytosis X): Immunophenotype and growth fraction. Hum Pathol 1993; 24:840.

198. Ruco LP, Pulford KAF, Mason DY, et al: Expression of macrophage-associated antigens in tissues involved by Langerhans cell histiocytosis (histiocytosis X). Am J Clin Pathol 1989; 92:273.

199. Wood GS, Freudenthal PS, Edinger A, et al: CD45 epitope mapping of human CD1a+ dendritic cells and peripheral blood dendritic cells. Am J Pathol 1991; 138:1451.

200. Ruco LP, Uccini S, Baroni CD: The Langerhans cells. Allergy 1989; 44:27.

201. The Writing Group of the Histiocyte Society: Histiocytosis syndromes in children. Lancet 1987; 1:208.

202. Lymphomas of the spleen, in Warnke RA, Weiss LM, Chan JKC, et al (eds): Atlas of Tumor Pathology: Tumors of the Lymph Nodes and Spleen, 3rd series, fascicle 14, p 348. Washington, DC, Armed Forces Institute of Pathology, 1995.

203. Wood C, Wood GS, Deneau DG, et al: Malignant histiocytosis X: Report of a rapidly fatal case in an elderly man. Cancer 1984; 54:347.

204. Ben-Ezra J, Bailey A, Azumi N, et al: Malignant histiocytosis X: A distinct clinicopathologic entity. Cancer 1991; 68:1050.

205. Scott RB, Robb-Smith AH: Histiocytic medullary reticulosis. Lancet 1939; ii:194.

206. Robb-Smith AH: Before our time: Half a century of histiocytic medullary reticulosis—a T-cell teaser? Histopathology 1990; 17:279.

207. Falini B, Pileri S, De Solas I, et al: Peripheral T-cell lymphoma associated with hemophagocytic syndrome. Blood 1990; 75; 434.

208. Rappaport H: Tumors of the hematopoietic system, in Atlas of Tumor Pathology, fascicle 8, p 48. Washington, DC, Armed Forces Institute of Pathology, 1966.

209. Zucker JM, Callaux JM, Vanel D, et al: Malignant histiocytosis in childhood, clinical study and therapeutic results in 22 cases. Cancer 1980; 45:2821.

210. Jurco S III, Starling K, Hawkins EP: Malignant histiocytosis in childhood: Morphologic considerations. Hum Pathol 1983; 14:1059.

211. Natelson EA, Lynch EC, Hettig RA, et al: Histiocytic medullary reticulosis: The role of phagocytosis in pancytopenia. Arch Intern Med 1968; 122:223.

212. Seligman BR, Rosner F, Lee SL, et al: Histiocytic medullary reticulosis: Fatal hemorrhage due to massive platelet phagocytosis. Arch Intern Med 1972; 129:109.

213. Byrne GE, Rappaport H: Malignant histiocytosis, in Akazaki K, Rappaport H, Berard CW, et al (eds): Malignant Diseases of the Hematopoietic System. Gann Monograph on Cancer Research 15, p 145. Tokyo, University of Tokyo Press, 1973.

214. Warnke RA, Kim H, Dorfman RF: Malignant histio-cytosis (histiocytic medullary reticulosis): A clinico-pathologic study of 29 cases. Cancer 1975; 35:215.

215. Ducatman BS, Wick MR, Morgan TW, et al: Malignant histiocytosis: A clinical, histologic, and immuno-histochemical study of 20 cases. Hum Pathol 1984; 15:368.

216. Sonneveld P, van Lom K, Kappers-Klunne M, et al: Clinicopathological diagnosis and treatment of ma-lignant histiocytosis. Br J Heamatol 1990; 75:511.

217. van Heerde P, Felkamp CA, Hart AA, et al: Malignant histiocytosis and related tumors: A clinicopathologic study of 42 cases using cytologic, histochemical and ultrastructural parameters. Hematol Oncol 1984; 2:13.

218. Vardiman JW, Byrne GE Jr, Rappaport H: Malignant histiocytosis with massive splenomegaly in asympto-matic patients: A possible chronic form of the dis-ease. Cancer 1975; 36:419.

219. Huhn D, Meister P: Malignant histiocytosis: Morpho-logic and cytochemical findings. Cancer 1978; 42:1341.

220. Lampert IA, Catovsky D, Bergier N: Malignant histio-cytosis: A clinicopathological study of 12 cases. Br J Haematol 1978; 40:65.

221. Risdall RJ, Brunning RD, Dehner LP, et al: Malignant histiocytosis: A light- and electron-microscopic and histochemical study. Am J Surg Pathol 1980; 4:439.

222. Goldman JM, Jacobsen BM: Splenectomy for histio-cytic medullary reticulosis. Postgrad Med J 1971; 47:671.

223. Wilson MS, Weiss ML, Gatter KC, et al: Malignant histiocytosis: A reassessment of cases previously re-ported in 1975 based on paraffin section immuno-phenotyping studies. Cancer 1990; 66:530.

224. Stein H, Mason DY, Gerdes J, et al: The expression of the Hodgkin's disease–associated antigen Ki-1 in reactive and neoplastic lymphoid tissue: Evidence that Reed-Sternberg cells and histiocytic malignan-cies are derived from activated lymphoid cells. Blood 1985; 66:848.

225. Pallesen G: Immunophenotypic markers for charac-terizing malignant lymphoma, malignant histio-cytosis and tumors derived from accessory cells. Can-cer Rev 1987; 8:1065.

226. Carbone A, Michaeu C, Caillaud JM, et al: A cyto-chemical and immunohistochemical approach to malignant histiocytosis. Cancer 1981; 47:2862.

227. Weiss LM, Trela MJ, Cleary ML, et al: Frequent immunoglobulin and T-cell receptor gene re-arrangements in "histiocytic" neoplasms. Am J Pa-thol 1985; 121:369.

228. Cattoretti G, Villa A, Vezzoni P, et al: Malignant histiocytosis: A phenotypic and genotypic investiga-tion. Am J Pathol 1990; 136:1009.

229. Isaacson PG, Spencer J, Connolly CH, et al: Malig-nant histiocytosis of the intestine: A T-cell lymphoma. Lancet 1985; 1:688.

230. Jaffe ES, Costa J, Fauci AS, et al: Malignant lym-phoma and erythrophagocytosis simulating malig-nant histiocytosis. Am J Med 1983; 75:741.

231. Chan JK, Ng CS, Hui PK, et al: Anaplastic large cell lymphoma: Delineation of two morphological types. Histopathol 1989; 15:11.

232. Nezelof C, Barbey S, Gogusev J, et al: Malignant histiocytosis in childhood: A distinctive CD30-positive clinicopathologic entity associated with a chromo-somal translocation involving 5q35. Semin Diagn Pa-thol 1992; 9:75.

233. Kaneko Y, Frizzers G, Edamura S, et al: A novel translocation t(2;5)(p23;q35) in childhood phago-cytic large T-cell lymphoma mimicking malignant histiocytosis. Blood 1989; 73:806.

234. Su IJ, Hsu YH, Lin MT, et al: Epstein-Barr virus containing T-cell lymphoma presents with hemopha-gocytic syndrome mimicking malignant histiocytosis. Cancer 1993; 72:2019.

235. Su IJ, Wang CH, Cheng AL, et al: Hemophagocytic syndrome in Epstein-Barr virus–associated T-lympho-proliferative disorders: Disease spectrum, pathogene-sis, and management. Leuk Lymphoma 1995; 19:401.

236. Huhn D, O'Connor NT, Spencer J, et al: Malignant histiocytosis of the intestine: A T-cell lymphoma. Lan-cet 1985; 2:688.

237. Chan JK, Ng CS, Law CK, et al: Reactive hemophago-cytic syndrome: A study of seven fatal cases. Pathol-ogy 1987; 19:43.

238. Wong KF, Chan JK: Hemophagocytic disorders: A review. Hematol Rev 1991; 5:5.

239. Wong KF, Chang JK: Reactive hemophagocytic syn-drome: A clinicopathologic study of 40 patients in an Oriental population. Am J Med 1992; 93:177.

240. Nichols CR, Roth BJ, Heerema N, et al: Hematologic neoplasia associated with primary mediastinal germ-cell tumors. N Engl J Med 1990; 322:1425.

241. DeMent SH, Eggleston JC, Spivak JL: Association between mediastinal germ cell tumors and hemato-logic malignancies. Am J Surg Pathol 1985; 9:23.

242. DeMent SH: Association between mediastinal germ cell tumors and hematologic malignancies: An up-date. Hum Pathol 1990; 21:699.

243. Takahashi S, Asamoto M, Nakazawa T, et al: Robb-Smith type malignant histiocytosis associated with a mediastinal germ cell tumor. Jpn J Clin Oncol 1994; 24:327.

244. Orazi A, Neiman RS, Ulbright TM, et al: Hematopoi-etic precursor cells within the yolk sac tumor compo-nent are the source of secondary hematopoietic ma-lignancies in patients with mediastinal germ cell tumors. Cancer 1993; 71:3873.

245. Ashby MA, Williams CJ, Buchanan RB, et al: Mediasti-nal germ cell tumor associated with malignant histio-cytosis and high rubella titres. Hematol Oncol 1986; 4:183.

246. Beasley SW, Tiedemann K, Howat A, et al: Precocious puberty associated with malignant thoracic teratoma and malignant histiocytosis in a child with Klinefel-ter's syndrome. Med Pediatr Oncol 1987; 15:277.

247. Landanyi M, Indrojit R: Mediastinal germ cell tu-mors and histiocytosis. Hum Pathol 1988; 19:586.

248. van der Volk P, te Velde J, Jansen J, et al: Malignant lymphoma of true histiocytic origin: Histiocytic sar-coma. Virchows Arch 1981; 391:249.

249. Isaacson P, Wright D, Jones DB: Malignant lym-phoma of true histiocytic (monocyte/macrophage) origin. Cancer 1983; 51:80.

250. Pileri S, Mazza P, Rivano MT: Malignant histiocytosis (true histiocytic lymphoma), clinicopathologic study of 25 cases. Histopathology 1985; 9:905.

251. Ralfkiaer E, Delsol G, O'Connor NT, et al: Malignant lymphomas of true histiocytic origin: A clinical, histo-logical, immunophenotypic and genotypic study. J Pathol 1990; 160:9.

252. Soria C, Orradre JL, Garcia-Almagro D, et al: True histiocytic lymphoma (monocytic sarcoma). Am J Dermatopathol 1992; 14:511.

253. Franchino C, Reich C, Distenfeld A, et al: A clinico-

pathological distinctive primary splenic histiocytic neoplasm: Demonstration of its histiocyte derivation by immunophenotypic and molecular genetic analysis. Am J Surg Pathol 1988; 12:398.

254. Gastineau DA, Banks PM, Knowles DM: Primary splenic neoplasm. Am J Surg Pathol 1989; 13:989.

255. Monda L, Warnke R, Rosai J: A primary lymph node malignancy with features suggestive of dendritic reticulum cell differentiation. Am J Pathol 1986; 122:562.

256. Perez-Ordonez B, Erlandson RA, Rosai J: Follicular dendritic cell tumor: Report of 13 additional cases of a distinctive entity. Am J Surg Pathol 1996; 20:944.

257. Chan JKC, Fletcher CDM, Nayler SJ, et al: Follicular dendritic cell sarcoma: Clinicopathologic analysis of 17 cases suggesting a malignant potential higher than currently recognized. Cancer 1997; 79:294.

258. Warnke RA: Tumors of lymph nodes and spleen, in Atlas of Tumor Pathology, 3rd series, fascicle 14, p 360. Washington, DC, Armed Forces Institute of Pathology, 1966.

259. Nakamura S, Koshikawa T, Kitoh K, et al: Interdigitating cell sarcoma: A morphologic and immunologic study of lymph node lesions in four cases. Pathol Int 1994; 44:374.

260. Miettinen M, Fletcher CD, Lasota J: True histiocytic lymphoma of small intestine: Analysis of two S-100 protein-positive cases with features of interdigitating reticulum cell sarcoma. Am J Clin Pathol 1993; 100:285.

261. Chan WC, Zaatari G: Lymph node interdigitating reticulum cell sarcoma. Am J Clin Pathol 1986; 85:739.

262. Lieu PK, Ho J, Ng HS: Primary malignant fibrous histiocytoma of the spleen and liver: A case report. Ann Acad Med 1993; 22:390.

263. Foucar E, Rosai J, Dorfman R: Sinus histiocytosis with massive lymphadenopathy (Rosai-Dorfman disease): Review of the entity. Semin Diagn Pathol 1990; 7:19.

264. Hernandez D, Gutierrez L, Duque H, et al: Association of sinus histiocytosis with massive lymphadenopathy and idiopathic hypereosinophilic syndrome. Histol Histopathol 1987; 2:239.

12

LEUKEMIAS

Both acute and chronic leukemias regularly involve the spleen; however, the degree varies with the type of leukemia and with the duration of the disease. In patients with acute leukemias, the spleen is usually not significantly enlarged, and morphologic evidence of involvement may be quite subtle. In patients with chronic leukemias, however, the degree of splenomegaly and of leukemic involvement of the organ is usually more pronounced. In some chronic leukemias, such as hairy cell leukemia, this degree may be dramatic and the presenting clinical feature.

Hypersplenism is a common occurrence in leukemias but may vary both in frequency and severity depending on the type and duration of the leukemia. For example, hypersplenism is a characteristic presenting feature of hairy cell leukemia but is rare in most cases of acute lymphoblastic leukemia. Splenectomy may be necessary in cases of leukemia in which hypersplenism results in severe cytopenias. Removal of the spleen may constitute effective therapy to ameliorate the cytopenias, but it usually does not affect the course of the underlying leukemia.

Although hyposplenism is not usually considered to occur in patients with acute leukemia, a recent study[1] demonstrated a deficiency in splenic function in more than 50 percent of patients with this disease, as measured by erythrocyte pit–counting methods. After successful treatment for the leukemia, splenic function returned to normal in all patients.

The cut surface of the spleen in leukemic disorders appears homogeneous, and the white pulp nodules are usually inconspicuous or absent (Color Plate 15). The color varies from gray to dark red, depending on the degree of congestion and white blood cell infil-

tration. Microscopically, the leukemic involvement is invariably in the red pulp (Fig. 12–1). However, peritrabecular and subendothelial leukemic infiltrates may be seen even in early stages of the disease. The leukemic cells usually appear localized primarily in the cords of Billroth of the red pulp, with secondary involvement of the sinuses. The white pulp is usually preserved to some degree until extensive involvement occurs. The presence or absence of residual white pulp is not a reliable differential morphologic feature to distinguish leukemic from nonleukemic disorders. Splenic rupture is a serious complication of the leukemias and is found to result either from infiltration of the trabecular framework and blood vessels by leukemic cells (Fig. 12–2) or by infarction within the organ.[2, 3] Splenic rupture more commonly occurs in the chronic leukemias, particularly chronic myeloid leukemia, than in the acute forms.[4, 5]

ACUTE MYELOID LEUKEMIA

Acute myeloid leukemia (AML) comprises several disorders derived from granulocytic, erythroid, monocytic, and megakaryocytic lineage. The disorders have been classified by the French-American-British (FAB) Cooperative Group into eight subtypes, M0 to M7 (Table 12–1).[6–9] The distinctions among the varying subtypes are based on cytologic and cytochemical examination of blood and bone marrow smears. These distinctions are usually difficult if not impossible in the spleen, even with touch imprints, and should rarely be attempted. However, it is usually possible to distinguish better differentiated forms of megakaryocytic, erythroid, and pure monocytic

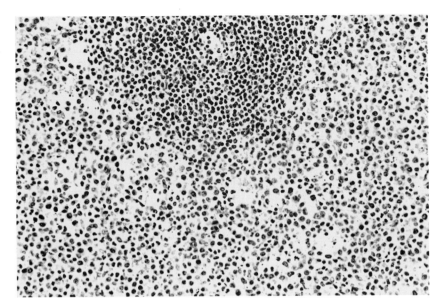

Figure 12–1. Leukemic infiltrations of the spleen, regardless of the cell of origin, involve the red pulp, as illustrated here. The white pulp may remain or be effaced by the infiltrate.

types of acute leukemia in the spleen from the M0 to M3 subtypes, but these latter subtypes may closely resemble one another when examined in tissue sections.

Splenic involvement in all types of AML may occur either "de novo" or as the "final common pathway" secondary to cytoxic therapy, the terminal phase or blast crisis of a chronic myeloproliferative disorder (MPD), or the acute transformation of myelodysplastic syn-

dromes. Distinction among these subtypes of acute leukemia in tissue sections of the spleen is usually impossible on morphologic grounds alone. However, in the examples of transformation of MPDs, the presence of hematopoietic cells of the other major cell lines (i.e. erythroid precursors, immature granulocytes, and megakaryocytes within the splenic red pulp) usually suggests that the disease has evolved from an MPD in chronic disease

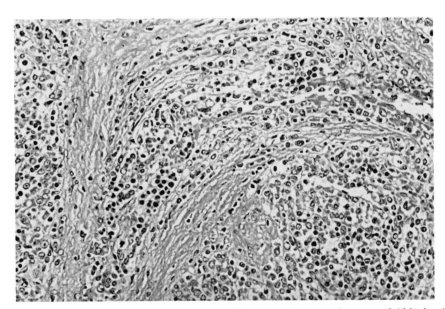

Figure 12–2. Infiltration of the trabecular vessels of the spleen in a case of acute myeloid leukemia.

Table 12–1. Modified French-American-British (FAB) Classification of Acute Myeloid Leukemias

AML-M0	Acute myeloblastic leukemia, minimally differentiated
AML-M1	Acute myeloblastic leukemia, without maturation
AML-M2	Acute myeloblastic leukemia, with maturation
AML-M3	Acute promyelocytic leukemia
	1. Hypergranular
	2. Microgranular
AML-M4	Acute myelomonocytic leukemia
AML-M5	Acute monocytic leukemia
	1. AML-M5a Acute monoblastic leukemia
	2. AML-M5b Acute monocytic leukemia, differentiated
AML-M6	Erythroleukemia
AML-M7	Acute megakaryoblastic leukemia

phase. It is unusual in the de novo acute leukemias for hematopoietic cells other than the leukemic line itself to be found in any significant numbers in the spleen, unless there is associated marrow fibrosis and leukoerythroblastosis in the peripheral blood.

Because splenectomy is rarely indicated in the acute leukemias, there are few published studies of the pathology of the spleen in these disorders. The following descriptions are therefore based largely on the authors' experience.

Acute Myeloid Leukemias (M0 to M3)

These subtypes of AML are neoplastic disorders involving the bone marrow in which the predominant proliferating cell is an immature granulocyte. The FAB Group defines four subsets of AML based on the percentage of maturing cells beyond the myeloblast stage. These range from myeloid leukemia minimally differentiated (M0) to promyelocytic leukemia (M3), in which the dominant cell is an abnormal promyelocyte. The distinction between subtypes, especially M1 and M2, is somewhat arbitrary, and in many cases a continuous spectrum of myeloid maturation is observed. The spleen in these disorders is usually only mildly to moderately enlarged. A cross section of the organ usually reveals a pale pink or salmon color but may also appear deeply congested. Acute myeloblastic leukemia (M1 and M2) is characterized by the presence of blast cells with round to slightly indented nuclei with fine chromatin and one or more distinct nucleoli. The cytoplasm in all four variants is

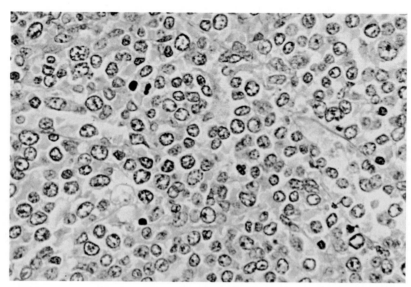

Figure 12–3. Acute myeloblastic leukemia. The leukemic cells appear to have little differentiation.

usually abundant and, with hematoxylin and eosin and periodic acid–Schiff (PAS) stains, appears finely granular and pink to red (Fig. 12–3). In touch imprints, nonspecific granules of promyelocytes and occasionally Auer rods may be noted. A monocytic component may be suggested by the presence of cells with folded or bean-shaped nuclei and pale cytoplasm, which may appear vacuolated (Fig. 12–4).[10] Cytochemical stains of touch imprints are positive for myeloperoxidase, Sudan black B, and/or chloroacetate esterase (CAE) in myeloid precursors.[11–14] Although CAE positivity may also be noted in tissue sections, CAE is no longer widely used, having been replaced by more reliable and more sensitive immunohistologic stains.

When immunophenotyping by flow cytometry is not available, immunohistochemistry is the most effective method for confirming the myeloid lineage of leukemic cells in tissue sections of the spleen as well as of other organs. The most widely used immunohistologic stains for myeloid cells in tissue sections such as those of the spleen are antimyeloperoxidase, antielastase, antilysozyme, CD15 (Leu-M1), and CD43 (DF-T1; Leu-22). Of these, only the first two are specific for cells of granulocytic lineage.[15, 16] CD43 is the least specific of these antigens, reacting with the blast cells of T-cell precursor, B-cell, or myeloid lineage.[17, 18] CD15 positivity has been reported in B- and T-cell lymphomas (as well as in Reed-Sternberg cells and nonhematologic malignancies).[19] CD15 has the disadvantage of being less sensitive and more variable in its positivity than other myeloid antigens.[19, 20] Antilysozyme is a useful marker for myeloid cells, but it also stains cells of the monocyte-macrophage series.[21] Antielastase is less sensitive than antimyeloperoxidase[16, 22, 23] because it appears later in the course of myeloid maturation than other enzymes such as myeloperoxidase.[16, 23] Our experience leads us to agree with Traweek et al[22] that myeloperoxidase is the single most useful antigen of the group in identifying AML in tissue sections. However, we believe that a battery of markers should be performed in order to maximize the positive yield in these cases.

The tumor cells in acute promyelocytic leukemia (M3)[24] usually contain more coarse granules and are more intensely pink in tissue sections, imparting a characteristic histologic appearance, particularly with the PAS stain (Fig. 12–5). In touch imprints numerous Auer rods may be seen.[25] However, a variant of acute promyelocytic leukemia, the microgranular variant, may have basophilic cytoplasm with granules so small that they may be seen only by electron microscopy.[26, 27] In tissue sections, this form of promyelocytic leukemia may be impossible to distinguish from the more usual forms of AML, M4 or M5 in particular. Acute eosinophilic[28] and acute basophilic leukemia[29, 30] are extremely rare disorders that may have splenic involvement.

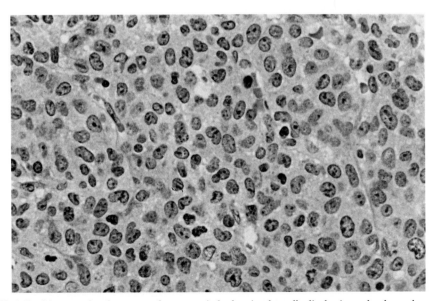

Figure 12–4. In this example of acute myelomonocytic leukemia, the cells display irregular, bean-shaped nuclei.

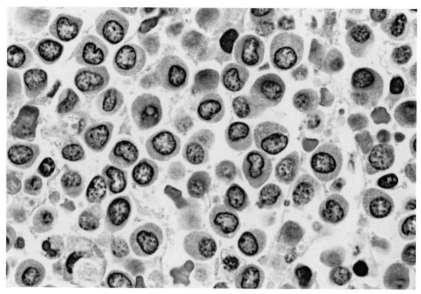

Figure 12–5. Acute promyelocytic leukemia (M3). Many of the cells have lobulated nuclei. Cytoplasm is abundant and granular.

Acute Myelomonocytic Leukemia (M4) and Acute Monoblastic Leukemia (M5a, M5b)

In the M4 subtype, the blast cells have characteristics of both the M2 subtype and acute monocytic leukemia. The proportion of promonocytes and monocytes is greater than 20 percent in the bone marrow or peripheral blood. Patients often present with extramedullary disease; gingival hypertrophy, leukemia cutis, and meningeal leukemia are more common than in the subtypes M0 to M3. Acute monoblastic leukemia is characterized by a monomorphous population of blast cells that show morphologic features of monoblasts with a variable degree of differentiation (Fig. 12–6). M5 is divided into two subtypes: a poorly differentiated monoblastic leukemia (M5a) and a differentiated monocytic leukemia (M5b).[31] Nuclear folding is often apparent, and the cytoplasm of the tumor cells may have pseudopods and may contain small vacuoles or fine azurophilic granules, although Auer rods are not seen. The leukemic cells may demonstrate phagocytosis of other blood elements.[32] The tumor cells stain positively with alpha-naphthyl acetate esterase, which is inhibited by sodium fluoride, and the butyrate esterase reaction. The cells usually demonstrate diffuse granular acid phosphatase. They do not stain for myeloperoxidase, CAE, and Sudan black B.[31, 33–35] The tumor cells may also express CD68 by immunohistochemistry. Acute monoblastic leukemia is often associated with a very high leukocyte count and extensive extramedullary involvement.[32, 35–37] Splenomegaly is the rule in acute monoblastic leukemia, often to a greater degree than in the other forms of acute leukemia, and infiltration of the organ by leukemic cells may be striking.

Erythroleukemia (M6)

DiGuglielmo[38] coined the term "erythremic myelosis" for a proliferation of immature erythroid cells resembling leukemia. Subsequently, he expanded the term to include cases involving a mixed proliferation of the erythroid and myeloid cell lines. Although the terminology in the literature is often confusing, "erythremic myelosis" has usually been reserved for a pure proliferation of erythroid elements, whereas "erythroleukemia" refers to a mixed proliferation of both erythroid and myeloid cells that terminates in an AML or myelomonocytic leukemia.[39] The varying disorders described by DiGuglielmo are now thought to fit in part into the group of myelodysplastic (preleukemic) syndromes. The diagnosis of M6 is based on revised criteria established by the FAB Group in 1985.[40] This diagnosis requires an erythroblastic component of at least 50 percent of all bone marrow nucleated cells and a myeloblastic cell compo-

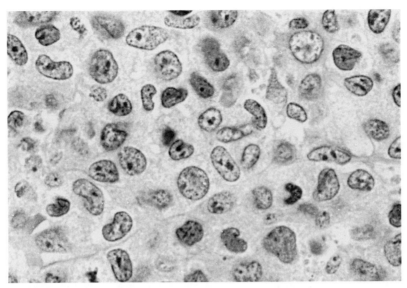

Figure 12–6. Monoblastic leukemia. Nuclear folding is apparent. The cells have copious cytoplasm that contains vacuoles, which may be faintly seen in tissue sections.

nent of at least 30 percent of the nonerythroid cells. In cases of AML in which erythroblasts are a prominent marrow finding and vary between 30 and 50 percent of nucleated marrow cells and myeloblasts number greater than 30 percent of the remaining cells, a diagnosis of erythroleukemia is warranted. If the erythroid percentage exceeds 50 percent, the diagnosis depends on the myeloblast percentage of the remaining nonerythroid cells. If it equals or exceeds 30 percent, the disorder should be termed erythroleukemia; if it is less than 30 percent, the disorder should be categorized as a myelodysplastic syndrome.[39]

The peripheral blood in erythroleukemia shows dysplastic nucleated erythroid cells that are usually macrocytic with basophilic stippling and polychromatophilia. The red cell population may be dimorphic with macro-ovalocytes and hypochromic microcytic forms. Thrombocytopenia with giant platelets showing abnormal granulation and neutropenia are common. Splenomegaly is often a feature of erythroleukemia and may be prominent in the chronic phase. In the few cases of splenic involvement in M6 we have seen, the spleen contains immature erythroid and myeloid cells but few or no megakaryocytes.

The morphologic features of the spleen in erythremic myelosis show involvement that appears preferentially sinusoidal, as opposed to the predominant involvement of the cords in the myeloid leukemias.[41] Large leukemia cells

tend to cluster in cohesive masses (Fig. 12–7). Multinucleated cells are frequent (Fig. 12–8). The mononuclear cells resemble megaloblasts in tissue sections, having grayish cytoplasm and round nuclei with single central nucleoli and fine chromatin typical of megaloblasts in the bone marrow. Occasionally, the erythroid nature of the more primitive erythroid cells can be recognized by the close association with mature normoblasts with pyknotic nuclei and copious pink or gray cytoplasm. In our experience as well as that of others, the erythroid nature of the blast cells can best be demonstrated with the immunoperoxidase technique using an antibody to hemoglobin.[41, 42] Other useful markers reactive in paraffin sections for erythroid cells include antiglycoprotein A[43] and C.[44] In cases of erythroleukemia, in addition to the erythroid infiltration there may be a variable degree of myeloid infiltration.

Acute Megakaryoblastic Leukemia (M7)

This subtype, in which at least 50 percent of the marrow blasts are of megakaryocytic lineage,[45] has distinctive morphologic features in the spleen (Fig. 12–9). Multinucleated cells resembling dysplastic megakaryocytes with megaloblastic-appearing, loosely lobulated nuclei and/or hyperchromatic pyknotic nuclei infiltrate cords and sinuses. Many of the blasts, termed "micromegakaryoblasts," appear mono-

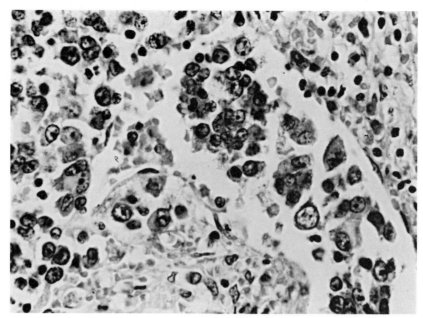

Figure 12–7. Acute erythroleukemia (M6). The erythroid nature of the blast cells in these cases may be surmised by their sinusoidal location and by the presence of associated more mature red cell precursors.

nuclear and are smaller than normal megakaryoblasts.[46] However, even the mononuclear variants contain copious, somewhat granular, PAS-positive cytoplasm that may have irregular borders as a manifestation of platelet shedding. However, megakaryopoiesis is ineffective, and the patients are usually thrombocytopenic. The dysplastic features of the nuclei and the presence of these cells in the red pulp of the spleen may mimic malignant histiocytosis. However, the clinical presentation; the absence of erythrophagocytosis; and the positive

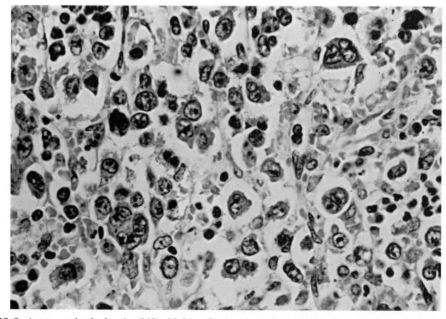

Figure 12–8. Acute erythroleukemia (M6). Multinucleation is a characteristic feature of erythroid leukemias and megakaryocytic leukemias. Such multinucleated cells are extremely uncommon in leukemias of myeloid origin.

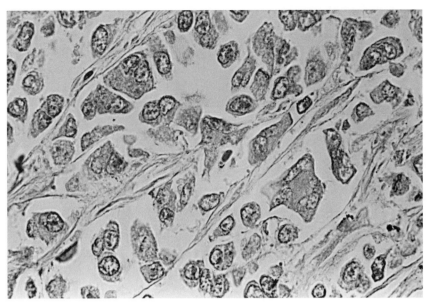

Figure 12-9. Acute megakaryoblastic leukemia (M7). Dysplastic megakaryocytes and promegakaryocytes infiltrate the cords.

staining with platelet factor VIII (von Willebrand factor)[47, 48] or platelet glycoproteins Ib, IIb/IIIa, and IIIa[49] as well as negative staining with such reagents as myeloperoxidase or lysozyme should allow the appropriate distinction between the two diseases. In addition, the tumor cells may stain positively with the alphanaphthyl acetate esterase reaction, which is partially inhibited by sodium fluoride. The demonstration of a platelet peroxidase using immunoelectron microscopy may also confirm the megakaryoblastic origin of the tumor cells.[50, 51] Antibodies to platelet glycoproteins are quite sensitive but not specific, having been reported to cross-react with leukemic erythroblasts in cases of M6 in patients with Down syndrome and to cross-react with monocytes.[52–54] In general, the factor VIII–related antigen (von Willebrand factor) is as sensitive for immature megakaryoblasts as is the antibody detected against platelet glycoprotein IIb to IIIa.[45, 55] In our experience, factor VIII staining represents the most useful marker for megakaryocytes and their precursors in tissue sections.

CHRONIC MYELOID LEUKEMIA

Chronic myeloid leukemia (CML) is associated with splenomegaly that may reach massive proportions.[56] The gross appearance of the spleen is solid and deep red without nodules (Color Plate 16). CML generally obliterates the white pulp, although occasionally small remnants of lymphoid follicles may persist. Fibrosis of the splenic cords may be prominent, particularly in prolonged illness or if the spleen has been irradiated. There may be subendothelial invasion of the splenic trabecular veins and infiltration of fibrous trabeculae, and infarcts are common. The cellular infiltrate is polymorphous, including myeloid cells at all stages of maturation (Fig. 12–10). The presence of eosinophilic myelocytes is often a useful aid in recognition of this tumor. Primitive granulocytes can be identified in tissue sections using the immunoperoxidase technique with an antimyeloperoxidase antibody.[15]

The majority of cases of CML terminate with the development of a clinical and morphologic disorder that resembles leukemia. This aggressive phase has been termed "transformation," "metamorphosis," "accelerated phase," or simply, "blast crisis."[57–61] Some researchers have subdivided this phenomenon into two forms: blast crisis and accelerated phase. Although blast transformation is most common and best characterized in CML, it may also occur in any of the other chronic MPDs (see Chapter 13). It has been stated that in a third of the cases of blast crisis, the clone giving rise to the blast cells arises in an extramedullary site, and the spleen appears to be

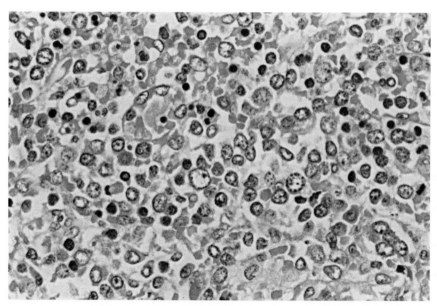

Figure 12–10. Chronic myeloid leukemia. Granulocytes in all stages of maturation are seen.

the most common of these extramedullary sites. Some investigators have reported that multiple cytogenetic abnormalities, including hyperdiploidy, may be found in the myeloid elements in the spleen before their appearance in the marrow, suggesting that an abnormal, more malignant clone arises in the spleen in some patients.[62-66] Gomez and colleagues[67] demonstrated an increased doubling time of the circulating immature cells following splenectomy in 9 of 14 patients, suggesting that a more rapidly proliferating clone existed in the spleen. Other studies have shown greater proliferative activity in the granulocytes from the spleen in CML than in marrow cells.[68-70]

The most common manifestation of splenic transformation of CML is a sudden and, in some cases, dramatic increase in the size of the organ. This may be accompanied by the development of pain because of pressure on the splenic capsule or because of infarction secondary to the proliferation of myeloid cells. Examination of the spleen in blast transformation shows a homogeneous cut surface. Occasionally, however, there may be nodules (Color Plate 17) composed largely of myeloblasts or of megakaryocytes. Histologically, clusters and aggregates of myeloblasts may be seen around trabeculae or forming ill-defined nodules of blastic cells in a spleen that in other locations shows maturation of granulocytic elements. Although occasionally evidence of trilinear hematopoiesis may be observed in CML, CML

can be distinguished from the myeloid metaplasia occurring in chronic idiopathic myelofibrosis or the spent phase of polycythemia vera in that in CML the erythroid and megakaryocytic maturation represents only a minority of the infiltrating cells. In the other two diseases, particularly in their later stages, the erythroid and megakaryocytic lineages appear dominant.

In approximately 25 to 35 percent of cases, the blast cells in the blastic phase of CML morphologically resemble lymphoblasts and contain the nuclear enzyme terminal deoxynucleotidyl transferase (TdT).[58, 59, 69, 71] In these cases the morphologic features of the blast cells in the spleen resemble the lymphoblasts in acute lymphoblastic leukemia or lymphoblastic lymphoma (Fig. 12–11). The lineage of the proliferating cells can best be characterized by immunohistologic stains for TdT, myeloperoxidase, hemoglobin, and factor VIII (von Willebrand) antigen.

Because of the high incidence of splenic blast transformation in CML, early prophylactic-therapeutic splenectomy has been advocated.[72-74] However, the role of splenectomy is controversial. Although it may be palliative in cases associated with hypersplenism,[75] an increased incidence of infectious and thrombotic complications may be associated with splenectomy.[75-79] Some investigators have suggested that elective splenectomy before blast crisis may decrease the incidence of transfor-

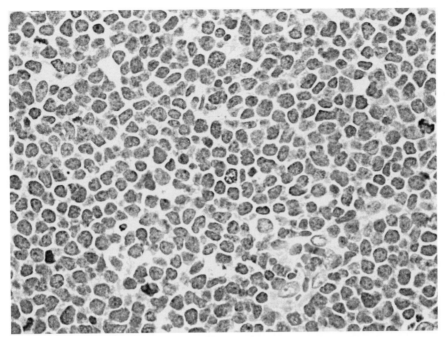

Figure 12–11. Lymphoblastic transformation of chronic myeloid leukemia. The cytologic features of the tumor cells are indistinguishable from those of lymphoblastic lymphoma or childhood acute lymphoblastic leukemia.

mation and prolong survival as well as ameliorate cytopenias resulting from hypersplenism.[73, 74, 80–82] Spiers et al[74] stated that the onset of blast crisis was delayed in splenectomized patients, and that during blast crisis splenectomized patients had an improved tolerance to chemotherapy. In contrast, Idhe and coworkers[73] and Wolf et al[82] found no delay in blast transformation or increased responsiveness to chemotherapy in splenectomized patients, although the former investigators did report a slightly prolonged survival among splenectomized patients once the disease entered blastic transformation. Splenectomy during blast crisis has not been shown to prolong survival.

Chronic Monocytic Leukemia

Chronic monocytic leukemia is a rare disorder. Five cases were reported by Bearman and colleagues.[83] The clinical course was similar in all patients, who presented with prominent splenomegaly and cytopenias. Peripheral blood and bone marrow monocytosis developed following splenectomy. The spleens were infiltrated by mature-appearing monocytes with folded or lobulated nuclei, fine chromatin, and gray cytoplasm with small vacuoles or granules. The monocytes demonstrated

phagocytosis of other blood elements. Following the appearance of the peripheral blood monocytosis, the disease tended to pursue a rapid course. These authors postulated that chronic monocytic leukemia is a distinct clinicopathologic entity in which prominent splenomegaly is a typical presenting manifestation.

LYMPHOID LEUKEMIAS

Acute Lymphoblastic Leukemia

Acute lymphoblastic leukemia (ALL) is predominantly a disease of childhood. Although enlargement of the spleen, liver, and peripheral lymph nodes often progresses during the course of the disease, organomegaly is not usually apparent at the time of diagnosis. When it is present, it is usually associated with adverse prognostic factors.[84]

ALL has been subdivided by both morphologic and immunologic parameters.[85] The most common type of ALL—L1, according to the FAB classification—is characterized by small lymphoblasts with round-to-oval nuclei, indistinct nucleoli, and scanty cytoplasm.[85, 86] The other forms of ALL include L2, composed of larger, more immature-appearing lymphoid cells with pleomorphic nuclei and prominent nucleoli; and L3, composed of tumor cells with deeply basophilic, often vacuolated cytoplasm resembling the cells of Burkitt lymphoma. Approximately 85 percent of cases of ALL are classified as L1 and 15 percent as L2 (L3 is a relatively rare variant[85]).

Immunophenotypically, ALL is divided into three main subtypes: precursor B-cell (early pre-B, pre-B), T-cell, and mature B-cell, which have been correlated by some to the FAB Group's L1, L2, and L3 subtypes, respectively. However, this correlation is weak, and many exceptions exist. The most common immunologic subtype of ALL, representing 70 to 80 percent of all cases, is precursor B-cell. This variant is the most frequent type in children. The lymphoblasts of precursor B-cell ALL lack the surface markers of mature B or T cells and express CD34, HLA-DR, CD10, CD19, and usually also TdT. The leukemic cells in approximately 25 percent of cases of precursor B-cell ALL contain cytoplasmic IgM, characteristic of pre-B lymphocytes.[86] Those cases of precursor B-cell ALL not expressing cytoplasmic IgM have also been termed "early pre–B-cell ALL," and those expressing this cytoplasmic heavy chain have been termed "pre–B-cell ALL."

The next most common subtype is T-cell ALL, representing approximately 15 percent of all cases. This subtype variably expresses T-cell antigens CD2, CD4, CD5, CD7, CD8, and CD10 as well as TdT. Attempts have been made to subclassify T-cell ALL according to the stage of thymocyte development, but this has been of limited value.

The third and least common form of ALL is the mature B-cell type. This type represents 5 percent or less of all cases of ALL, and it expresses such B-cell antigens as CD20 and monoclonal surface immunoglobulin. It is the leukemic counterpart of malignant lymphoma, small noncleaved cell, or Burkitt, type. Most investigators believe that acute leukemia of mature B-cell type is a disseminated form of Burkitt lymphoma, because both conditions share common cytogenetic, molecular genetic, immunologic, cytologic, and clinical features.[87]

Cytochemical study of ALL cells, regardless of the subtype, reveals the absence of myeloperoxidase, nonspecific esterase, and Sudan black staining. In addition, most ALL cells contain either fine or coarse PAS-positive granules. Some cases of T-cell ALL also may demonstrate perinuclear acid phosphatase positivity. However, in our experience, this is not specific because we have seen it in precursor B-cell ALL cases as well.

Splenomegaly occurs in only about 10 percent of ALL cases and is most frequent in the T-cell subtype. Morphologic studies of splenic involvement in ALL are rare because splenectomy is rarely, if ever, performed. In the few cases we have seen, the patterns of splenic involvement are identical in all cases, regardless of subtype. The infiltrate is sparse and invariably in the red pulp. In precursor B-cell and T-cell ALL, the tumor cells in tissue sections resemble those of lymphoblastic lymphoma. In mature B-cell ALL, the cells have cytologic features of small noncleaved B lymphocytes. Demonstration of these cells in tissue section may be difficult on morphologic grounds alone. We have found the utilization of anti-TdT and CD99 (013) immunostains[88, 89] to be of value in the diagnosis of cases of pre B-cell and T-cell ALL. These stains are negative in mature B-cell ALL.

Chronic Lymphocytic Leukemia

Splenomegaly may be an early feature of chronic lymphocytic leukemia (CLL) but more often is a hallmark of more aggressive, high-stage disease. Splenomegaly in CLL is rarely as massive as it is in CML. A palpable spleen has been reported in 50 percent of patients at the time of diagnosis, with massive splenomegaly in 10 to 15 percent.[90] Occasional cases of CLL have been reported in which the spleen was extremely enlarged at the time of diagnosis, while peripheral blood lymphocytosis was mild or absent.[91] Such cases overlap with malignant lymphoma small lymphocytic type described in Chapter 8.

Grossly, the follicular markings of the spleen may be accentuated due to expansion of the malpighian corpuscles or may be obliterated due to diffuse involvement (Color Plate 18). CLL is unique in that it is the only leukemia in which the splenic white pulp is involved. The white pulp involvement is characterized by infiltration and replacement by morphologically mature small lymphocytes forming irregular small nodules (Fig. 12–12). There are no germinal centers or distinct mantle zones. The tumor cells have coarse chromatin, and nucleoli are not apparent. Mitoses are rare. In the early stages, the tumor may be difficult to distinguish from the immunologically unstimulated adult spleen. These small cells may be associated with larger lymphoid cells with vesicular nuclei and distinct nucleoli, analogous

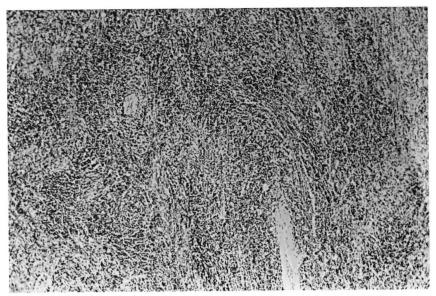

Figure 12–12. Chronic lymphocytic leukemia. Involvement of the spleen is unique among leukemias in that it affects both red and white pulp.

to the prolymphocytes or paraimmunoblasts described in lymph nodes involved with small lymphocytic lymphoma/CLL.[91–93] The lymphocytes usually infiltrate the red pulp as well (Fig. 12–13). In advanced disease the diffuse red pulp involvement may become striking, often obscuring the white pulp. Infiltration of the trabecular veins is a common finding, occasionally leading to splenic rupture.[94] The morphologic diagnosis can be confirmed by immunophenotyping. The typical small lymphocytic lymphoma/CLL phenotype has been described (see Chapter 8).

Splenic enlargement in CLL may result in secondary hypersplenism, which may necessitate splenectomy.[95] A more frequent cause of cytopenias is autoimmune hemolytic anemia or thrombocytopenia, which complicates CLL in 5 to 10 percent of cases.[96, 97]

Marked splenomegaly, particularly when associated with severe anemia or thrombocytopenia, has been recognized as a poor prognostic sign in CLL.[98] Rai and coworkers[99] devised a clinical staging system based on the belief that CLL is a progressive accumulative disease. Stage II, with palpable splenomegaly, was asso-

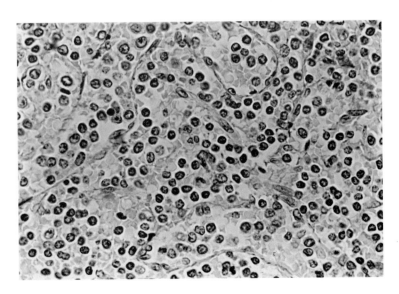

Figure 12–13. Chronic lymphocytic leukemia. Tumor cells infiltrate the cords and sinuses of the red pulp.

ciated with a median survival of 71 months in their series, compared with 150 months for stage 0 (lymphocytosis only) and 101 months for stage I (enlarged lymph nodes). Patients with thrombocytopenia or anemia, or both, had a median survival of only 19 months. A simpler staging system has been established by an international study group.[100] Patients who have splenomegaly but lack cytopenias are usually treated with single-agent chemotherapy. Splenectomy is usually reserved for patients with advanced disease and severe cytopenias. Adler and associates[101] reported an improvement in hematologic parameters following splenectomy in 80 percent of patients with advanced disease and hypersplenism. In addition, patients who responded to splenectomy also had an increased tolerance to further chemotherapy and irradiation. These investigators found that failure to demonstrate sequestration in the spleen of ^{51}Cr-labeled erythrocytes did not preclude favorable response to splenectomy. The effect of splenectomy in overall survival in advanced CLL is a subject of controversy. In a single-institution study of 50 cases from the Mayo Clinic, Neal et al[102] found that splenectomy was effective in relieving refractory cytopenias secondary to splenomegaly. Although the perioperative mortality rate was quite low, there was no proven effect on overall survival. A more recent study from Australia, however, demonstrated that splenectomy was associated with a strong trend for improved overall survival in Rai stage IV patients.[103] Local irradiation may be useful in patients with CLL with marked splenomegaly who are poor surgical risks for splenectomy.[104]

Prolymphocytoid Transformation of CLL

In most cases of CLL, a variable but small number of prolymphocytes are noted in the blood. These cells are characterized by larger size than those of typical CLL cells; coarse nuclear chromatin with a typically prominent, central nucleolus with condensation of chromatin around it; and a moderate amount of cytoplasm. In typical CLL these cells constitute less than 10 percent of the circulating lymphocytes. However, in 10 percent of cases over a variable chronic period stated to be from 1.3 to 5 years, prolymphocytoid transformation occurs. This is characterized by the presence of an increasing number and percentage of prolymphocytes in the blood and the development of splenomegaly and lymphadenopa-thy.[105] The prolymphocytes in these cases usually retain the immunophenotype of the original CLL cells but frequently display more intense surface immunoglobulin and may lose their CD5 coexpression.

Examination of the spleen in prolymphocytoid transformation reveals an infiltrate similar in pattern to that in typical CLL but with many of the infiltrating lymphocytes displaying the morphologic characteristics of prolymphocytes.

Some patients may present with 11 to 54 percent prolymphocytes in the blood, prominent lymphadenopathy, and splenomegaly. These cases should be designated CLL/prolymphocytic leukemia.[106] Involvement of the spleen in these cases is indistinguishable from that in prolymphocytoid transformation.

Richter Transformation of CLL

In a small number of CLL cases, a complication occurs characterized by the development of a high-grade B-cell lymphoproliferative disease with systemic symptoms (so-called Richter transformation). This transformation may be in the form of a diffuse large cell lymphoma, diffuse small cleaved cell lymphoma, or lymphoblastic lymphoma/leukemia. The spleen may be involved by this transformation. Although it is commonly thought that Richter transformation represents dedifferentiation of the lymphocytes of the underlying CLL, this issue is not resolved.[106] Although most studies have revealed similar characteristics in both the underlying CLL cells and the transformed cells in some cases,[107, 108] differences between the two-cell populations have also been reported.[109–111]

CLL, T-Cell Type

A small number of lymphocytic leukemias of CD4- and CD8-positive subtypes have been sporadically reported for some years.[112–123] Many of these subtypes have displayed overlapping clinical and laboratory features with a disorder characterized by neutropenia and T-cell lymphocytosis.[118–131] These cases are now termed large granular lymphocytic (LGL) leukemia. We have had the opportunity to study the spleen in several cases of CLL of confirmed T-cell type that do not bear the morphologic hallmarks of LGL. As in B-cell CLL, there was a diffuse infiltrate of small lymphocytes in cords and sinuses of the red pulp. In contrast to B-cell CLL, there was no involvement of the white pulp.

Prolymphocytic Leukemia

Prolymphocytic leukemia (PLL) is an uncommon variant of CLL in which more than 55 percent of the lymphocytes in the blood are prolymphocytes.[132, 133] Although the original cases described were of B-cell immunophenotype, it is now recognized that a T-cell counterpart also exists.[134, 135]

Approximately three quarters of the reported cases of PLL are of B-cell immunophenotype. The disease occurs in older patients and most commonly affects males.[133] It is characterized by extremely high white blood cell counts, with frequent anemia and thrombocytopenia. Splenomegaly is usually marked, and lymphadenopathy not commonly present.[133, 135, 136]

The tumor cells are larger than the small lymphocytes of CLL and have vesicular nuclei that are round to oval or slightly irregular, often with a single prominent nucleolus (Fig. 12–14). The chromatin is usually coarser than that of lymphoblasts, and mitoses are rare. The cytoplasm is abundant and pale blue and lacks granules. Occasional cells appear more blastic. Immunophenotypically, the cells of B-PLL express strong surface immunoglobin of either IgM or IgD or both. The cells also express CD19, CD20, and CD24; they usually do not express CD5, CD11c, CD22, or CD23.

Clinically, T-PLL is more heterogenous than B-PLL.[137] Although the median-age incidence is similar to that of B-cell CLL, cases have been reported in younger patients. A striking lymphocytosis also occurs in T-cell PLL. Cytologically, the T prolymphocytes may display greater morphologic variability than do B-PLL cells and may demonstrate nuclear irregularities. Splenomegaly, hepatomegaly, lymphadenopathy, and skin lesions are characteristic. T prolymphocytes are characterized by the expression of T-cell markers CD2, CD3, CD5, and CD7. The majority also express CD4, a minority may express both CD4 and CD8, and a minority may express CD8 alone. The majority of patients with T-PLL have cytogenetic abnormalities associated with chromosomes 14 or 8. In the few cases we have studied of T-PLL involving the spleen, the pattern of involvement is similar to that of B-PLL.

The degree of splenomegaly in PLL is usually much more marked than in CLL. Patterns of infiltration, however, are similar to that of CLL. PLL may affect the splenic white pulp primarily. Bearman and colleagues[136] described a prominent nodular pattern in the spleen resulting from both nodular and diffuse replacement of the white and red pulp in cases that showed B-cell markers, whereas their single T-cell case revealed diffuse infiltration of the red pulp only. Despite the primitive appearance of the cells, mitotic activity is usually low; but occasional cases with a high mitotic rate occur.[138] Splenic irradiation has little

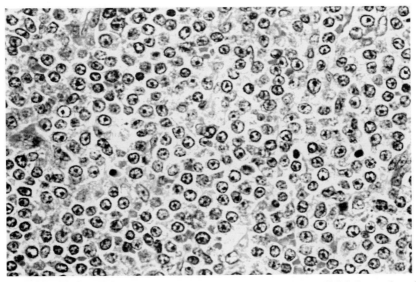

Figure 12–14. Prolymphocytic leukemia. Tumor cells infiltrating the red pulp are slightly larger than the lymphocytes of chronic lymphocytic leukemia and contain more cytoplasm. Note the characteristic single prominent nucleoli.

effect on splenic size in patients with this disorder.[137] Splenectomy may be palliative for the cytopenias but has no lasting effect on the circulating lymphocyte count. The response to chemotherapy is usually poor and survival quite short.

Hairy Cell Leukemia

Perhaps the most characteristic leukemic disorder involving the spleen is hairy cell leukemia (HCL). It is typically a disease of middle-aged males who present with massive splenomegaly; cytopenias, especially monocytopenia; and inconspicuous lymphadenopathy.[139-142] Leukemic cells are usually scarce in the peripheral blood, and the presence of an increased bone marrow reticulin content often results in an inability to aspirate the marrow. Although bone marrow biopsy is frequently a successful diagnostic procedure,[143] splenectomy is often performed for diagnosis.

The spleen in HCL grossly appears homogeneous, dark red, and firm with occasional infarcts (Color Plate 19). The white pulp is inconspicuous, and tumor nodules are not seen. The tumor cells infiltrate the red pulp cords and sinuses, obliterating the normal architecture, and the white pulp (Fig. 12–15).[144-146] Cytologically the cells have round, oval, or bean-shaped nuclei with delicate chromatin, inconspicuous nucleoli, and abundant cytoplasm with indistinct cell borders (Fig. 12–16). Mitoses are vanishingly rare. Subendothelial

invasion of trabecular veins is prominent; and predominant localization of the leukemic infiltrate around fibrous trabeculae or subendothelial regions of the trabecular veins is frequent in spleens with early involvement. On purely morphologic grounds, HCL and large granular lymphocytic leukemia may closely resemble one another in tissue sections and in touch imprints as well as in clinical presentation. They are easily separable on immunologic grounds, however: hairy cells are B cells, and large granular lymphocytes are either T or NK cells. The pattern of splenic involvement in HCL resembles that of malignant histiocytosis. However, the tumor cells in HCL lack the cytologic atypia and phagocytic activity of the neoplastic cells of malignant histiocytosis. The splenic infiltrate in HCL may also superficially resemble that of myeloid leukemia, from which it can be differentiated by either the lack of a polymorphous infiltrate or eosinophilic myelocytes or evidence of mitotic activity in the latter disorder. Finally, HCL must be differentiated from mast cell disease. Both the cytologic appearance and pattern of involvement of mast cell disease may mimic HCL, because mast cell infiltrates are frequently composed of round cells with fairly abundant cytoplasm and occasional spindle-shaped variants. However, mast cells contain metachromatic granules that can be demonstrated with Giemsa or toluidine-blue stains and may also be demonstrated by the CAE (Leder) reaction. In addition, immunohistochemical stains in mast cell disease reveal KP-

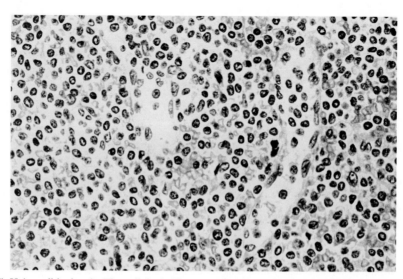

Figure 12–15. Hairy cell leukemia. The cellular infiltrate involves the red pulp and affects both cords and sinuses.

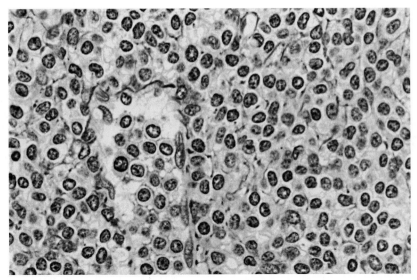

Figure 12–16. The tumor cells of hairy cell leukemia have round-to-oval nuclei and virtually no mitotic activity. The cells appear set apart from one another because of the large amount of cytoplasm, which in tissue sections is often inconspicuous because of the relative lack of cytoplasmic organelles.

1 (CD68) positivity and a lack of reactivity with CD20 and DBA.44.

Although not entirely specific,[147, 148] an important diagnostic feature in HCL is the tartrate-resistant acid phosphatase positivity of the tumor cells, which can be demonstrated cytochemically in the majority in blood or marrow smears or on touch imprints of the spleen[147, 149–151] or immunohistologically in sections of bone marrow or spleen.[152, 153] Cytoplasmic projections, originally seen in phase contrast microscopy and responsible for the term "hairy cell,"[154] may also be seen in blood smears (Fig. 12–17) but are usually not well demonstrated on touch imprints. Ultrastructural examination of the tumor cells reveals distinctive structures termed "ribosome-lamellar complexes" (Fig. 12–18).[145, 155] Although characteristic of HCL, these structures may be difficult to find and are not unique to the disease, having also been reported in cases of CLL and other lymphomas with leukemic dissemination.[148, 156–158]

A characteristic feature in the spleen in HCL is the presence of pseudosinuses or blood lakes in the red pulp (Fig. 12–19).[159] The pseudosinuses range in size from slightly larger than the normal splenic sinuses to large, distended, grossly visible structures that may resemble a hemangioma. Similar angiomatous lesions may be seen in the portal areas of the liver. The pseudosinuses lack ring fibers and are lined by hairy cells. In an electron micro-scopic study, Pilon and coworkers[146] reported that some red pulp sinuses in HCL were lined by hairy cells that attach by their processes to the sinus lining cells. These authors postulated that the tumor cells damage the sinus lining cells, causing their degeneration and leaving the abnormal blood-filled spaces lined by tumor cells. On occasion, the marked congestion of the red pulp and resultant dispersal of hairy cells make recognition of the tumor difficult (Fig. 12–20).

Hypersplenism in HCL results from widening of the pulp cords by tumor cells and from proliferating cordal macrophages. Lewis and associates[160] reported that radioisotope scans in HCL demonstrated a greater degree of splenic red cell pooling compared with other MPDs and lymphoproliferative disorders with comparable degrees of splenomegaly. This phenomenon parallels the morphologic finding of prominent blood lakes in the red pulp. Electron microscopic studies have revealed no evidence of phagocytosis by the tumor cells.[145]

Splenectomy is an effective treatment for HCL and was once the treatment of choice, resulting in remission of the cytopenias and long-term survival without adjuvant therapy in approximately two thirds of cases.[161–163] Splenectomy was usually performed once symptomatic cytopenias developed. Relapse in one third of patients after splenectomy has prompted the search for more effective modalities of therapy. Interferons were the first effec-

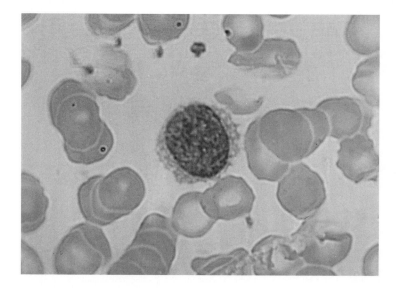

Figure 12–17. A diagnostic hairy cell in the peripheral blood. The hairy projections in this photomicrograph are not always visible in peripheral blood smears and may be seen in lymphocytes that have been allowed to sit at room temperature before the blood smear is made.

tive therapeutic agents[164–168]; and most recently deoxycoformycin[169] and 2-chlorodeoxyadenosine[170–172] have demonstrated dramatic therapeutic effect. One result of this therapeutic advance is that splenectomy is much less frequently performed in this disease.

The cell of origin of HCL was once a subject of controversy. It was originally thought to be of monocyte-macrophage derivation, as the original term for the disorder, "leukemic reticuloendotheliosis," implies.[139, 140] However, HCL is now recognized as a tumor of B lymphocytes.[173–178] The tumor cells exhibit monotypic surface immunoglobulin and B-cell antigens such as CD19, CD20, CD22, and DBA.44. They are CD5-negative, CD10-negative, and CD21-negative and CD25-positive, CD11c-positive, CD68 (KP-1)-positive, and HLA-DR–positive. Following splenectomy, hairy cells are virtually absent from the peripheral blood and inconspicuous in marrows that still contain significant hematopoiesis, suggesting that HCL may originate from a cell line within the spleen.[178] It has been suggested that monocy-

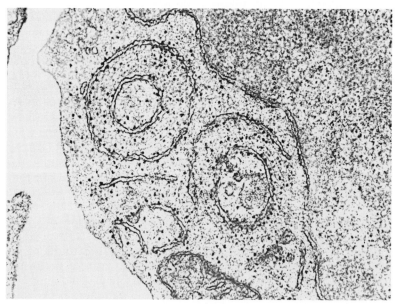

Figure 12–18. A ribosome-lamellar complex in the cytoplasm of a hairy cell. Although characteristic of hairy cell leukemia, these ultrastructural features may be seen in other lymphoid cells.

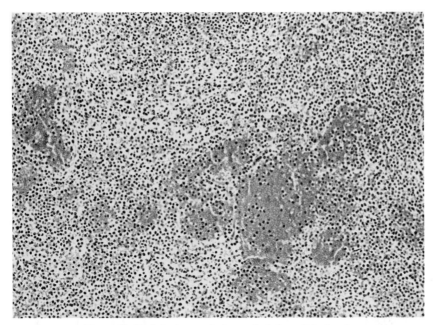

Figure 12–19. Splenic pseudosinuses in hairy cell leukemia.

toid B lymphocytes in lymph nodes share morphologic and immunophenotypic characteristics with hairy cells.[179] However, the existence of monocytoid B lymphocytes has not been documented in human spleens. Moreover, there is an immunohistologic difference between hairy cells and monocytoid B lymphocytes, which are CD25-negative. Hairy cells also resemble splenic marginal zone cells, and it is interesting to note that early involvement of hairy cell disease involves the zones of the spleen in which splenic marginal zone cells normally occur. However, splenic marginal zone cells are CD11c-negative.

Several authors have described a variant of HCL (HCL-V) based on morphologic and

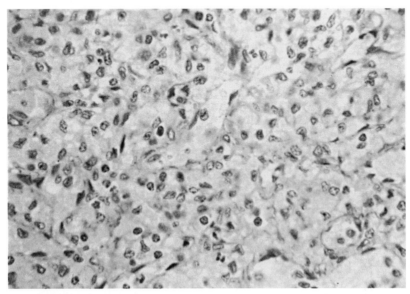

Figure 12–20. Hairy cell leukemia. The marked congestion of the red pulp with resultant dispersal of the hairy cells occasionally creates an appearance that resembles a vascular tumor and makes the diagnosis of hairy cell leukemia difficult.

prognostic features.[180–185] In the few cases we have studied, the pattern of splenic involvement is similar to that of classic hairy cell disease. The cytology of the infiltrating cells is different, however, reflecting the described differences in the morphology of the tumor cells; there appears to be little or no formation of splenic pseudosinuses. In contrast to typical hairy cells, HCL-V cells do not react with CD25 and are less consistently CD11c-positive. A rare T-cell variant of HCL has also been reported.[186]

Large Granular Lymphocytic Leukemia

"Leukemia of large granular lymphocytes (LGL)" is the preferred term for a group of disorders characterized by the proliferation of lymphoid cells with large amounts of cytoplasm containing characteristic azurophilic granules. Other terms used to describe this disorder include "chronic T-cell lymphocytosis with neutropenia,"[124, 130, 187] "T8 CLL,"[123] "T-cell CLL,"[121] "granulated T-cell lymphocytosis with neutropenia,"[188] "neutropenia with T lymphocytosis,"[189] "T-suppressor CLL,"[126] "suppressor T-cell CLL,"[190] "T-gamma lymphocytosis,"[191] and "erythrophagocytic T-gamma lymphoproliferative disease."[192]

As has been mentioned, the existence of a CLL of T-cell type has been recognized for some years.[112–123] A disorder characterized by the presence of circulating lymphoid cells with the characteristic morphologic features of LGL and associated with chronic neutropenia was described in the 1970s. However, it was not clear at that time whether the proliferation represented a benign or malignant disorder.[193, 194] In 1985, Loughran et al[195] documented the presence of clonal cytogenetic abnormalities in lymphocytes from patients with this disorder. An increased number of large granular lymphocytes may occur in the blood of normal patients and may be seen in association with a variety of neoplastic and non-neoplastic processes, as well as in patients with acquired aplastic anemia, rheumatoid arthritis, or other autoimmune disorders.[196, 197] In a survey from England,[198] it was determined that more than 31 percent of adult blood samples analyzed revealed an increased absolute number of large granular lymphocytes or NK-associated cells (either greater than 25 percent of total lymphocyte count or greater than 1.0 × 10⁹ LGL cells per liter). Fewer than 10 percent of the patients in this series were found to have clonal disease by molecular

studies, despite the fact that more than 80 percent of the patients studied had persistence of large granular lymphocytosis for more than 6 months. The presence of neutropenia is common in most published series but does not appear to have prognostic significance or to define clonal disease. Because distinct criteria for differentiating benign from malignant processes have not been determined with certainty, an international study group has proposed that a granular lymphocytosis of greater than 2 × 10⁹ per liter occurring for more than 6 months must be present to satisfy diagnostic criteria for the disease.[196] Recently, however, it has been shown, using combined molecular and immunologic techniques, that clonal (malignant) disease may be present in patients who do not meet these criteria.[199]

LGL leukemia has been divided into two subtypes distinguished from one another by their immunophenotype and, to some degree, by their clinical presentation.[196, 200, 201] The subtype of LGL leukemia referred to as CD3-positive or T-LGL, is CD3-positive, CD8-positive, CD16-positive, and CD57-positive and usually CD56-negative. The other subtype, referred to as CD3-negative or NK-LGL, is CD3-negative, CD4-negative, CD8-negative, and CD57-negative and CD16-positive and CD56-positive.

T-LGL may occur in patients at any age, but it is unusual in the pediatric age group. The median age of incidence is in the 6th decade of life. The disease affects males and females equally. The most characteristic presenting manifestation is the development of recurrent bacterial infections because of the neutropenia that characteristically occurs in this disease. Patients also have a high incidence of rheumatoid arthritis.

Examination of the peripheral blood in T-LGL usually reveals only a modest absolute lymphocytosis accompanied by neutropenia that is often severe. The reason for the neutropenia is difficult to assess. Although there is usually infiltration of the bone marrow, the degree of involvement cannot account for the significant decrease in granulocytes; an autoimmune mechanism has been postulated. Anemia and thrombocytopenia are less frequent and usually less severe. Hepatosplenomegaly occurs quite frequently, but lymphadenopathy is rare. The incidence of splenic involvement is approximately 50 percent.

The majority of cases of T-LGL are quite indolent, with many patients requiring no specific chemotherapy. A study of 68 patients reported a median survival of 161 months.[202] However, an aggressive variant of T-LGL has been reported[203] in which patients present with a rapidly progressive disease that appears resistant to cytotoxic therapy. These patients are characterized by a clinical presentation of rapidly increasing splenomegaly, lymphadenopathy, and the presence of B-cell symptoms.

The clinical features of NK-LGL are somewhat different from those of T-LGL.[196, 197] The median age in NK-LGL is lower than that in T-LGL, with a median incidence in the 4th decade. The disorder occurs equally in males and females. Cytopenias are less severe, and recurrent infections are much less common. Fever without an infectious cause and B-cell symptoms are common. Hepatosplenomegaly is almost invariable in this subtype of LGL and is frequently massive. In addition, peripheral blood large granular lymphocyte counts may increase rapidly and are frequently quite high. The clinical course of NK-LGL is more rapid than that of T-LGL, and the majority of patients die within a year of diagnosis of progressive disease, despite aggressive multiagent chemotherapy.

Splenic involvement in both types of LGL leukemia is similar and is predominantly confined to the red pulp. LGL cells infiltrate cords and sinuses (Fig. 12–21). Plasmacytosis in the red pulp is also frequent.[204] The histopathologic features of LGL leukemia may closely simulate those of HCL; however, the blood lakes characteristic of HCL are not present in LGL leukemia. Definite distinction between the two disorders can be made by immunohistologic stains, which document the B-cell nature of HCL and the T-cell or NK-cell cause of LGL leukemia. The massive splenic involvement occurring in NK-LGL may also mimic PLL. However, the differential diagnosis again should be straightforward because of the difference in immunophenotype between the two disorders and the characteristic morphologic features of each of these diseases in the peripheral blood.

Adult T-Cell Leukemia/Lymphoma

Adult T-cell leukemia/lymphoma (ATL) was first described in Japan,[205, 206] where a particular clustering of cases in the southwestern part of the country, around the island of Kyushu, was noted. However, other cases have been reported in the Caribbean and West Africa,[207] and sporadic cases have been described in the United States. The tumor is caused by a retrovirus termed "human T-cell leukemia virus type I (HTLV-1)."[208] The disease is usually subacute or chronic, although it often follows a rapid terminal course. Hepatosplenomegaly, lymphadenopathy, and skin involvement are common findings. The peripheral lymphocytosis is usually striking and is characterized by

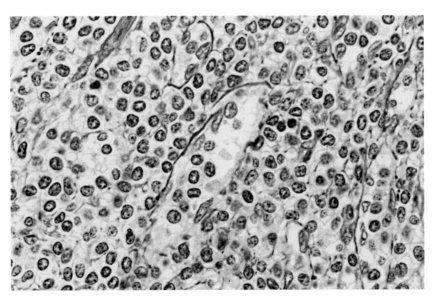

Figure 12–21. Large granular lymphocytic leukemia. The morphologic similarity of these cells to hairy cells is striking. However, the cells of large granular lymphocytic leukemia are either T cells or NK cells, whereas hairy cells are B cells.

the presence of bizarre lymphocytes with markedly hyperlobated nuclei, which have been called "flowerlike."

The proliferating cells in ATL are T cells, which express the pan T-cell antibodies CD2, CD3, and CD5. They usually express CD4, but occasional cases may express CD8. Their post-thymic nature is also characterized by their being TdT-negative. In contrast to the cells in T-PLL, which are usually CD7-positive, the tumor cells in ATL are negative for this antigen.

A subclassification of ATL, based on the degree of leukemic cells in the blood and the presence of lymphadenopathy, has been proposed.[209] Patients with 10 percent or more cells in the blood and no detectible lymphadenopathy are considered to have leukemia. Patients with lymphadenopathy and few or no leukemic cells in the blood are considered to have lymphoma. However, an intermediate, or mixed, group has been described.[209] Splenomegaly has been reported to occur in 40 to 50 percent of the cases and is thought to be due to infiltration of the spleen by leukemic cells.[210, 211] However, very few reports of the pathologic features of splenic involvement have been described. In the few cases we have had the opportunity to study, there has been a variable degree of infiltration of the red pulp of the spleen by lymphoid cells.

Generalized Mastocytosis

Generalized mastocytosis,[212–216] or systemic mast cell disease,[217–219] is a disorder characterized by a proliferation of mast cells that may involve skin,[220] bone marrow,[221, 222] spleen,[223–226] liver,[224, 227] and lymph nodes.[226] Several classifications of mast cell proliferations have been proposed.[219, 226, 228] Despite variations, all classifications recognize localized or diffuse cutaneous forms (urticaria pigmentosa), a benign systemic mastocytosis (usually associated with skin involvement), and a clinically aggressive systemic form of the disease (usually not associated with skin involvement). Additional subtypes include mast cell leukemia[228, 229] and mast cell sarcoma.[228, 230] Disseminated forms of mastocytosis, which represent approximately 10 percent of all mast cell diseases, can be subdivided into those cases with cutaneous involvement, which are usually indolent with good prognosis (systemic mastocytosis), and those without cutaneous involvement, which pur-

sue an aggressive course (malignant mastocytosis)[221, 226, 231] and have an association with MPDs and myelodysplastic disorders, acute leukemias, and other secondary malignancies.[232–236]

Mastocytosis is usually a disease of middle-aged adults. There is no gender predilection. Patients commonly present with symptoms of flushing, diarrhea, and generalized bone disease. Splenomegaly is noted at the time of presentation in one half to three quarters of cases and may occur as the presenting feature of the disease in patients without cutaneous involvement.[229] Peripheral adenopathy is uncommon.[216]

Splenic infiltration by mast cells is the cause of splenomegaly in almost all cases of systemic mast cell disease, even in the absence of mast cell leukemia. The degree of splenomegaly is usually mild to moderate. The splenic capsule is often thickened. The cut surface reveals prominent fibrous streaks and irregular nodularity, and calcification may be present.[226] A broad spectrum of morphologic patterns may occur.[216, 218, 219, 225, 226] Most investigators have reported a diffuse infiltration of the red pulp, although Brunning et al[216] reported that nodular perivascular aggregates may also occur. Others[219, 225] have stated that focal perifollicular involvement is also common. In six cases seen in our laboratory, we have noted striking involvement of the marginal zone in the white pulp, resulting in a concentric rimming of the lymphoid follicles. The mast cell infiltrate is usually associated with a variable degree of fibrosis similar to that seen in involved bone marrows (Fig. 12–22) and may be associated with eosinophils, especially at the periphery of the mast cell aggregates.[234] Mast cell infiltrates in the spleen are associated with significant sclerosis, and in spleens with significant involvement, fibrous tissue may dominate, with mast cells becoming less conspicuous. The mast cells show a variable cytology (Fig. 12–23). Some appear typically cuboidal with large pale nuclei and grayish cytoplasm in hematoxylin and eosin–stained sections. Others are spindle-shaped, and some may resemble histiocytes. Mast cell granules are basophilic in Wright-Giemsa–stained sections and are metachromatic with toluidine blue. The granules also stain with the CAE (Leder) stain. In addition, they are tartrate-resistant acid phosphatase–positive by immunohistologic staining in most cases.[153] It has also been shown that the mast cells in mastocytosis stain well with tryptase.[236a]

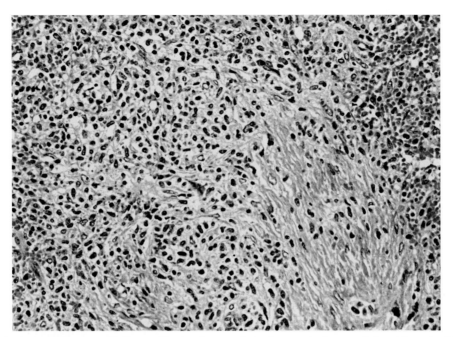

Figure 12–22. Systemic mast cell disease. The involvement is in the marginal zone of the white pulp. Fibrosis is a characteristic accompanying feature.

Diebold et al[237] have reported that the topographic and histologic pattern of splenic involvement correlates with the subtype of mast cell disease. The larger series of Horny et al,[225] however, did not confirm these findings. Splenic involvement in mastocytosis may occasionally produce cytopenias due to secondary hypersplenism.[216, 219] Splenectomy has been re-

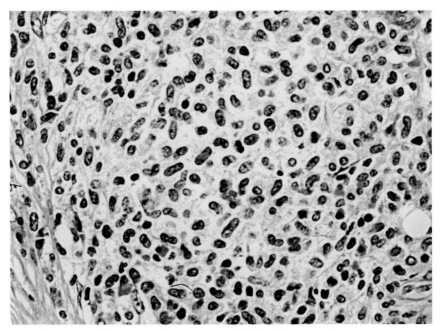

Figure 12–23. Mast cells have round or bean-shaped nuclei with abundant cytoplasm. Occasional nucleoli may be spindle-shaped. Mast cells may resemble hairy cells. However, the distribution within the spleen differs. Mast cells may also be mistaken for histiocytes.

ported to ameliorate the cytopenias in several cases.[219]

REFERENCES

1. Simoes BP, Tone LG, Zago MA, et al: Splenic function in acute leukemia. Acta Haematol 1995; 94:123.
2. Flood MJ, Carpenter RA: Spontaneous rupture of the spleen in acute myeloid leukaemia. Br Med J 1961; 1:35.
3. Serur D, Terjanian T: Spontaneous rupture of the spleen as the initial manifestation of acute myeloid leukemia. N Y State J Med 1992; 92:160.
4. Greenfield MM, Lund H: Spontaneous rupture of the spleen in chronic myeloid leukemia. Ohio Med J 1944; 40:950.
5. Sarin LR, Sarin JC: Spontaneous rupture of the spleen in chronic myeloid leukemia. J Ind Med Assoc 1957; 29:286.
6. Bennett JM, Catovsky D, Daniel MT, et al: Proposals for the classification of the acute leukemias: French-American-British (FAB) Cooperative Group. Br J Haematol 1976; 33:451.
7. Bennett JM, Catovsky D, Daniel MT, et al: Proposed revised criteria for the classification of acute myeloid leukemia. Ann Intern Med 1985; 103:626.
8. Bennett JM, Catovsky D, Daniel MT, et al: Criteria for the diagnosis of acute leukemia of megakaryocyte lineage (M_7). Ann Intern Med 1985; 103:460.
9. Lee EJ, Pollak A, Leavitt RD, et al: Minimally differentiated acute nonlymphocytic leukemia: A distinct entity. Blood 1987; 70:1400.
10. Fenaux P, Jovet JP, Zandecki M, et al: Chronic and subacute myelomonocytic leukemia in the adult: A report of 60 cases with special reference to prognostic factors. Br J Haematol 1985; 65:101.
11. Li CY, Lam KW, Yam LT: Esterase in human leukocytes. J Histochem Cytochem 1973; 21:1.
12. Moloney WC, McPherson K, Fliegelman L: Esterase activity in leukocytes demonstrated by the use of naphthol AS-D chloroacetate substrate. J Histochem Cytochem 1960; 8:200.
13. Schmalzl F, Braunsteiner H: The application of cytochemical methods to the study of acute leukemia. Acta Haematol 1971; 45:209.
14. Yam LT, Li CY, Crosby WH: Cytochemical identification of monocytes and granulocytes. Am J Clin Pathol 1971; 55:283.
15. Pinkus GS, Pinkus JL: Myeloperoxidase: A specific marker for myeloid cells in paraffin sections. Mod Pathol 1991; 4:733.
16. Pulford KAF, Erber WN, Crick JA, et al: Use of monoclonal antibody against human neutrophil elastase in normal and leukemic myeloid cells. J Clin Pathol 1988; 41:853.
17. Said JW, Stoll PN, Shintaku P, et al: Leu-22: A preferential marker for T-lymphocytes in paraffin sections. Am J Clin Pathol 1989; 91:542.
18. Segal GH, Stoler MH, Tubbs RR: The "CD43 only" phenotype: An aberrant, nonspecific immunophenotype requiring comprehensive analysis for lineage resolution. Am J Clin Pathol 1992; 98:861.
19. Arber DA, Weiss LM: CD15: A Review. Appl Immunohistochem 1993; 1:17.
20. Holowiecki J, Lutz D, Krezemien S, et al: CD15 antigen detected by VIM-D5 monoclonal antibody for prediction of ability to achieve complete remission in acute non-lymphocytic leukemia. Acta Haematol 1986; 76:16.
21. Pinkus GS, Said JW: Profile of intracytoplasmic lysozyme in normal tissues, myeloproliferative disorders, hairy cell leukemia, and other pathologic processes: An immunoperoxidase study of paraffin sections and smears. Am J Pathol 1997; 89:351.
22. Traweek ST, Arber DA, Rappaport H, et al: Extramedullary myeloid cell tumors: An immunohistochemical and morphologic study of 28 cases. Am J Surg Pathol 1993; 17:1011.
23. Traweek ST: Immunophenotypic analysis of acute leukemia. Am J Clin Pathol 1993; 99:504.
24. Stone RM, Mayer TJ: The unique aspects of acute promyelocytic leukemia. J Clin Oncol 1990; 8:1913.
25. Breton-Gorius J, Houssay D: Auer bodies in acute promyelocytic leukemia: Demonstration of their fine structure and peroxidase localization. Lab Invest 1973; 28:135.
26. Golomb HM, Rowley JD, Vardiman JW, et al: "Microgranular" acute promyelocytic leukemia: A distinct clinical, ultrastructural, and cytogenetic entity. Blood 1980; 55:253.
27. McKenna RW, Parkin J, Bloomfield CD, et al: Acute promyelocytic leukaemia: A study of 39 cases with identification of a hyperbasophilic microgranular variant. Br J Haematol 1982; 50:201.
28. Benvenisti DS, Ultmann JE: Eosinophilic leukemia: Report of five cases and review of the literature. Ann Intern Med 1969; 71:731.
29. Wick MR, Li CY, Pierre RV: Acute nonlymphocytic leukemia with basophilic differentiation. Blood 1982; 60:38.
30. Peterson LC, Parkin JL, Arthur DC, et al: Acute basophilic leukemia: A clinical, morphologic and cytogenetic study of eight cases. Am J Clin Pathol 1991; 96:160.
31. Brunning RD, McKenna RW: Tumors of the Bone Marrow, in Atlas of Tumor Pathology, series 3, fascicle 9, p 56. Washington DC, Armed Forces Institute of Pathology, 1994.
32. Straus DJ: The acute monocytic leukemias. Medicine 1980; 59:409.
33. Byrnes RK, Golomb HM, Desser RK, et al: Acute monocytic leukemia: Cytologic, histologic, cytochemical, ultrastructural and cytogenetic observations. Am J Clin Pathol 1976; 65:471.
34. McKenna RW, Bloomfield CD, Nesbit M, et al: Nonspecific esterase-positive acute leukemia: A distinctive cytologic and clinical entity. Proc Am Assoc Cancer Res/Am Soc Clin Oncol 1975; 11:61.
35. Tobelem G, Jacquillat C, Chastang C, et al: Acute monoblastic leukemia: A clinical and biologic study of 74 cases. Blood 1980; 55:71.
36. Cuttner J, Conjalka MS, Reilly M, et al: Association of monocytic leukemia in patients with extreme leukocytosis. Am J Med 1980; 69:555.
37. Peterson L, Dehner LP, Brunning RD: Extramedullary masses as presenting features of acute monoblastic leukemia. Am J Clin Pathol 1981; 75:140.
38. DiGuglielmo G: Ricerche di ematologia. I. Un caso di eritroleucemia. Folia Med 1917; 3:386.
39. Brunning, RD, McKenna RW: Tumors of the Bone Marrow, in Atlas of Tumor Pathology, series 3, fascicle 9, p 67. Washington DC, Armed Forces Institute of Pathology, 1994.
40. Bennett JM, Catovsky D, Daniel MT, et al: Proposed

revised criteria for the classification of acute myeloid leukemia. Am Intern Med 1985; 103:620.

41. Neiman RS: Erythroblastic transformation in myeloproliferative disorders: Confirmation by an immunohistologic technique. Cancer 1980; 46:1636.

42. Pinkus GS, Said JW: Intracellular hemoglobin—a specific marker for erythroid cells in paraffin sections: An immunoperoxidase study of normal, megaloblastic, and dysplastic erythropoiesis, including erythroleukemia and other myeloproliferative disorders. Am J Pathol 1971; 102:308.

43. Greaves MF, Sieff C, Edwards PA: Monoclonal antiglycophorin as a probe for erythroleukemias. Blood 1983; 61:645.

44. Thiele J, Meuter RB, Titius RB, et al: Proliferating cell nuclear antigen expression by erythroid precursors in normal bone marrow, in reactive lesions and in polycythaemia rubra vera. Histopathology 1993; 22:429.

45. Bennett, JM, Catovsky D, Daniel M-T, et al: Criteria for the diagnosis of acute leukemia of megakaryocyte lineage (M7). Ann Intern Med 1985; 103:460.

46. Brunning RD, McKenna RW: Tumors of the Bone Marrow, in Atlas of Tumor Pathology, series 3, fascicle 9. Washington DC, Armed Forces Institute of Pathology, 1994.

47. Huang MJ, Li CY, Nichols WL, et al: Acute leukemia with megakaryocytic differentiation: A study of 12 cases identified immunocytochemically. Blood 1984; 64:427.

48. Innes DJ Jr, Mills SE, Walter GK: Megakaryocytic leukemia: Identification using anti-factor VIII immunoperoxidase. Am J Clin Pathol 1982; 77:107.

49. Gatter KC, Cordell JL, Turley H, et al: The immunohistological detection of platelets, megakaryocytes, and thrombi in routinely processed specimens. Histopathology 1988; 13:257.

50. Breton-Gorius J, Vanhaeke D, Pryzwansky KB, et al: Simultaneous detection of membrane markers with monoclonal antibodies and peroxidatic activities in leukaemia: Ultrastructural analysis using a new method of fixation preserving the platelet peroxidase. Br J Haematol 1984; 58:447.

51. Breton-Gorius J, Reyes F, Duhamel G, et al: Megakaryoblastic acute leukemia: Identification by the ultrastructural demonstration of platelet peroxidase. Blood 1978; 51:45.

52. Breton-Gorius J, Villeval JL, Kieffer N, et al: Limits of phenotypic markers for the diagnosis of megakaryoblastic leukemia. Blood Cells 1989; 15:259.

53. Ohata M, Sugiura K, Otsuka S, et al: Acute erythroblastic leukemia presenting as FAB M6 with surface marker positive for megakaryocytic and erythroid: Report of a case (Japanese). Jpn J Clin Hematol 1994; 35:127.

54. Debili N, Kieffer N, Mitjavila MT, et al: Expression of platelet glycoproteins by erythroid blasts in four cases of trisomy 21. Leukemia 1989; 3:669.

55. Erber WN, Breton-Gorius J, Villeval JL, et al: Detection of cells of megakaryocytic lineage in haematological malignancies by immunoalkaline phosphatase labeling cell smears with a panel of monoclonal antibodies. Br J Haematol 1987; 65:87.

56. Medical Research Council's Working Party for Therapeutic Trials in Leukaemia: Chronic granulocytic leukaemia: Comparison of radiotherapy and busulfan therapy. Br Med J 1968; 1:201.

57. Kantarjian HM, Keating MJ, Talpaz M, et al: Chronic myelogenous leukemia in blast crisis: Analysis of 242 patients. Am J Med 1987; 83:445.

58. Muehleck SD, McKenna RW, Arthur DC, et al: Transformation of chronic myelogenous leukemia: Clinical, morphologic, and cytogenetic features. Am J Clin Pathol 1984; 82:1.

59. Kantarjian HM, Deisseroth A, Kurzrock R, et al: Chronic myelogenous leukemia: A concise update. Blood 1993; 82:691.

60. Canellos GP: Clinical characteristics of the blast phase of chronic granulocytic leukemia. Hematol Oncol Clin North Am 1990; 4:359.

61. Shaw MT, Bottomley RH, Grozea PN, et al: Heterogeneity of morphological, cytochemical, and cytogenetic features in the blastic phase of chronic granulocytic leukemia. Cancer 1975; 35:199.

62. Baccarani M, Zaccaria A, Santucci AM, et al: A simultaneous study of bone marrow, spleen, and liver in chronic myeloid leukemia: Evidence for differences in cell composition and karyotypes. Ser Haematol 1975; 8:81.

63. Mitelman F: Comparative cytogenetic studies of bone marrow and extramedullary tissues in chronic myeloid leukaemia. Ser Haematol 1975; 8:113.

64. Stoll C, Oberling F, Flori E: Chromosome analysis of spleen and/or lymph nodes of patients with chronic myeloid leukaemia. Blood 1978; 52:328.

65. Mitelman F, Brandt L, Nilsson PG: Cytogenetic evidence for splenic origin of blastic transformation in chronic myeloid leukaemia. Scand J Haematol 1974; 13:87.

66. Zaccaria A, Baccarani M, Barbieri E, et al: Differences in marrow and spleen karyotype in early chronic myeloid leukemia. Eur J Cancer 1975; 11:123.

67. Gomez GA, Sokal JE, Mittelman A, et al: Splenectomy for palliation of chronic myelocytic leukemia. Am J Med 1976; 61:14.

68. Brandt L, Schnell CR: Granulopoiesis in bone marrow and spleen in chronic myeloid leukaemia. Scand J Haematol 1969; 6:65.

69. Brandt L: Differences in the proliferative activity of myelocytes from bone marrow, spleen, and peripheral blood in chronic myeloid leukaemia. Scand J Haematol 1969; 6:65.

70. Brandt L: Difference in uptake of tritiated thymidine by myelocytes from bone marrow and spleen in chronic myeloid leukaemia. Scand J Haematol 1973; 11:23.

71. Rosenthal S, Canellos GP, Whang-Peng J, et al: Blast crisis of chronic granulocytic leukemia: Morphologic variants and therapeutic implications. Am J Med 1977; 63:542.

72. Gomez GA, Hossfeld DK, Sokal JE: Removal of abnormal clone of leukaemic cells by splenectomy. Br Med J 1975; 2:421.

73. Idhe DC, Canellos GP, Schwartz JH, et al: Splenectomy in the chronic phase of chronic granulocytic leukemia: Effects in 32 patients. Ann Intern Med 1976; 84:17.

74. Spiers ASD, Baikie AG, Galton DAG, et al: Chronic granulocytic leukaemia: Effect of elective splenectomy on the course of disease. Br Med J 1975; 1:175.

75. Canellos GP, Nordland J, Carbone PP: Splenectomy for thrombocytopenia in chronic granulocytic leukemia. Cancer 1972; 29:660.

76. Fisher JH, Welch CS, Dameshek W: Splenectomy in leukemia and leukosarcoma. N Engl J Med 1952; 246:477.

77. Meeker WR Jr, DePerio JM, Grace JT Jr, et al: Role of splenectomy in malignant lymphoma and leukemia. Surg Clin North Am 1967; 47:1163.

78. Mittelman A, Elias EG, Wieckowska W, et al: Splenectomy in patients with malignant lymphoma or chronic leukemia. Cancer Bull 1970; 22:10.

79. Strumia MM, Strumia PV, Bassert D: Splenectomy in leukemia: Hematologic and clinical effects on 34 patients and review of 299 published cases. Cancer Res 1966; 26:519.

80. Brodsky L, Fusculdo KE, Kahn SB, et al: Chronic myelogenous leukaemia: A clinical and experimental evaluation of splenectomy and intensive chemotherapy. Ser Haematol 1975; 8:143.

81. Tura S, Baccarani M, Gugliotta L, et al: Italian Cooperative Study Group on chronic myeloid leukaemia: A clinical trial of early splenectomy, hydroxyurea, and cyclic arabinosyl cytosine, vincristine, and prednisone in chronic myeloid leukaemia. Ser Haematol 1975; 8:121.

82. Wolf DJ, Silver RT, Coleman M: Splenectomy in chronic myeloid leukemia. Ann Intern Med 1978; 89:684.

83. Bearman RM, Kjeldsberg CR, Pangalis GA, et al: Chronic monocytic leukemia in adults. Cancer 1981; 48:2239.

84. Crist W, Boyett J, Pullen J, et al: Clinical and biological features predict poor prognosis in acute lymphoid leukemias in children and adolescents: A Pediatric Oncology Group review. Med Pediatr Oncol 1986; 14:135.

85. Bennett JM, Catovsky D, Daniel MT, et al: The French-American-British (FAB) Cooperative Group: The morphological classification of acute lymphoblastic leukemia—concordance among observers and clinical correlations. Br J Haematol 1981; 47:553.

86. Vogler LB, Crist WM, Bockman DE, et al: Pre–B-cell leukemia: A new phenotype of childhood lymphoblastic leukemia. N Engl J Med 1978; 298:872.

87. Magrath IT, Ziegler JL: Bone marrow involvement in Burkitt's lymphoma and its relationship to acute B-cell leukemia. Leuk Res 1980; 4:33.

88. Orazi A, Cotton J, Cattoretti G, et al: Terminal deoxynucleotidyl transferase staining in acute leukemia and normal bone marrow using routinely processed paraffin sections. Am J Clin Pathol 1994; 102:640.

89. Robertson PB, Neiman RS, Worapongpaiboon S, et al: 013 (CD99) positivity in hematologic proliferations correlates with TdT positivity. Mod Pathol 1997; 10:277.

90. Hansen MM: Chronic lymphocytic leukaemia: Clinical studies based on 189 cases followed for a long time. Scand J Haematol 1973; suppl 18:3.

91. Pangalis GA, Nathwani BN, Rappaport H: Malignant lymphoma, well-differentiated lymphocytic: Its relationship with chronic lymphocytic leukaemia and macroglobulinemia of Waldenström. Cancer 1977; 39:999.

92. Dick FR, Maca RD: The lymph node in chronic lymphocytic leukemia. Cancer 1978; 41:283.

93. Evans HL, Butler JJ, Youness EL: Malignant lymphoma, small lymphocytic type: A clinicopathologic study of 84 cases with suggested criteria for intermediate lymphocytic lymphoma. Cancer 1978; 41:1440.

94. Stites TB, Ultmann JE: Spontaneous rupture of the spleen in chronic lymphocytic leukemia. Cancer 1966; 19:1587.

95. Christensen BE: Effects of an enlarged splenic erythrocyte pool in chronic lymphocytic leukaemia: Mechanism of erythrocyte sequestration in the spleen and liver. Scand J Haematol 1971; 8:92.

96. Kaden BR, Rosse WF, Hauch TW: Immune thrombocytopenia in lymphoproliferative diseases. Blood 1979; 53:545.

97. Young LE, Miller G, Christian RM: Clinical and laboratory observations on autoimmune hemolytic disease. Ann Intern Med 1951; 35:507.

98. Binet JL, Leporrier M, Dighiero G, et al: A clinical staging system for chronic lymphocytic leukemia: Prognostic significance. Cancer 1977; 40:855.

99. Rai KR, Sawitsky A, Cronkite EP, et al: Clinical staging of chronic lymphocytic leukemia. Blood 1975; 46:219.

100. Binet JL, Auquier A, Dighiero G, et al: A new prognostic classification of chronic lymphocytic leukemia derived from a multivariate survival analysis. Cancer 1981; 48:198.

101. Adler S, Stutzman L, Sokal JE, et al: Splenectomy for hematologic depression in lymphocytic lymphoma and leukemia. Cancer 1975; 35:521.

102. Neal TF Jr, Tefferi A, Witzig TE, et al: Splenectomy advances chronic lymphocytic leukemia: A single institution experience with 50 patients. Am J Med 1992; 93:435.

103. Seymour JF, Cusack JD, Lerner SA, et al: Case/control study of the role of splenectomy in chronic lymphocytic leukemia. J Clin Oncol 1997; 15:52.

104. Byhardt RW, Brace KC, Wiernik PH: The role of splenic irradiation in chronic lymphocytic leukemia. Cancer 1975; 35:1621.

105. Enno A, Catovsky D, O'Brien M, et al: Prolymphocytoid transformation of chronic lymphocytic leukaemia. Br J Haematol 1979; 41:9.

106. Dighiero G, Travade P, Chevret S, et al: B-cell chronic lymphocytic leukaemia: Present status and future directions. Blood 1991; 78:1901.

107. Traweck ST, Liu J, Johnson RM, et al: High-grade transformation of chronic lymphocytic leukemia and low-grade non-Hodgkin's lymphoma: Genotypic confirmation of clonal identity. Am J Clin Pathol 1993; 100:519.

108. Nakamine H, Masih AS, Sanger WG, et al: Richter's syndrome with different immunoglobulin light chain types: Molecular and cytogenetic features indicate a common clonal origin. Am J Clin Pathol 1992; 97:656.

109. McDonnell JM, Beschorner WE, Staal SP, et al: Richter's syndrome with two different B-cell clones. Cancer 1986; 58:2031.

110. Suster S, Rywlin AM: A reappraisal of Richter's syndrome: Development of two phenotypically distinctive cell lines in a case of chronic lymphocytic leukemia. Cancer 1987; 59:1412.

111. Matolcsy A, Inghirami G, Knowles DM: Molecular genetic demonstration of the diverse evolution of Richter's syndrome (chronic lymphocytic leukemia and subsequent large cell lymphoma). Blood 1994; 83:1363.

112. Brouet JC, Flandrin G, Sasportes M, et al: Chronic lymphocytic leukemia of T-cell origin: Immunological and clinical evaluation in eleven patients. Lancet 1975; 2:890.

113. Catovsky D, Pittman S, O'Brien M, et al: Multiparameter studies in lymphoid leukemias. Am J Clin Pathol 1979; 72:736.

114. Marks SM, Yanovich S, Rosenthal DS, et al: Multipa-

rameter analysis of T-cell chronic lymphocytic leukemia. Blood 1978; 51:435.

115. Reinherz EL, Nadler LM, Rosenthal DS, et al: T-cell subset characterization of human T-CLL. Blood 1979; 53:1066.

116. Sumiya M, Mizoguchi H, Hosaka K, et al: Chronic lymphocytic leukaemia of T cell origin? Lancet 1973; 2:910.

117. Yodoi J, Takatsuki K, Aoki N, et al: Chronic lymphocytic leukemia of T-cell origin: Demonstration in two cases by the use of antithymocyte membrane antiserum. Acta Haematol Jpn 1974; 37:46.

118. Yodoi J, Takatsuki K, Masuda T: Two cases of T-cell chronic lymphocytic leukemia in Japan. N Engl J Med 1974; 290:572.

119. Pandoli F, DeRossi G, Semenzato G, et al: Immunologic evaluation of T chronic lymphocyte leukemia cells: Correlations among phenotype, functional activities and morphology. Blood 1982; 59:688.

120. Matutes E, Brito-Babapulle V, Foroni L, et al: The nature of T-chronic lymphocytic leukaemia. Br J Haematol 1986; 62:402.

121. Phyliky RL, Li CY, Yam LT: T-cell chronic lymphocytic leukemia with morphologic and immunologic characteristics of cytotoxic/suppressor phenotype. Mayo Clin Proc 1983; 58:709.

122. Aisenberg AC, Wilkes BM, Harris NL, et al: T-cell chronic lymphocytic leukemia: Report of a case studied with monoclonal antibody. Am J Med 1982; 72:695.

123. Brisbane JU, Berman LD, Osband ME, et al: T_8 chronic lymphocytic leukemia: A distinctive disorder related to T_8 lymphocytosis. Am J Clin Pathol 1983; 80:391.

124. Newland AC, Catovsky D, Linch D, et al: Chronic T cell lymphocytosis: A review of 21 cases. Br J Haematol 1984; 58:433.

125. Brody JI, Burningham RA, Nowell PC, et al: Persistent lymphocytosis with chromosomal evidence of malignancy. Am J Med 1975; 58:547.

126. Bakri K, Ezdinli EZ, Wasser LP, et al: T-suppressor cell chronic lymphocytic leukemia: Phenotypic characterization by monoclonal antibodies. Cancer 1984; 54:284.

127. Pizzoli G, Chilosi M, Cetto GL, et al: Immunohistological analysis of bone marrow involvement in lymphoproliferative disorders. Br J Haematol 1982; 50:95.

128. Delforge A, Bron D, Stryckmans P: Neutropenia associated with excess of T lymphocytes. Br J Haematol 1981; 49:488.

129. Linch DC, Cawley JC, Worman CP, et al: Abnormalities of T cell subsets in patients with neutropenia and an excess of lymphocytes in the bone marrow. Br J Haematol 1981; 48:137.

130. Aisenberg AC, Wilkes BM, Harris NL, et al: Chronic T-cell lymphocytosis with neutropenia: Report of a case studied with monoclonal antibody. Blood 1981; 58:818.

131. McKenna RW, Parkin J, Kersey JH, et al: Chronic lymphoproliferative disorder with unusual clinical, morphologic, ultrastructural and membrane surface marker characteristics. Am J Med 1977; 62:588.

132. Catovsky D: Hairy-cell leukaemia and prolymphocytic leukaemia. Clin Haematol 1977; 6:245.

133. Galton DAG, Goldman JM, Wiltshaw E, et al: Prolymphocytic leukaemia. Br J Haematol 1974; 27:7.

134. Catovsky D, Galetto J, Okos A, et al: Prolymphocytic leukaemia of B and T cell type. Lancet 1973; 2:232.

135. Stone RM: Prolymphocytic leukemia. Hematol Oncol Clin North Am 1990; 4:457.

136. Bearman RM, Pangalis GA, Rappaport H: Prolymphocytic leukemia: Clinical, histopathologic, and cytochemical observations. Cancer 1978; 42:2360.

137. Matutes E, Brito-Babapulle V, Swansbury J, et al: Clinical and laboratory features of 78 cases of T-prolymphocytic leukemia. Blood 1991; 78:3269.

138. Owens MR, Strauchen JA, Rowe JM, et al: Prolymphocytic leukemia: Histologic findings in atypical cases. Hematol Oncol 1984; 2:249.

139. Bouroncle BA, Wiseman BK, Doan CA: Leukemic reticuloendotheliosis. Blood 1958; 13:609.

140. Catovsky D, Pettit JE, Galton DAG, et al: Leukaemic reticuloendotheliosis (hairy cell leukaemia): A distinct clinicopathological entity. Br J Haematol 1974; 26:9.

141. Flandrin G, Sigaux F, Sebahoun G, et al: Hairy cell leukemia: Clinical presentation and follow-up of 211 patients. Semin Oncol 1984; 11:458.

142. Brunning RD, McKenna RW: Tumors of the Bone Marrow, in Atlas of Tumor Pathology, series 3, fascicle 9, p 276. Washington DC, Armed Forces Institute of Pathology, 1994.

143. Burke JS: The value of bone-marrow biopsy in the diagnosis of hairy cell leukemia. Am J Clin Pathol 1978; 70:876.

144. Burke JS, Byrne GE Jr, Rappaport H: Hairy cell leukemia (leukemic reticuloendotheliosis). I. A clinical pathologic study of 21 patients. Cancer 1974; 33:1399.

145. Burke JS, MacKay B, Rappaport H: Hairy cell leukemia (leukemic reticuloendotheliosis). II. Ultrastructure of the spleen. Cancer 1976; 37:2267.

146. Pilon VA, Davey FR, Gordon GB, et al: Splenic alterations in hairy cell leukemia. II. An electron microscopic study. Cancer 1982; 49:1617.

147. Katayama I, Yang JPS: Reassessment of a cytochemical test for differential diagnosis of leukemic reticuloendotheliosis. Am J Clin Pathol 1977; 86:163.

148. Neiman RS, Sullivan AL, Jaffe R: Malignant lymphoma simulating leukemic reticuloendotheliosis: A clinicopathologic study of ten cases. Cancer 1979; 43:329.

149. Mover S, Li CY: Semiquantitative evaluation of tartrate-resistant acid phosphatase activity in human blood cells. J Lab Clin Med 1972; 80:711.

150. Yam LT, Li CY, Lam KW: Tartrate-resistant acid phosphatase isoenzyme in the reticulum cells of leukemic reticuloendotheliosis. N Engl J Med 1971; 284:357.

151. Yam LT, Janckila AJ, Li CY, et al: Cytochemistry of tartrate-resistant acid phosphatase: 15 years' experience. Leukemia 1987; 1:285.

152. Janckila AJ, Cradwell EM, Yam LT, et al: Hairy cell identification by immunohistochemistry of tartrate-resistant acid phosphatase. Blood 1995; 85:2839.

153. Hoyer JD, Li C-Y, Yam LT, et al: Immunohistochemical demonstration of acid phosphatase isoenzyme 5 (tartrate-resistant) in paraffin sections of hairy cell leukemia and other hematologic disorders. Am J Clin Pathol 1997; 108:308.

154. Schrek R, Donnelly WJ: "Hairy" cells in blood in lymphoreticular neoplastic disease and "flagellated" cells of normal lymph nodes. Blood 1966; 27:199.

155. Katayama I, Schneider GB: Further ultrastructural characterization of hairy cells in leukemic reticuloendotheliosis. Am J Pathol 1977; 86:163.

156. Anday GJ, Goodman JR, Tishkoff GH: An unusual

cytoplasmic ribosomal structure in pathologic lymphocytes. Blood 1973; 41:439.

157. Brunning RD, Parkin J: Ribosome-lamella complexes in neoplastic hematopoietic cells. Am J Pathol 1975; 79:565.

158. Zucker-Franklin D: Virus-like particles in the lymphocytes of a patient with chronic lymphocytic leukemia. Blood 1963; 21:509.

159. Nanba K, Soban EJ, Bowling MC, et al: Splenic pseudosinuses and hepatic angiomatous lesions: Distinctive features of hairy cell leukemia. Am J Clin Pathol 1977; 67:415.

160. Lewis SM, Catovsky D, Hows JM, et al: Splenic red cell pooling in hairy cell leukaemia. Br J Haematol 1977; 35:351.

161. Golomb HM, Catovsky D, Golde DW: Hairy cell leukemia: A clinical review based on 71 cases. Ann Intern Med 1978; 89:677.

162. Jansen J, Hermans JO: Splenectomy in hairy cell leukemia: A retrospective multicenter analysis. Cancer 1981; 47:2066.

163. Van Norman AS, Nagorney DM, Martin JK, et al: Splenectomy for hairy cell leukemia: A clinical review of 63 patients. Cancer 1986; 57:644.

164. Bardawil RG, Groves C, Ratain MJ, et al: Changes in peripheral blood and bone marrow specimens following therapy with recombinant alpha$_2$ interferon for hairy cell leukemia. Am J Clin Pathol 1986; 85:194.

165. Castaigne S, Sigaux F, Cantell K, et al: Interferon alpha in the treatment of hairy cell leukemia. Cancer 1986; 57:1681.

166. Quesada JR, Gutterman JU, Hersh EM: Treatment of hairy cell leukemia with alpha interferons. Cancer 1986; 57:1678.

167. Quesada JR, Reuben J, Manning JT, et al: Alpha interferon for induction of remission in hairy cell leukemia. N Engl J Med 1984; 310:15.

168. Ratain MJ, Golomb HM, Vardiman JW, et al: Treatment of hairy cell leukemia with recombinant alpha$_2$ interferon. Blood 1985; 65:644.

169. Spiers AS, Moore D, Cassileth PA, et al: Remissions in hairy-cell leukemia with Pentostatin (2'-deoxycoformycin). N Engl J Med 1987; 316:825.

170. Piro LD, Carrera CJ, Carson DA, et al: Lasting remissions in hairy-cell leukemia induced by a single infusion of 2-chlorodeoxyadenosine. New Engl J Med 1990; 322:1117.

171. Estey EH, Kurzrock R, Kantarjian HM, et al: Treatment of hairy cell leukemia with 2-chlorodeoxyadenosine (2-CdA). Blood 1992; 79:882.

172. Beutler E, Carson DA: 2-Chlorodeoxyadenosine: Hairy cell leukemia takes a surprising turn. Blood Cells 1993; 19:559.

173. Hsu SM, Yang K, Jaffe ES: Hairy cell leukemia: A B-cell neoplasm with a unique antigenic profile. Am J Clin Pathol 1983; 80:421.

174. Jansen J, LeBain TW, Kersey JH: The phenotype of the neoplastic cells of hairy-cell leukemia studied with monoclonal antibodies. Blood 1982; 59:609.

175. Worman CP, Brooks DA, Hogg N, et al: The nature of hairy cells: A study with a panel of monoclonal antibodies. Scand J Haematol 1983; 30:223.

176. Korsmeyer SJ, Greene WC, Cossman J, et al: Rearrangement and expression of immunoglobulin genes and expression of Tac antigen in hairy cell leukemia. Proc Natl Acad Sci U S A 1983; 80:4522.

177. Cleary ML, Wood GS, Warnke R, et al: Immunoglob-

178. Cawley JC, Worman CP: Hairy-cell leukaemia. Br J Haematol 1985; 60:213.

179. Burke JS, Sheibani K, Brownell MD: Reactive and neoplastic monocytoid B lymphocytes share immunophenotypic characteristics with hairy cell leukemia. Lab Invest 1987; 56:9A.

180. Bartl R, Frisch B, Hill W, et al: Bone marrow histology in hairy cell leukemia: Identification of subtypes and their prognostic significance. Am J Clin Pathol 1983; 79:531.

181. Catovsky D, O'Brien M, Melo JV, et al: Hairy cell leukemia (HCL) variant: An intermediate disease between HCL and B prolymphocytic leukemia. Semin Oncol 1984; 11:362.

182. Cawley JC, Burns GF, Hayhoe FGJ: A chronic lymphoproliferative disorder with distinctive features: A distinct variant of hairy-cell leukaemia. Leuk Res 1980; 4:547.

183. Diez Martin JL, Li CY, Banks PM: Blastic variant of hairy-cell leukemia. Am J Clin Pathol 1987; 87:576.

184. Jansen J, Schuit HRE, Schreuder GMT, et al: Distinct subtypes within the spectrum of hairy cell leukemia. Blood 1979; 54:459.

185. Sainati L, Matutes E, Mulligan S, et al: A variant form of hairy cell leukemia resistant to alpha-interferon: Clinical and phenotypic characteristics of 17 patients. Blood 1990; 76:157.

186. Saxon A, Stevens RH, Golde DW: T-lymphocyte variant of hairy-cell leukemia. Ann Intern Med 1978; 88:323.

187. Herrod HG, Wang WC, Sullivan JL: Chronic T-cell lymphocytosis with neutropenia: Its association with Epstein-Barr virus infection. Am J Dis Child 1985; 139:405.

188. McKenna RW, Arthur DC, Gajl-Peczalska KJ, et al: Granulated T cell lymphocytosis with neutropenia: Malignant or benign chronic lymphoproliferative disorder? Blood 1985; 66:259.

189. Chan WC, Check I, Schick C, et al: A morphologic and immunologic study of the large granular lymphocyte in neutropenia with T lymphocytosis. Blood 1984; 63:1133.

190. Palutke M, Eisenberg L, Kaplan J, et al: Natural killer and suppressor T-cell chronic lymphocytic leukemia. Blood 1983; 62:627.

191. Reynolds CW, Foon KA: T-gamma lymphoproliferative disease and related disorders in humans and experimental animals: A review of the clinical, cellular, and functional characteristics. Blood 1984; 64:1146.

192. Kadin ME, Kamoun M, Lamberg J: Erythrophagocytic T-gamma lymphoma: A clinicopathologic entity resembling malignant histiocytosis. N Engl J Med 1981; 304:648.

193. Okuno SH, Tefferi A, Hannson CA, et al: Spectrum of diseases associated with increased proportions or absolute numbers of peripheral blood natural killer cells. Br J Haematol 1996; 93:810.

194. Maciejewski JP, Hibbs JR, Anderson S, et al: Bone marrow and peripheral blood lymphocyte phenotype in patients with bone marrow failure. Exp Hematol 1994; 22:1102.

195. Loughran TP Jr, Kadin ME, Starkebaum G, et al: Leukemia of large granular lymphocytes: Association with clonal chromosomal abnormalities and autoimmune neutropenia, thrombocytopenia and hemolytic anemia. Ann Intern Med 1985; 102:169.

196. Loughran P Jr: Clonal diseases of large granular lymphocytes. Blood 1993; 82:1.
197. Semenzato G, Pandolfi F, Chisesi T, et al: The lymphoproliferative disease of granular lymphocytes: A heterogeneous disorder ranging from indolent to aggressive conditions. Cancer 1987; 60:2971.
198. Scott CS, Richards SJ, Sivakumaran M, et al: Transient and persistent expansions of large granular lymphocytes (LGL) and NK-associated (NKa) cells: the Yorkshire Leukaemia Group study. Br J Haematol 1993; 83:504.
199. Semenzato G, Zambello R, Starkebaum G, et al: The lymphoproliferative disease of granular lymphocytes: Updated criteria for diagnosis. Blood 1997; 89:256.
200. Chan WC, Link S, Mawie A, et al: Heterogeneity of large granular lymphocyte proliferations: Delineation of two major subsets. Blood 1986; 68:1142.
201. Pandolfi F, Loughran TP Jr, Starkebaum G, et al: Clinical course and prognosis of the lymphoproliferative disease of granular lymphocytes: A multicenter study. Cancer 1990; 65:341.
202. Dhodapkar MV, Li CY, Lust JA, et al: Clinical spectrum of clonal proliferations of T-large granular lymphocytes: A T-cell clonopathy of undetermined significance? Blood 1994; 84:1620.
203. Gentile TC, Uner AH, Hutchinson RE, et al: CD3+, CD56+ aggressive variant of large granular lymphocyte leukemia. Blood 1994; 84:2315.
204. Agnarsson BA, Loughran TP Jr, Starkebaum G, et al: The pathology of large granular lymphocyte leukemia. Hum Pathol 1989; 20:643.
205. Uchiyama T, Yodoi J, Sagawa K, et al: Adult T-cell leukemia: Clinical and hematologic features of 16 cases. Blood 1977; 50:481.
206. Shimoyama M, Minato K, Saito H, et al: Comparison of clinical, morphologic and immunologic characteristics of adult T-cell leukemia-lymphoma and cutaneous T-cell lymphoma. Jpn J Clin Oncol 1979; 9:357.
207. Catovsky D, Greaves MF, Rose M, et al: Adult T-cell lymphoma-leukaemia in blacks from the west Indies. Lancet 1982; 1:639.
208. Yoshida M, Miyoshi I, Hinuma Y: Isolation and characterization of retrovirus from cell lines of human adult T-cell leukemia and its implication in the disease. Proc Natl Acad Sci U S A 1981; 78:6476.
209. Shimamoto Y, Yamaguchi M, Miyamoto Y, et al: The differences between lymphoma and leukemia type of adult T-cell leukemia. Leuk Lymphoma 1990; 1:101.
210. Tajima K: The T- and B-cell Malignancy Study Group: The fourth nationwide study of adult T-cell leukemia/lymphoma (ATL) in Japan—estimates of risk of ATL and its geographical and clinical features. Int J Cancer 1990; 45:247.
211. Kinoshita K, Kamihira S, Ikeda S, et al: Clinical, hematologic and pathologic features of leukemic T-cell lymphoma. Cancer 1982; 50:1554.
212. Demis DJ: The mastocytosis syndrome: Clinical and biologic studies. Ann Intern Med 1963; 59:194.
213. Sagher F, Even-Paz Z: Mastocytosis and the Mast Cell. Chicago, Year Book Medical Publishers, 1967.
214. Cryer PE, Kissane JM: Systemic mastocytosis. Am J Med 1976; 61:671.
215. Fishman RS, Fleming CR, Li CY: Systemic mastocytosis: With a review of gastrointestinal manifestations. Mayo Clin Proc 1979; 54:51.
216. Brunning RD, McKenna RW, Rosai J, et al: Systemic

mastocytosis extracutaneous manifestations. Am J Surg Pathol 1983; 7:425.
217. Mutter RD, Tannenbaum M, Ultmann JE: Systemic mast cell disease. Ann Intern Med 1963; 59:887.
218. Szveda JA, Abraham JP, Fine G, et al: Systemic mast cell disease: A review and report of three cases. Am J Med 1967; 32:227.
219. Webb TA, Li CY, Yam LT: Systemic mast cell disease: A clinical and hematopathologic study of 26 cases. Cancer 1982; 49:927.
220. Mihm MC, Clark WH, Reed RJ, et al: Mast cell infiltrates of the skin and the mastocytosis syndrome. Hum Pathol 1973; 4:231.
221. Travis WD, Li CY, Bergstralh J, et al: Systemic mast cell disease: Analysis of 58 cases and literature review. Medicine 1988; 67:345.
222. Horny HP, Parwaresch MR, Lennert K: Bone marrow findings in systemic mastocytosis. Hum Pathol 1985; 16:808.
223. Ende N, Cherniss EI: Splenic mastocytosis. Blood 1958; 13:631.
224. Gonnella JS, Lipsey AI: Mastocytosis manifested by hepatosplenomegaly: Report of a case. N Engl J Med 1964; 271:533.
225. Horny H-P, Ruck MT, Kaiserling E: Spleen findings in generalized mastocytosis. Cancer 1992; 70:459.
226. Travis WD, Li CY: Pathology of the lymph node and spleen in systemic mast cell disease. Mod Pathol 1988; 1:4.
227. Horny H-P, Kaiserling E, Campbell M, et al: Liver findings in generalized mastocytosis: A clinicopathologic study. Cancer 1989; 63:532.
228. Lennert K, Parwaresch MR: Mast cells and mast cell neoplasia: A review. Histopathology 1979; 3:349.
229. Travis WD, Li C-Y, Hoagland HC, et al: Mast cell leukemia: Report of a case and review of the literature. Mayo Clin Proc 1986; 61:957.
230. Parwaresch MR, Horny HP, Lennert K: Tissue mast cells in health and disease. Pathol Res Pract 1985; 179:439.
231. Katsuda S, Okada Y, Oda Y, et al: Systemic mastocytosis without cutaneous involvement. Acta Pathol Jpn 1987; 37:167.
232. Travis W, Li C-Y, Yam LT, et al: Significance of systemic mast cell disease with associated hematologic disorders. Cancer 1988; 62:965.
233. Travis WD, Li C-Y, Bergstralh EJ: Solid and hematologic malignancies in 60 patients with systemic mast cell disease. Arch Pathol Lab Med 1989; 113:365.
234. Yam LT, Yam C-F, Li CY: Eosinophilia in systemic mastocytosis. Am J Clin Pathol 1980; 73:48.
235. Horny HP, Ruck M, Wehrmann M, et al: Blood findings in generalized mastocytosis: Evidence of frequent simultaneous occurrence of myeloproliferative disorders. Br J Haematol 1990; 76:186.
236. Wong KF, Chan JK, Chan JC, et al: Concurrent acute myeloid leukemia and systemic mastocytosis. Am J Hematol 1991; 38:243.
236a. Horny H-P, Sillaber C, Menke D, et al: Diagnostic value of immunostaining for tryptase in patients with mastocytosis. Am J Surg Pathol 1998; 22:1132.
237. Diebold J, Riviere O, Gosselin B, et al: Different patterns of spleen involvement in systemic and malignant mastocytosis: A histological and immunohistochemical study of three cases. Virchows Arch 1991; 419:273.

13

MYELOPROLIFERATIVE DISORDERS

The myeloproliferative disorders or myeloproliferative syndromes are a group of interrelated chronic diseases that include essential thrombocythemia (ET), polycythemia vera (PV), chronic idiopathic myelofibrosis (CIMF), and chronic myelogenous leukemia (CML). Although all of these disorders are recognized as clonal disorders of the hematopoietic stem cell, they vary in their presenting clinical, laboratory, and morphologic findings.[1, 2] Each syndrome has characteristic diagnostic clinical, laboratory, and morphologic features established by group studies of these diseases.[2] However, distinguishing between them is not always easy, particularly in early stages of the disease. Moreover, some cases do not fit into a single diagnostic category, and many patients evolve from one myeloproliferative disease to another during the course of their illness. All patients with myeloproliferative disorders have an increased risk of development of acute leukemia. This risk is highest in patients who are treated with certain therapeutic modalities, but the incidence of leukemic transformation or evolution is significantly higher in all patients with myeloproliferative diseases than in a control population, regardless of the type of therapy. Splenomegaly is a frequent occurrence in all of the myeloproliferative disorders; however, its incidence varies with the disease process. In addition, the pathogenesis of the splenomegaly and the morphologic findings in the spleen vary in the different syndromes. This chapter includes a discussion of the splenic disorders in ET, PV, and CIMF. CML was discussed in Chapter 12.

ESSENTIAL THROMBOCYTHEMIA

Essential thrombocythemia (essential thrombocytosis, hemorrhagic or primary thrombocy-themia) (ET)[3–6] is a chronic myeloproliferative disorder characterized by a persistent elevation of the platelet count, usually above 1,000,000/μL,[7] and associated with hemorrhagic and/or thromboembolic phenomena. The updated diagnostic criteria for essential thrombocythemia are listed in Table 13–1.[8] Most patients with ET are middle-aged or elderly. However, a separate peak incidence occurs in younger females,[9] who appear to have a particularly benign course.

The diagnosis of ET is largely one of exclusion. The platelet count must be at least 600,000/μL, and all causes of reactive thrombocytosis, such as those that may be seen in some patients with acute infection, malignant tumors, or iron deficiency anemia, must be eliminated.[8] Because striking increases in the platelet count may be the predominant or sole presenting manifestation in all of the other chronic myeloproliferative diseases, as well as in some types of myelodysplastic syndromes

Table 13–1. Diagnostic Criteria: Essential Thrombocythemia

1. Platelet count >600,000 μL
2. Hematocrit count <40, or normal red blood cell mass (males <36 mL/kg, females <32 mL/kg)
3. Stainable iron in marrow, normal serum ferritin, or normal red blood cell mean corpuscular volume
4. No Philadelphia chromosome or *bcr/abl* gene rearrangement
5. Collagen fibrosis of marrow
   A. Absent or
   B. <1/3 biopsy area without both marked splenomegaly and leukoerythroblastic reaction
6. No cytogenetic or morphologic evidence for a myelodysplastic syndrome
7. No cause for reactive thrombocytosis

such as the 5q minus syndrome, the criteria for the diagnosis also include elimination of these other diseases by morphologic, clinical, or cytogenetic criteria.[3–6, 10–12]

Using G-6PD isoenzyme studies, Fialkow et al[13] have demonstrated that ET is a clonal disorder.[13] However, conventional cytogenetic studies have documented the presence of karyotypic abnormalities in only approximately 5 percent of cases.[14] More recent studies using molecular techniques have revealed a higher incidence of clonal hematopoiesis in ET.[15–17]

The peripheral blood in patients with ET is characterized by thrombocytosis with platelets that vary greatly in size, often with bizarre forms. Fragments of megakaryocytes occasionally occur.[1, 3, 4, 8, 18] A hypochromic microcytic anemia secondary to blood loss, and neutrophilic leukocytosis, sometimes associated with mild eosinophilia or basophilia, are often present. The bone marrow reveals a marked increase in the number of megakaryocytes and prominent platelet masses, frequently associated with an increase in granulopoiesis and erythropoiesis.[11, 12, 18] There may be an increase in marrow reticulin as well.[19] The hemorrhagic diathesis that may be associated with ET is related to qualitative platelet defects, which include abnormal platelet aggregation and adhesiveness, defective release of platelet factor III, and decrease in platelet serotonin content.[20–22] Recurrent hemorrhages occur mainly from mucous membranes, particularly the gastrointestinal and genitourinary tracts. Thrombotic complications usually result from occlusion of the microvasculature, which may lead to cerebrovascular accidents, peripheral gangrene, or skin lesions.[23]

Mild to moderate splenomegaly occurs in approximately 40 percent of patients with ET.[24] The degree of splenomegaly is less marked than that in the other chronic myeloproliferative diseases. Because platelets are normally sequestered in the spleen, splenectomy is contraindicated in patients with ET. Removal of the spleen may result in a marked increase in the peripheral platelet count. Because of the spleen's ability to sequester large numbers of platelets, the organ provides a protective effect in this disorder because platelet sequestration partially ameliorates the thrombocytosis. Studies of splenic pathology in ET are few. However, we have had the opportunity to study several spleens removed from patients with ET because of traumatic rupture of that organ. In these cases the pulp cords are widened and appear relatively hypocellular because of sequestration of large numbers of platelets (Fig. 13–1). Platelets also may be seen in the sinuses. Sequestration and destruction of platelets are best demonstrated using splenic touch imprints but may be noted in splenic sections in many cases (Fig. 13–2). In advanced cases, however, the spleen often becomes atrophic and nonfunctional, probably resulting from infarction secondary to massive platelet pooling or possibly from splenic vein thrombosis.[25]

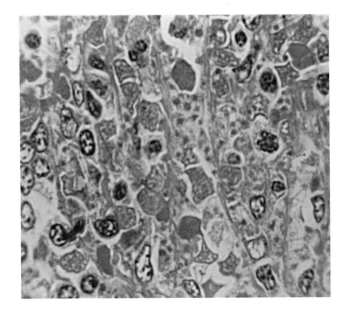

Figure 13–1. Essential thrombocythemia. Thick plastic-embedded section of red pulp. Numerous platelets are sequestered within the cords.

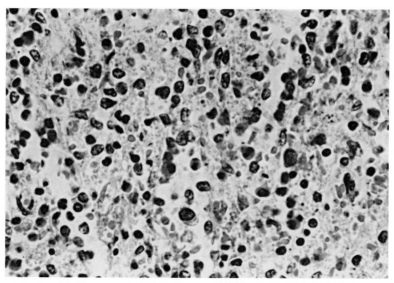

Figure 13–2. Platelets accumulate in the red pulp in essential thrombocythemia and can be appreciated as granular debris.

Such spleens show fibrosis and Gamna-Gandy bodies similar to those in the advanced stages of sickle cell disease. Functional asplenia may be detected by the appearance of Howell-Jolly bodies and target cells in the peripheral blood.

ET is a relatively benign disease, with a medium survival period of approximately 10 years.[4, 8, 19, 26, 27] Death in untreated patients is usually related to thrombotic complications.[8, 19, 26, 28–30] An overall risk of 2 to 5 percent of developing acute leukemia has been reported. However, a higher incidence of the development of leukemia has been reported in patients who are treated with radioactive phosphorus or alkylating agents.[8]

POLYCYTHEMIA VERA

Polycythemia vera (PV) is a chronic myeloproliferative disorder in which an elevated red blood cell mass occurs in the absence of hypoxic stimulation.[31] It is usually accompanied by leukocytosis and thrombocytosis. This disorder must be distinguished from erythrocytosis secondary to hypoxemia or to erythropoietin (EPO) production by a malignant neoplasm and from relative erythrocytosis due to hypovolemia.[31] In contrast to secondary erythrocytosis, EPO levels in PV are not increased.[32] This has led to the hypothesis that the marrow cells in PV have an increased responsiveness to hematopoietic growth factors such as EPO.[33, 34]

This hypothesis is supported by in vitro marrow culture studies that have shown that PV marrow has a higher cloning efficiency than normal marrow when grown in either in the presence of or without exogenous EPO.[35, 36] The fact that these colonies are of mixed hematopoietic lineage provides evidence that primitive hematopoietic progenitor cells are also more responsive to growth factors and suggests that in PV an abnormal marrow clone is present.

We now know that Dameshek's thesis that PV, as well as other MPDs, is a neoplastic (clonal) disorder is correct.[37] Evidence that PV is a clonal disorder of the marrow stem cell was first provided by analysis of G6PD isoenzymes.[38] The clonal nature of the disorder has been confirmed by molecular techniques[39, 40] and involves B lymphocytes as well as the myeloid, erythroid, and megakaryocytic lineages.[41]

Conventional cytogenetic studies have confirmed the presence of chromosome abnormalities in only about half of PV cases.[42–48] However, it appears that the incidence of cytogenetic abnormalities increases with the evolution of the disease,[47] having been reported in 15 to 20 percent of patients at diagnosis but in one third to one half of cases upon follow-up. In patients in whom acute leukemia eventually develops, chromosome abnormalities have been documented in well over three quarters of the cases.[49] There is no single characteristic chromosome abnormality in PV, and multiple abnormalities involving chromosomes 1, 5, 7, 8, 9, 12, 13, and 20 have been detected. The most frequently observed chromosome abnormalities at diagnosis are trisomy 8 and 9 and 20qminus.[50] Cytogenetic abnormalities most frequently associated with progression of the disease are 1qminus, 12qminus, and 13qminus. Additional chromosome abnormalities involving chromosomes 5 and 7 are frequently associated with chemotherapy.[42, 49]

The clinical evolution of PV has been divided into four phases.[31, 51, 52] The first phase, in which patients are "asymptomatic," is characterized by the presence of either isolated erythrocytosis or thrombocytosis and splenomegaly. The second, or "erythrocytotic" phase is characterized by erythrocytosis, thrombocytosis, and leukocytosis as well as clinical evidence of hemorrhagic or thrombotic complications. The thrombotic phenomena are caused by increased blood viscosity secondary to the high hematocrit level and by the thrombocytosis; hemorrhagic phenomena are caused by defective platelet function and may also occur secondary to thrombosis.[31, 52, 53] The third, or "stable" phase is characterized by a return to normal in the peripheral blood counts. The fourth phase, termed "spent phase" or "postpolycythemic myeloid metaplasia (PPMM)," is characterized by anemia, leukoerythroblastosis, progressive splenomegaly, and systemic symptoms of fever and weight loss.[31, 51, 52, 54–56] PPMM may be clinically indistinguishable from CIMF. All patients with PV have an increased incidence of development of acute leukemia in comparison to normal patients.[52, 57] However, the incidence of acute leukemia varies, depending on the development of PPMM and the type of therapy used.[57–65]

The bone marrow in PV usually shows trilinear hyperplasia of the hematopoietic elements, without any significant increase in reticulin, and characteristically contains no hemosiderin (storage iron).[66, 67] However, in 10 to 15 percent of cases marrow cellularity is normal, or the reticulin appears increased.[66–68]

Although palpable splenomegaly occurs in up to three quarters of patients and is one of the major criteria for diagnosis[31, 52] (Table 13–2), the spleen is rarely available for study in uncomplicated PV. Splenectomy is contraindicated because it leads to even greater thrombocytosis and may result in life-threatening thrombotic complications. Moreover, at the time of autopsy the disease has often evolved into the spent phase or into acute leukemia.[52]

The degree of splenomegaly in PV is usually mild or moderate. Smaller spleens are associated with disease of shorter duration.[69–71] The size of the spleen may be transiently decreased following myelosuppressive therapy or radioactive phosphorus (^{32}P). Gross examination reveals congested parenchyma with inconspicuous white pulp, often with foci of hemorrhage or infarction.[71, 72] Because of the scarcity of splenectomy specimens for study, speculation about the cause of the splenomegaly in PV has been controversial. Investigators have stated that extramedullary hematopoiesis and increased reticulin deposition are responsible for the splenic enlargement.[51, 56, 69] Ward and Block[51] stated that the spleen in early PV shows trilinear extramedullary hematopoiesis identical to that in agnogenic myeloid metaplasia. Rappaport,[72] on the other hand, stated that splenomegaly in PV is due primarily to congestion and that if significant extramedullary hem-

Table 13–2. Criteria for the Diagnosis of Polycythemia Vera

Categories

A1. Increased red cell mass:
    greater than or equal to 36 mL/kg (male)
    greater than or equal to 36 mL/kg (female)
or: Hematocrit greater than 60%

A2. Normal arterial O_2 saturation (greater than or equal to 92%)

A3. Splenomegaly

B1. Thrombocytosis greater than 400,000 per μL

B2. Leukocytosis greater than 12,000 per μL (no fever or infection)

B3. Leukocyte alkaline phosphatase greater than 100 (no fever or infection)
Serum B_{12} greater than 900 pg/mL,
              or:
unbound B_{12} binding capacity greater than 2,200 pg/mL

Diagnosis established if following combinations are present: A1 + A2 + A3; A1 + A2 + any two from category B.

atopoiesis is present, it probably indicates a transition to postpolycythemic myeloid metaplasia. Review of the studies reporting splenic myeloid metaplasia in PV reveals that the bone marrow in these cases usually showed some degree of fibrosis or that the peripheral blood showed leukoerythroblastosis, features that suggest that the disorder had evolved to the spent phase (i.e., postpolycythemic myeloid metaplasia). Two studies of splenic aspirates reported the absence of myeloid metaplasia in uncomplicated PV,[56, 73] and one postulated that aggregates of platelets were responsible for the splenomegaly.[73]

In a review of 22 spleens obtained at autopsy from patients with uncomplicated PV, Wolf and colleagues[71] found minimal extramedullary hematopoiesis by conventional examination of histologic sections and by immunohistologic techniques (Fig. 13–3). In contrast, spleens from 20 patients in the spent phase of PV—as manifested by increasing splenomegaly, leukoerythroblastosis, normalization of the red blood cell mass, and increased bone marrow reticulin—showed a significant degree of trilinear extramedullary hematopoiesis (Fig. 13–4). These findings prove that splenomegaly in uncomplicated PV is due primarily to congestion associated with the plethora that is characteristic of the disease. The presence of significant numbers of hematopoietic precur-

sors in the spleen of patients with PV correlates with the transition to PPMM.

CHRONIC IDIOPATHIC MYELOFIBROSIS

Among the myeloproliferative disorders, both the incidence and the degree of splenomegaly is greatest in chronic idiopathic myelofibrosis (CIMF). This disorder has been referred to by a large number of terms, including "agnogenic myeloid metaplasia," "myelofibrosis with myeloid metaplasia," "idiopathic myeloid metaplasia," "myelosclerosis with myeloid metaplasia," "leukoerythroblastic anemia," and "chronic nonleukemic myelosis."[1, 2, 51, 74–79] CIMF is a chronic disorder, with an average survival after diagnosis of about 5 years. However, survival may range from 1 to more than 30 years.[78] The rate of progression of the disease may vary.[80] However, prognostic factors also appear related to the point in the progression of the disease in which the diagnosis is made.[81–84] CIMF may share clinical, laboratory, and morphologic features with other myeloproliferative diseases.[2, 78, 80, 85–87] However, characteristic diagnostic features are reticulin deposition and fibrosis in the bone marrow, leukoerythroblastosis with giant platelets, megakaryo-

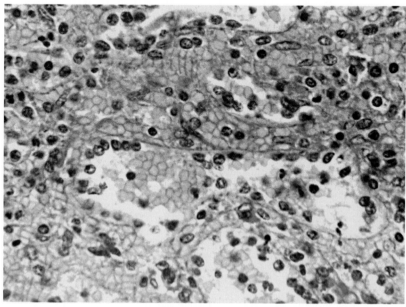

Figure 13–3. Representative example of the morphology of the spleen in a patient dying of unrelated causes during the erythrocytotic phase of polycythemia vera. Note that the red pulp is engorged with mature erythrocytes and that there is no significant extramedullary hematopoiesis.

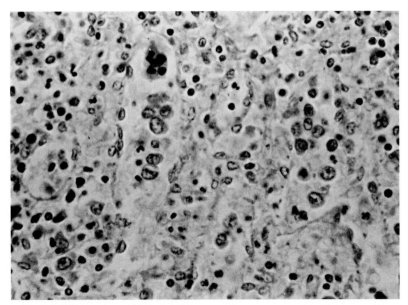

Figure 13–4. The spleen in the spent phase of polycythemia vera shows extramedullary hematopoiesis identical to that in chronic idiopathic myelofibrosis.

cyte fragments and anisocytosis and poikilocytosis with teardrop-shaped erythrocytes in the peripheral blood, and proliferation of trilinear hematopoietic precursor cells in the spleen. The disease may arise de novo or may evolve from PV, in which case it has been termed "postpolycythemic myeloid metaplasia (PPMM)" or "spent phase PV."[31, 51, 52, 54–56] CIMF most commonly occurs in middle-aged to elderly individuals. However, it has been reported on rare occasions in pediatric patients.[88]

As is the case with the other myeloproliferative disorders, CIMF is a clonal disorder of the bone marrow stem cell.[42, 89–92] The marrow fibrosis has been shown to be a secondary reaction. The fibroblasts of the bone marrow have been shown to be cytogenetically normal[93, 94] and having the physical and proliferative characteristics of normal marrow fibroblasts.[94–97] Evidence has been provided that growth factors released from the neoplastic clone of hematopoietic cells in CIMF are the probable source of the fibroblastic proliferation. The megakaryocyte appears to be the primary source of these factors.[98, 99] Platelet-derived growth factor, transforming growth factor-β, and epidermal growth factor have all been considered to be involved in this process.[100–105] It has been demonstrated that the fibroblasts in CIMF are more sensitive to growth factors than are normal marrow fibroblasts.[106]

Approximately one half of patients with CIMF have karyotypic abnormalities.[107–112] No abnormality specific to this disorder has been identified. However, the most common abnormalities involve trisomy 1q, 8, 9, 21, and 13q.[107–112]

Bone marrow morphology varies widely in cases of CIMF.[1, 51, 80, 113–115] Although all biopsy samples show a patchy increase in reticulin, the degree is extremely variable.[51, 80, 113–115] Marrow cellularity ranges from almost 100 percent, with only a slight increase in reticulin, to virtual depletion of the hematopoietic elements associated with extensive collagenous fibrosis. In spite of this variability, there are several constant features.[113] The hematopoietic cellularity is always trilinear, although in some cases one cell line may predominate. However, increased numbers of megakaryocytes are always seen and characteristically appear dysplastic with bizarre nuclear configurations, including hyposegmented and hyperchromatic hypersegmented forms. In addition, several studies[113, 114] have noted that all cases show increased numbers of distended bone marrow sinusoids that frequently contain hematopoietic precursors, a feature we believe is important in the pathogenesis of the leukoerythroblastosis and the splenomegaly in this disorder.

Progressive splenomegaly is typical of CIMF, although the splenic enlargement may be temporarily arrested by splenic irradiation or chemotherapy and may vary in the rate of enlargement.[1, 51, 80, 113, 114] We have shown that the degree of splenomegaly correlates with the duration of disease.[113] Ward and Block[51] estimated that the splenic size increases clinically by approximately 1.0 cm per year. Massive splenomegaly is the rule in advanced disease, and splenic weights of 5000 g or greater are not uncommon. Splenomegaly may be the presenting feature of this disorder, resulting in pressure symptoms, early satiety, or pain from infarction. It is not unusual for massive splenomegaly to be found at routine physical examination in asymptomatic patients.[78]

The gross appearance of the spleen in CIMF is essentially indistinguishable from that of the acute leukemias (Color Plate 20). The organ may appear deep red, from marked congestion of the red pulp, or pale because of the infiltration of hematopoietic cells. The white pulp markings are usually indistinct. Infarcts at varying stages of organization are common. Microscopic examination of the spleen reveals hematopoietic precursors in the red pulp (Fig. 13–5). The hematopoiesis is trilinear and contains cells at all stages of maturation.[51, 113, 116] Although some authors[51] have stated that the hematopoietic cells are found only in the sinuses, Tavassoli and Weiss,[117] using electron microscopy, demonstrated hematopoietic cells

in the cords of Billroth as well. Normoblasts are easily recognized in routinely stained sections because of their tendency to cluster in erythroid islands within red pulp sinuses. Megakaryocytes showing the same dysplastic features seen in the bone marrow are also readily identifiable both within sinusoids and the cords of Billroth.[113] Myeloid precursors are usually more difficult to discern because they tend to preferentially infiltrate the pulp cords where they may be mistaken for cordal macrophages. They may also aggregate around trabeculae. Immature hematopoietic precursors of the myeloid, erythroid, and megakaryocytic cell lines can be identified by the immunoperoxidase technique using antibodies to myeloperoxidase, hemoglobin, and platelet factor VIII, respectively. Phagocytosis of hematopoietic precursors and nuclear debris by cordal macrophages are common findings.[113, 117] A variable degree of fibrosis of the cords of Billroth may occur, particularly later in the course of the disease.[51, 113]

In some cases, relatively pure aggregates of megakaryocytes (Fig. 13–6), or less commonly of immature erythroid or myeloid cells, may be found. These aggregates may sometimes form grossly visible nodules that have been termed "plums" (Fig. 13–7) (see Color Plate 17). This formation may occur in the chronic

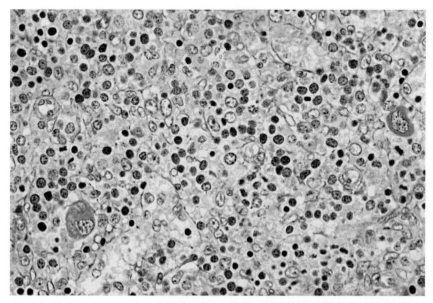

Figure 13–5. Extramedullary hematopoiesis in chronic idiopathic myelofibrosis. Dysplastic megakaryocytes are easily identified, as are clusters of normoblasts and immature hematopoietic cells. Granulocyte precursors are usually more difficult to discern because they are preferentially located in the pulp cords, where they may be mistaken for cordal macrophages, and in peritrabecular spaces, where they mimic large lymphoid cells.

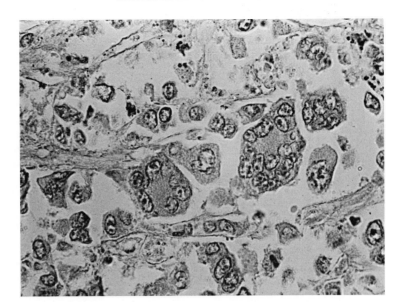

Figure 13–6. Dysplastic cells of megakaryocytic lineage form a tumor mass of chronic idiopathic myelofibrosis.

phase of the disorder or may represent an extramedullary manifestation of the transformation of CIMF to acute leukemia.

It was formerly believed that progressive fibrosis occurs in the bone marrow in the course of CIMF and that this fibrosis resulted in compensatory hematopoiesis in the spleen.[51, 85] This belief was supported by the observation that hypercellular marrows were often found in patients with mild splenomegaly, and fibrotic marrows were often associated with mas-

sive splenomegaly. However, recent studies have indicated that there is controversy regarding whether the fibrosis that occurs in CIMF is in fact progressive.[51, 80, 85, 113, 114, 118–121] Progression in fibrosis was documented in a study by Thiele et al.[118] However, in a study of 35 cases of CIMF, Wolf and Neiman found that hypercellular marrows were obtained in some cases from patients with symptoms of many years' duration and with prominent splenomegaly.[113] In addition, hypocellular fibrotic biopsy sam-

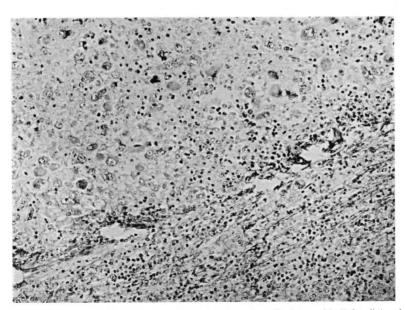

Figure 13–7. A nodule composed predominantly of megakaryocytic cells forms this "plum" in chronic idiopathic myelofibrosis.

ples were sometimes taken from patients with a short history and only mild splenomegaly. We were unable to demonstrate a relationship between splenic size and the degree of medullary fibrosis. Our findings were similar to those previously published by Pitcock et al[119] and by Lohman and Beckman,[120] who reported a reversion of some cases to polycythemia vera, and by a more recent study of Thiele et al.[80] We have concluded that although progression in marrow fibrosis does occur in many cases, it is variable in both its rate and in different marrow sites and that it is probably reversible in certain cases.

There is also controversy regarding whether the size of the spleen at presentation has prognostic significance. Although Ward and Block[51] and Varki et al[82] indicated that there was a correlation between the size of the spleen at presentation and overall survival, Barosi et al[83] and Visani et al[84] have not found this to be the case.

Although the number, degree of immaturity, and the relative proportions of the hematopoietic cells in the spleen do not appear to correlate with the degree of bone marrow fibrosis, we have observed that both the number and immaturity increase in the latter stages of the disease (Fig. 13–8) and that these findings appear to correlate with the likelihood of developing acute leukemic transformation.

Progressive enlargement of the spleen in CIMF results in a number of complications. In addition to the physical symptoms such as pain, abdominal distension, and loss of appetite due to massive splenomegaly, there are hematologic complications, attributable to anemia, bleeding, or thrombocytopenia, due to increasing hypersplenism in the presence of a failing bone marrow.[122] Splenic irradiation and treatment with cytoxic agents have been used to shrink the spleen. The results of splenic irradiation with or without concomitant chemotherapy have been transient.[123–128]

The role of splenectomy in the management of CIMF is controversial.[129–136] Intuitively, it seems to make little sense to remove the major hematopoietic organ in this disease, and early investigators stated that splenectomy was contraindicated, in part because one would remove the major hematopoietic organ and because of a high incidence of postoperative infectious complications.[133] However, others suggested that the hematopoiesis in the spleen was ineffective and proposed that splenectomy be performed immediately at the time of diagnosis, believing that the operation was better tolerated early in the course of the disease before the development of massive splenomegaly or severe cytopenias.[129] Splenectomy is currently performed in cases in which secondary hypersplenism results in severe anemia or thrombocytopenia or in which the enlarged spleen causes intractable pressure symptoms.[130, 134, 136] Because of the high operative morbidity and mortality rates,[133] some have advised ferrokinetic studies to determine the relative values of blood production versus destruction in the spleen. However, these studies have proved to be of little value in predicting

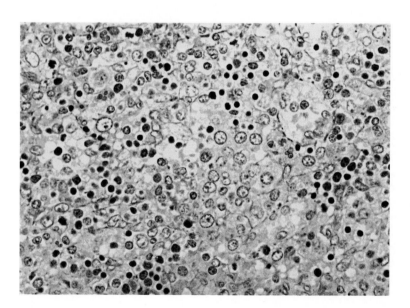

Figure 13–8. In this example of long-standing chronic idiopathic myelofibrosis (CIMF), there are numerous blastic cells in addition to normoblasts. More primitive hematopoietic precursors occur most frequently in long-standing cases of CIMF and may indicate extramedullary blast transformation of the disease.

the outcome of splenectomy.[130, 136] Splenectomy most usually results in the remission of cytopenias,[135] although it does not alter the course of the disease. However, some patients with CIMF may have thrombocytosis, which is a contraindication to splenectomy because, postoperatively, the thrombocytosis may be aggravated, resulting in thromboembolic complications. Occasionally, striking enlargement and dysfunction of the liver has been observed following splenectomy, most likely due to the liver assuming the role of filtering hematopoietic precursors of the blood.[137, 138] In addition, we have noted an increased incidence of the development of extramedullary hematopoiesis and extramedullary hematopoietic tumors in other sites in patients following splenectomy. One study has reported an increased incidence of the development of leukemic transformation after splenectomy.[136] Because of the high degree of morbidity and mortality associated with splenectomy in CIMF,[133] partial splenectomy has recently been employed.[139] Other therapeutic modalities have been sought, and interferons have been used; therapeutic results, however, have been variable. Although positive responses have been obtained, they are associated with some serious side effects.[140–143]

One of the major causes of death in CIMF and one of the most dreaded complications is the development of acute leukemia. This has been estimated to occur in 5 to 22 percent of cases.[51, 78, 81, 82, 144–149] Patients who have received therapy with alkylating agents or radiotherapy appear to be at highest risk.[83, 87, 148–156] There appears to be an unusually high incidence of megakaryoblastic transformation in patients with CIMF.[149] Because of the widespread distribution of hematopoietic cells into other organs in this disease, extramedullary transformation is fairly common in CIMF. As might be expected, the spleen is the most common site of this transformation.

Three theories have been advanced to explain the extramedullary hematopoiesis in CIMF.[51] First, early investigators postulated that CIMF was a neoplastic disorder or a form of leukemia. Ward and Block[51] dismissed this theory because they believed that the trilinear hematopoiesis clearly differs from the destructive proliferation of one cell line that occurs in the leukemias. In favor of this theory, however, are the facts that the hematopoietic cells are clonal and that there is progressive accumulation and proliferation of these cells with

frequent predominance of primitive cells of a single line. Second, the compensatory theory states that splenic hematopoiesis occurs in compensation for a progressively failing bone marrow.[51] This hypothesis is clearly disproved by the observation of striking splenic hematopoiesis in patients whose bone marrows are markedly hypercellular.[113, 114]

The third theory regarding the cause of splenic extramedullary hematopoiesis in CIMF, and the one accepted by Ward and Block,[51] is the myelostimulatory theory. Dameshek first postulated a "myelostimulatory factor" that causes proliferation not only of marrow elements but also of potential hematopoietic precursors present in sites of embryonic hematopoiesis.[37] Splenic "myeloid metaplasia" would therefore recapitulate the hematopoiesis that is believed to occur in the human fetal spleen.[51] However, recent studies from our laboratory and others (see Chapter 2) have indicated that the human fetal spleen does not usually function as an active site of hematopoiesis,[157, 158] nor is it an active site for erythropoietic and granulopoietic growth factors.[158] If the human spleen is not normally a hematopoietic organ, the origin of the hematopoietic cells found there in CIMF must be extrasplenic. We believe that splenic "myeloid metaplasia" in CIMF results from filtration and entrapment of circulating hematopoietic precursors. Numerous studies have confirmed the intuitive notion that there is a significant increase in circulating hematopoietic precursor cells in CIMF.[159–164] The invariable presence in CIMF of distended bone marrow sinusoids containing intravascular hematopoietic cells explains the leukoerythroblastosis characteristic of this disorder.[55] The altered marrow stroma may provide a mechanism for these cells to gain access to the blood.[113] This hypothesis is consistent with our observation that the progression of splenomegaly does not correlate with the extent of bone marrow fibrosis in CIMF because the accumulation of hematopoietic cells in the spleen would, therefore, be a function of duration of disease rather than the degree of medullary fibrosis.[113] The thesis that the presence of splenic hematopoietic cells in CIMF is the result of filtration of an increased number of circulating hematopoietic precursor cells released from the bone marrow because of alterations in the marrow stroma is supported by data in experimental animals in which chemically induced myelofibrosis produces a disease almost identical to

CIMF.[165] This theory is also supported by the observations of Neiman and colleagues in patients with carcinoma with marrow metastasis.[166] In that study, we noted that intravascular hematopoiesis in the bone marrow, leukoerythroblastosis, and the presence of hematopoietic cells in the spleen coexist in these patients in a manner virtually identically to that in CIMF. A similar mechanism probably exists in another unrelated disease, osteopetrosis (marble bone disease).[167] It is therefore clear that the triad of intravascular hematopoiesis, leukoerythroblastosis, and the presence of hematopoietic precursor cells in the spleen may occur in widely differing conditions, including those in which clonal evolution in an extramedullary site cannot be the likely mechanism and in which the common denominator is alteration in the bone marrow stroma (Table 13–3).

ACUTE MYELOFIBROSIS

In 1963 Lewis and Szur described a disorder that they termed "malignant myelosclerosis," characterized by an acute clinical course, rapid development of peripheral blood cytopenias with leukoerythroblastosis, and no detectable splenomegaly.[168] Bone marrow findings in their study were considered to be identical with those in classic CIMF. A number of subse-

Table 13–3. Conditions Associated with Splenic Extramedullary Hematopoiesis

1. Neoplastic (clonal)
   A. Idiopathic myelofibrosis
   B. Spent-phase polycythemia vera ("postpolycythemic myeloid metaplasia")
   C. Other myeloproliferative disorders associated with marrow fibrosis
   D. Some myelodysplastic disorders, usually associated with marrow fibrosis
   E. Hematologic neoplasms associated with mediastinal germ cell tumors
2. Non-neoplastic (nonclonal)
   A. Severe hemolytic processes (primarily or exclusively erythropoiesis)
      1. Hemoglobinopathies (most notably thalassemia)
      2. Autoimmune hemolytic anemias
      3. Thrombotic thrombocytopenic purpura
   B. Hemophagocytic syndromes
   C. Immune thrombocytopenic purpura
   D. Cytokine administration
   E. Post–bone marrow transplantation
   F. Marrow involvement by metastatic carcinomas
   G. Osteopetrosis
   H. Splenic vascular tumors

quent studies have described a similar disorder that has been termed "acute myelofibrosis," "acute myelosclerosis," "acute megakaryocytic myelofibrosis," and "acute myelodysplasia with myelofibrosis."[169–172] Most cases are characterized by a fibrotic bone marrow with trilinear hypoplasia of immature hematopoietic elements and conspicuous megakaryocytes showing variable degrees of atypia. The peripheral blood usually shows pancytopenia with occasional circulating blast cells and lacks the anisocytosis and poikilocytosis of CIMF. Splenomegaly is minimal or absent, and myeloid metaplasia is not a prominent feature. The course is rapidly fatal, often terminating in acute leukemia of myeloid, megakaryocytic, or lymphoblastic type, in which splenomegaly may result from leukemic infiltration.[173–175] The disease usually occurs in adults, but rare cases have been described in children.[176] The true nature of acute myelofibrosis is not understood. It is known that fibroblastic proliferation in the bone marrow is a common finding in many myeloproliferative and myelodysplastic disorders. Moreover, the presence of fibrosis in the bone marrow has made immunologic, molecular, and cytogenetic studies difficult. The few studies that are available do not indicate that there is a characteristic cytogenetic abnormality in cases called acute myelofibrosis.[177–180] As a result, there is lack of unanimity as to the nature of this disorder. Some believe that it is a variant of acute myeloid leukemia.[175, 181–183] Others consider it to be equivalent to acute megakaryocytic leukemia (M7).[175, 181, 182] Yet others believe that it is an acute variant of myelodysplastic syndromes,[183–187] a group of disorders in which myelofibrosis can also be observed.[188]

Splenomegaly is not a characteristic feature of acute myelofibrosis, and there are no studies of the organ in this disease, except for those in which the disorder has evolved into an acute leukemia. In the few such cases we have studied, the spleen reveals the characteristic features of acute leukemia.

ACUTE LEUKEMIA AND THE CHRONIC MYELOPROLIFERATIVE DISORDERS

The development of acute leukemia is a long-term complication in all the myeloproliferative disorders. The incidence of leukemic transformation appears to be significantly affected by the type of therapy given the patient. However, all the myeloproliferative diseases appear to have an increased incidence of development of leukemia over that of control patients regardless of the therapy given. The development of acute leukemia appears to be highest in CIMF and has been reported to range from 5 to 22 percent.[78] The next highest incidence occurs in PV, in which an overall leukemia rate appears to range from 8 to 10 percent.[57, 189, 190] The lowest incidence appears to be in ET.[8] In all diseases, an increased incidence of acute leukemia appears to be directly related to the prior usage of alkalizing agents, radiotherapy, or ^{32}P.[8, 81, 147, 148, 189, 190] In the case of ET, it would appear that the incidence of acute leukemia is rare in patients who have not been treated with ^{32}P or an alkylating agent.[8, 191] In the case of PV, the findings are more complicated. Even in those patients treated long-term with hydroxyurea and pipobroman, the risk rate of leukemia approximates 10 percent.[192, 193] The incidence of acute leukemia in polycythemia vera is also, in part, determined by the development of postpolycythemic myeloid metaplasia, being higher in those patients who progress to this disorder. In CIMF, it has been shown that patients with greater than 10 percent white blood precursors in the peripheral blood and a hemoglobin level of less than 10 g/dL have a higher incidence of leukemic conversion than patients without these hematologic parameters.[83, 84] In contrast to patients with ET and PV, only approximately one half of patients who develop acute leukemia following CIMF have received previous alkalining agents or radiation therapy, suggesting that there is an increased likelihood of developing acute leukemia as an underlying characteristic of the disease in CIMF.[78]

The leukemic transformation occurring in the myeloproliferative diseases may be of any of the FAB subtypes, presumably because all three disorders represent stem cell abnormalities.[148] Megakaryoblastic transformation is particularly common in CIMF, although other subtypes can also occur.[149] An association between acute myelofibrosis and lymphoblastic transformation has been recently reported.[174]

The early stages of transformation to acute leukemia may be difficult to recognize morphologically. This is particularly true in CIMF, in which increased numbers of blasts may occur in the bone marrow and in the peripheral blood in the stable phase of the disorder. In these circumstances, the documentation of acute leukemia rests on a comparison of serial bone marrow or peripheral blood samples or both. In approximately one third to one half of cases, the acute leukemic transformation occurs in an extramedullary site. The spleen is the most common of these sites.[194, 195] This occurrence is usually characterized clinically by a sudden increase in splenic size with pain, due either to increased pressure on the splenic capsule or to infarction. Splenectomy is frequently undertaken to ameliorate the symptoms or to alleviate the hypersplenism that may occur because of a relatively rapid increase in splenic size. In these cases, histologic examination of the spleen may provide the first clue that the patient has entered a transformation to acute leukemia. Evidence of the underlying myeloproliferative disorder may be present, in particular trilinear extramedullary hematopoiesis in either the spent phase of PV or in CIMF. However, careful examination of histologic sections in splenic blast transformation usually reveals that there is a replacement of the trilinear hematopoietic proliferation by a predominant cell line and that there is less differentiation in that cell line.

REFERENCES

1. Dickstein JI, Vardiman JW: Hematopathologic findings in the myeloproliferative disorders. Semin Oncol 1995; 22:355.
2. Dickstein JI, Vardiman JW: Issues in the pathology and diagnosis of the chronic myeloproliferative disorders and the myelodysplastic syndromes. Am J Clin Pathol 1993; 99:513.
3. van Genderen PJ, Michiels JJ: Primary thrombocythemia: Diagnosis, clinical manifestations and management. Ann Hematol 1993; 67:57.
4. Tefferi A, Silverstein MN, Hoagland HC: Primary thrombocythemia. Semin Oncol 1995; 22:334.
5. Kwong YL, Liang RH, Chiu EK, et al: Essential thrombocythemia: A retrospective analysis of 39 cases. Am J Hematol 1995; 49:39.
6. Tefferi A, Hoagland HC: Issues in the diagnosis and management of essential thrombocythemia. Mayo Clin Proc 1994; 69:651.
7. Murphy S, Iland H, Rosenthal D, et al: Essential thrombocythemia: An interim report from the polycythemia vera study group. Semin Hematol 1986; 23:177.
8. Murphy S, Peterson P, Iland H, et al: Experience of the polycythemia vera study group with essential thrombocythemia: A final report on diagnostic criteria, survival, and leukemic transition by treatment. Semin Hematol 1997; 34:29.
9. McIntyre KJ, Hoagland HC, Silverstein MN, et al: Essential thrombocythemia in young adults. Mayo Clin Proc 1991; 66:149.
10. Stroll DB, Peterson P, Exten R, et al: Clinical presen-

tation and natural history of patients with essential thrombocythemia and the Philadelphia chromosome. Am J Hematol 1988; 27:77.

11. Thiele J, Moedder B, Kremer B, et al: Chronic myeloproliferative disorders with an elevated platelet count (in excess of 1,000,000/μL): A clinicopathological study on 46 patients with special emphasis on primary (essential) thrombocythemia. Hematol Pathol 1987; 1:227.

12. Thiele J, Schneider G, Hoeppner B, et al: Histomorphometry of bone marrow biopsies in chronic myeloproliferative disorders with associated thrombocytosis: Features of significance for the diagnosis of primary (essential) thrombocythaemia. Virchows Arch 1988; 413:407.

13. Fialkow PJ, Faguet FB, Jacobson RJ, et al: Evidence that essential thrombocythemia is a clonal disorder with origin in a multipotent stem cell. Blood 1981; 58:916.

14. Report on Essential Thrombocythemia: Third international workshop on chromosomes in leukemia. Cancer Genet Cytogenet 1981; 4:138.

15. Yang L, Elkassar N, Gardin C, et al: Clonality assays and megakaryocyte culture techniques in essential thrombocythemia. Leuk Lymphoma 1996; 1:31.

16. Kassar NE, Hetet G, Li Y, et al: Clonal analysis of haemopoietic cells in essential thrombocythaemia. Br J Haematol 1995; 90:131.

17. el-Kassar N, Hetet G, Briere J, et al: Clonality analysis of hematopoiesis in essential thrombocythemia: Advantages of studying T lymphocytes and platelets. Blood 1997; 89:128.

18. Buss DH, O'Connor ML, Woodruff RD, et al: Bone marrow and peripheral blood findings in patients with extreme thrombocytosis: A report of 63 cases. Arch Pathol Lab Med 1991; 115:475.

19. Hehlmann R, Jahn M, Baumann B, et al: Essential thrombocythemia: Clinical characteristics and course of 61 cases. Cancer 1988; 61:2487.

20. Sehayek E, Ben-Yosef N, Modan M, et al: Platelet parameters and aggregation in essential and reactive thrombocytosis. Am J Clin Pathol 1988; 90:431.

21. Mitus AJ, Barbui T, Shulman LN, et al: Hemostatic complications in young patients with essential thrombocythemia. Am J Med 1990; 88:371.

22. Haznedaroglu IC, Ertenli I, Ozcebe OI, et al: Megakaryocyte-related interleukins in reactive thrombocytosis versus autonomous thrombocythemia. Acta Haematol 1996; 95:107.

23. Singh AK, Wetherley-Mein G: Microvascular occlusive lesions in primary thrombocythaemia. Br J Haematol 1977; 36:553.

24. Murphy S, Iland H: Thrombocytosis, in Laszlo J, Schafer A (eds): Thrombosis and Hemorrhage, p 597. Cambridge, Mass, Blackwell Scientific, 1994.

25. Marsh GW, Lewis SM, Szur L: The use of 51Cr-labeled heat-damaged red cells to study splenic function. II. Splenic atrophy in thrombocythaemia. Br J Haematol 1966; 12:167.

26. Bellucci S, Janvier M, Tobelem G, et al: Essential thrombocythemias: Clinical evolutionary and biological data. Cancer 1986; 58:2440.

27. Fenaux P, Simon M, Caulier MT, et al: Clinical course of essential thrombocythemia in 147 cases. Cancer 1990; 66:549.

28. Geller SA, Shapiro E: Acute leukemia as a natural sequel to primary thrombocythemia. Am J Clin Pathol 1982; 77:353.

29. Sedlacek SM, Curtis JL, Weintraub J, et al: Essential thrombocythemia and leukemic transformation. Medicine 1986; 65:353.

30. Shibata K, Shimamoto Y, Suga K, et al: Essential thrombocythemia terminating in acute leukemia with minimal myeloid differentiation: A brief review of recent literature. Acta Haematol 1994; 91:84.

31. Berlin NI: Classification of the polycythemias and initial clinical features in polycythemia vera, in Wasserman LR, Berk PD, Berlin NI (eds): Polycythemia and the Myeloproliferative Disorders, p 22. Philadelphia, WB Saunders, 1995.

32. Koeffler HP, Goldwasser E: Erythropoietin radioimmunoassay in evaluating patients with polycythemia. Ann Intern Med 1981; 94:44.

33. Dai CH, Krantz SB, Means RT Jr, et al: Polycythemia vera blood burst-forming units-erythroid are hypersensitive to interleukin-3. J Clin Invest 1991; 87:391.

34. Zanjani ED, Lutton JD, Hoffman R, et al: Erythroid colony formation by polycythemia vera bone marrow in vitro: Dependence on erythropoietin. J Clin Invest 1977; 59:841.

35. Fauser AA, Messner HA: Pluripotent hemopoietic progenitors (CFU-GEMM) in polycythemia vera: Analysis of erythropoietin requirement and proliferative activity. Blood 1981; 58:1224.

36. Ash RC, Detrick RA, Sanjani ED: In vitro studies of human pluripotent hematopoietic progenitors in polycythemia vera. J Clin Invest 1982; 69:1112.

37. Dameshek W: Some speculations on the myeloproliferative syndromes. Blood 1951; 6:372.

38. Adamson JW, Fialkow PJ, Murphy S, et al: Polycythemia vera: Stem-cell and probable clonal origin of the disease. N Engl J Med 1976; 295:913.

39. Gilliland DG, Glanchard KL, Levy J, et al: Clonality in myeloproliferative disorders: Analysis by means of the polymerase chain reaction. Proc Natl Acad Sci U S A 1991; 88:6848.

40. Lucas GS, Padua RA, Masters GS, et al: The application of X chromosome gene probes to the diagnosis of myeloproliferative disease. Br J Haematol 1989; 72:530.

41. Raskind WH, Jacobson R, Murphy S, et al: Evidence of the involvement of B lymphoid cells in polycythemia vera and essential thrombocythemia. J Clin Invest 1985; 75:1388.

42. Testa Jr, Kanofsky JR, Rowley JA, et al: Karyotypic patterns and their clinical significance in polycythemia vera. Am J Hematol 1981; 11:29.

43. Rege-Chambrin G, Mecucci C, Tricot G, et al: A chromosomal profile of polycythemia vera. Cancer Genet Cytogenet 1987; 25:233.

44. Wurster-Hill D, Whang-Peng J, McIntyre OR, et al: Cytogenetic studies in polycythemia vera. Semin Hematol 1976; 13:13.

45. Swolin B, Weinfield A, Westin J: Trisomy 1q in polycythemia vera and its relation to disease transition. Am J Hematol 1986; 22:155.

46. Johnson DD, DeWald GW, Pierre RV, et al: Deletions of chromosome 13 in malignant hematologic disorders. Cancer Genet Cytogenet 1985; 18:235.

47. Swolin B, Weinfeld A, Westin J: A prospective long-term cytogenetic study in polycythemia in relationship to treatment and clinical course. Blood 1988; 72:386.

48. Diez-Martin JL, Graham DL, Petitt RM, et al: Chromosome studies in 104 patients with polycythemia vera. Mayo Clin Proc 1991; 66:287.

49. Groupe Francaise de Cytogenetique Hematologique: Cytogenetics of acutely transformed chronic myeloproliferative syndromes without a Philadelphia chromosome. Cancer Genet Cytogenet 1988; 32:157.

50. Aatola M, Armstrong E, Teerenhovi L, et al: Clinical significance of the del(20q) chromosome in hematologic disorders. Cancer Genet Cytogenet 1992; 62:75.

51. Ward HP, Block MH: The natural history of agnogenic myeloid metaplasia (AMM) and a critical evaluation of its relationship with the myeloproliferative syndrome. Medicine 1971; 50:357.

52. Peterson P, Wasserman LR: The natural history of polycythemia vera, in Wasserman LR, Berk PD, Berlin NI (eds): Polycythemia and the Myeloproliferative Disorders, p 14. Philadelphia, WB Saunders, 1995.

53. Murphy S: Megakaryocytes, platelets, and coagulation in the myeloproliferative disease. In Wasserman LR, Berk PD, Berlin NI (eds): Polycythemia and the Myeloproliferative Disorders, p 102. Philadelphia, WB Saunders, 1995.

54. Silverstein MN: The evolution into and treatment of late stage polycythemia vera. Semin Hematol 1976; 13:79.

55. Silverstein MN: Postpolycythemia myeloid metaplasia. Ann Intern Med 1975; 134:113.

56. Ikkala E, Rapola J, Kotilaninen M: Polycythaemia vera and myelofibrosis. Scand J Haematol 1967; 4:453.

57. Landaw SA: Acute leukemia in polycythemia vera, in Wasserman LR, Berk PD, Berlin NI (eds): Polycythemia and the Myeloproliferative Disorders, p 154. Philadelphia, WB Saunders, 1995.

58. Berk PD, Goldberg JD, Silverstein MN, et al: Increased incidence of acute leukemia in polycythemia vera associated with chlorambucil therapy. N Engl J Med 1981; 304:441.

59. Lawrence JH, Winchell HS, Donald WG: Leukemia in polycythemia vera: Relationship to splenic myeloid metaplasia and therapeutic radiation dose. Ann Intern Med 1969; 70:763.

60. Modan B, Lilienfeld AM: Polycythemia vera and leukemia: The role of radiation treatment—a study of 1,222 patients. Medicine 1965; 44:305.

61. Berk PD, Goldberg JD, Donovan PB, et al: Therapeutic recommendations in polycythemia vera based on polycythemia vera study group protocols. Semin Hematol 1986; 23:132.

62. Wasserman LR, Goldberg JD, Balcerzak SP, et al: Influence of therapy on causes of death in polycythemia vera. Clin Res 1981; 29:573.

63. Nand S, Messmore H, Fisher SG, et al: Leukemic transformation in polycythemia vera: Analysis of risk factors. Am J Hematol 1990; 34:32.

64. Landaw SA: Acute leukemia in polycythemia vera. Semin Hematol 1986; 23:157.

65. Fruchtman SM, Kaplan ME, Peterson P, et al: Hydroxyurea (HU) in the management of polycythemia vera (PV): Analysis of long-term leukemogenic potential. Clin Res 1992; 40:281.

66. Ellis JT, Silver RT, Coleman M, et al: The bone marrow in polycythemia vera. Semin Hematol 1975; 12:433.

67. Peterson P, Ellis, JT: The bone marrow in polycythemia vera, in Wasserman LR, Berk PD, Berlin NI (eds): Polycythemia and the Myeloproliferative Disorders, p 31. Philadelphia, WB Saunders, 1995.

68. Ellis JT, Peterson P, Geller SA, et al: Studies of the bone marrow in polycythemia vera and the evolution

69. of myelofibrosis and second hematologic malignancies. Semin Hematol 1986; 23:144.

69. Westin J, Lanner L-O, Larsson A, et al: Spleen size in polycythemia: A clinical and scintigraphic study. Acta Med Scand 1972; 191:263.

70. Tinney WS, Hall BE, Giffin HZ: The liver and spleen in polycythemia vera. Mayo Clin Proc 1943; 18:46.

71. Wolf BC, Banks PM, Mann RB, et al: Splenic hematopoiesis in polycythemia vera: Morphologic and immunohistologic study. Am J Clin Pathol 1988; 89:69.

72. Rappaport H: Tumors of the hematopoietic system, in Atlas of Tumor Pathology, section 3, fascicle 8, p 285. Washington, DC, Armed Forces Institute of Pathology, 1966.

73. Berg B, Stahl E, Soderstrom N: The cytology of spleen aspiration in uncomplicated polycythaemia vera. Scand J Haematol 1973; 10:59.

74. Heller EL, Lewisohn MG, Palin WE: Aleukemic myelosis, chronic nonleukemic myelosis, agnogenic myeloid metaplasia, osteosclerosis, leukoerythroblastic anemia, and synonymous designations. Am J Pathol 1947; 23:327.

75. Bouroncle BA, Doan CA: Myelofibrosis: Clinical, hematologic and pathologic study of 110 patients. Am J Med Sci 1962; 243:697.

76. Rosenthal DS, Maloney WC: Myeloid metaplasia: A study of 98 cases. Postgrad Med J 1969; 45:136.

77. Reich C, Rumsey W Jr: Agnogenic myeloid metaplasia of the spleen. JAMA 1942; 118:120.

78. Hoffman R, Silverstein MN: Agnogenic myeloid metaplasia, in Hoffman R, Benz EJ, Shattil SJ, et al (eds): Hematology Basic Principles and Practice, 2nd ed, p 1160. New York, Prentice-Hall, 1995.

79. Tefferi A, Silverstein MN, Noel P: Agnogenic myeloid metaplasia. Semin Oncol 1995; 22:327–333.

80. Thiele J, Kvasnicka H-M, Werden C, et al: Idiopathic primary osteo-myelofibrosis: A clinicopathological study on 208 patients with special emphasis on evolution of disease features, differentiation from essential thrombocythemia and variables of prognostic impact. Leuk Lymph 1996; 22:303.

81. Silverstein MN, Linman JW: Causes of death in agnogenic myeloid metaplasia. Mayo Clin Proc 1969; 44:36.

82. Varki A, Lottenberg R, Griffith R, et al: The syndrome of idiopathic myelofibrosis: A clinicopathologic review with emphasis on the prognostic variables predicting survival. Medicine 1983; 62:353.

83. Barosi G, Berzuini C, Liberato LN, et al: A prognostic classification of myelofibrosis with myeloid metaplasia. Br J Haematol 1988; 70:397.

84. Visani G, Finelli C, Castelli U, et al: Myelofibrosis with myeloid metaplasia: Clinical and haematological parameters predicting survival in a series of 133 patients. Br J Haematol 1990; 75:4.

85. Buyssens N, Bourgeois NH: Chronic myelocytic leukemia versus idiopathic myelofibrosis: A diagnostic problem in bone marrow biopsies. Cancer 1977; 40:1548.

86. Adamson JW, Fialkow PJ: The pathogenesis of myeloproliferative syndromes. Br J Haematol 1979; 38:299.

87. Hoyle CF, de Bastos M, Wheatley K, et al: AML associated with previous cytotoxic therapy, MDS or myeloproliferative disorders: Results from the MRC's 9th AML trial. Br J Haematol 1989; 72:45.

88. Tobin MS, Tan C, Argano SA: Myelofibrosis in the pediatric age group. N Y State J Med 1969; 69:1080.

89. Jacobson RJ, Salo A, Fialkow PJ: Agnogenic myeloid

metaplasia: A clonal proliferation of hematopoietic stem cells with secondary myelofibrosis. Blood 1978; 51:189.

90. Buschle M, Janssen JWG, Drexler H, et al: Evidence of pluripotent stem cell origin of idiopathic myelofibrosis: Clonal analysis of a case characterized by an *N-ras* gene mutation. Leukaemia 1988; 2:658.

91. Anger B, Janssen JWG, Schrezenmeier H, et al: Clonal analysis of chronic myeloproliferative disorders using X-linked DNA polymorphisms. Leukemia 1990; 4:258.

92. Kreipe H, Jaquet K, Felgner J, et al: Clonal granulocytes and bone marrow cells in the cellular phase of agnogenic myeloid metaplasia. Blood 1991; 78:1814.

93. Greenburg BR, Woo L, Veomett IC, et al: Cytogenetics of bone marrow fibroblastic cells in idiopathic chronic myelofibrosis. Br J Haematol 1987; 66:487.

94. Wang JC, Lang H-D, Lichter S, et al: Cytogenetic studies of bone marrow fibroblasts cultured from patients with myelofibrosis and myeloid metaplasia. Br J Haematol 1992; 80:184.

95. Castro-Malaspina H, Gay RE, Jhanwar SC: Characteristics of bone marrow fibroblast colony-forming cells (CFU-F) and their progress in patients with myeloproliferative disorders. Blood 1982; 59:1046.

96. Wang JC: Myelopoietic effect of bone marrow fibroblasts cultured from patients with myelofibrosis. Am J Hematol 1988; 27:235.

97. Hirata J, Takahira H, Kaneko S, et al: Bone marrow stromal cells in myeloproliferative disorders. Acta Haematol 1989; 82:35.

98. Groopman JE: The pathogenesis of myelofibrosis in myeloproliferative disorders. Ann Intern Med 1980; 92; 857.

99. Castro-Malaspina H, Rabellino EM, Yen A, et al: Human megakaryocyte stimulation of proliferation of bone marrow fibroblasts. Blood 1981; 57:781.

100. Kimura A, Katoh O, Kuramoto A: Effect of platelet derived growth factor, epidermal growth factor and transforming growth factor-B on the growth of human marrow fibroblasts. Br J Haematol 1988; 69:9.

101. Katoh O, Kimura A, Kuramoto A: Platelet derived growth factor is decreased in patients with myeloproliferative disorders. Am J Hematol 1988; 27:276.

102. Kimura A, Katoh O, Hyodo H, et al: Transforming growth factor-B regulates growth as well as collagen and fibronectin synthesis of human marrow fibroblasts. Br J Haematol 1989; 72:486.

103. Burstein SA, Malpass TW, Yee E: Platelet factor 4 excretion in myeloproliferative disease: Implications for the etiology of myelofibrosis. Br J Haematol 1989; 51:383.

104. Martyre MC, Magdelenat H, Bryckaert MC, et al: Increased intraplatelet levels of platelet-derived growth factor and transforming growth factor-beta in patients with myelofibrosis with myeloid metaplasia. Br J Haematol 1991; 77:80.

105. Martyre MC, Romquin N, Le Bousse-Kerdiles MC, et al: Transforming growth factor-B and megakaryocytes in the pathogenesis of idiopathic myelofibrosis. Br J Haematol 1994; 88:9.

106. Kimura A, Katoh O, Kuramoto A: Marrow fibroblasts from patients with myeloproliferative disorders show increased sensitivity to human serum mitogens. Br J Haematol 1989; 69:153.

107. Whang-Peng J, Lee E, Knutson T, et al: Cytogenetic studies in patients with myelofibrosis and myeloid metaplasia. Leuk Res 1978; 2:41.

108. Miller JB, Testa JR, Lindgren V, et al: The pattern and clinical significance of karyotypic abnormalities in patients with idiopathic and postpolycythemic myelofibrosis. Cancer 1985; 55:582.

109. Castoldi G, Cuneo A, Tomas P, et al: Chromosome abnormalities in myelofibrosis. Acta Haematol 1987; 78:104.

110. Lawler SD, Swansberg GJ: Cytogenetic studies in myelofibrosis and related conditions, in Lewis SM (ed): Myelofibrosis Pathophysiology and Clinical Management, p 167. New York, Marcel Dekker, 1987.

111. Dewald GW, Pierre RV: Cytogenetic studies in neoplastic hematologic diseases, in Fairbanks VF (ed): Current Hematology and Oncology, vol 6, p 231. Chicago, Year Book Medical, 1988.

112. Demory JL, Dupriez B, Fenaux P, et al: Cytogenetic studies and their prognostic significance in agnogenic myeloid metaplasia: A report on 47 cases. Blood 1988; 72:855.

113. Wolf BC, Neiman RS: Myelofibrosis with myeloid metaplasia: Pathophysiologic implications of the correlation between bone marrow changes and progression of splenomegaly. Blood 1985; 65:803.

114. Thiele J, Zankovich R, Steinberg T, et al: Agnogenic myeloid metaplasia (AMM) correlation of bone marrow lesions with laboratory data: A longitudinal clinicopathologic study on 114 patients. Hematol Oncol 1989; 7:327.

115. Thiele J, Rompcik V, Wagner S, et al: Vascular architecture and collagen type IV in primary myelofibrosis and polycythaemia vera: An immunomorphometric study on trephine biopsies of the bone marrow. Br J Haematol 1992; 80:227.

116. Jackson J Jr, Parker F Jr, Lemon HM: Agnogenic myeloid metaplasia of the spleen: A syndrome simulating other more definite hematologic disorders. N Engl J Med 1940; 222:985.

117. Tavassoli M, Weiss L: An electron microscopic study of spleen in myelofibrosis with myeloid metaplasia. Blood 1973; 42:267.

118. Thiele J, Hoeppner B, Zankovich R, et al: Histomorphometry of bone marrow biopsies in primary osteomyelofibrosis/sclerosis (agnogenic myeloid metaplasia): Correlations between clinical and morphological features. Virchows Arch 1989; 415:191.

119. Pitcock JA, Reinhard EH, Justus BW, et al: A clinical and pathologic study of seventy cases of myelofibrosis. Ann Intern Med 1962; 57:73.

120. Lohman TP, Beckman EN: Progressive myelofibrosis in agnogenic myeloid metaplasia. Arch Pathol 1983; 107:593.

121. Hasselbalch H, Lisse I: A sequential histological study of bone marrow fibrosis in idiopathic myelofibrosis. Eur J Haematol 1991; 46:285.

122. Nathan DG, Berlin NI: Studies of the production and life span of erythrocytes in myeloid metaplasia. Blood 1959; 14:668.

123. Szur L, Pettit JC: The effect of radiation on splenic function in myelosclerosis: Studies with ^{52}Fe and ^{99m}Tc. Br J Radiol 1973; 46:295.

124. Parmentier C, Charbord P, Tibi M, et al: Splenic irradiation in myelofibrosis: Clinical findings and ferrokinetics. Int J Radiat Oncol Biol Phys 1975; 2:1075.

125. Silverstein MN: Control of hypersplenism and painful splenomegaly in myeloid metaplasia by irradiation. In J Radiat Oncol Biol Phys 1977; 2:1221.

126. Greenberger JS, Chaffey JT, Rosenthal DS, et al: Irradiation for control of hypersplenism and painful

splenomegaly in myeloid metaplasia. Int J Radiat Oncol Biol Phys 1977; 2:1083.

127. Koeffler HP, Cline MJ, Golde DW: Splenic irradiation in myelofibrosis: Effect on circulating myeloid progenitor cells. Br J Haematol 1979; 43:69.

128. Wagner H Jr, McKeough PG, Desforges J, et al: Splenic irradiation in the treatment of patients with chronic myelogenous leukemia or myelofibrosis with myeloid metaplasia: Effects of daily and intermittent fractionation with or without concomitant hydroxyurea. Cancer 1986; 58:1204.

129. Crosby WH: Splenectomy in hematologic disorders. N Engl J Med 1972; 286:1533.

130. Milner JR, Geary CG, Wadswoth LD, et al: Erythrokinetic studies as a guide to the value of splenectomy in primary myeloid metaplasia. Br J Haematol 1973; 25:467.

131. Mulder H, Steenbergen J, Haanen C: Clinical course and survival after elective splenectomy in 19 patients with primary myelofibrosis. Br J Haematol 1977; 35:419.

132. Silverstein MN, ReMine WH: Splenectomy in myeloid metaplasia. Blood 1979; 53:515.

133. Benbassat J, Penchas S, Ligumski M: Splenectomy in patients with agnogenic myeloid metaplasia: An analysis of 321 published cases. Br J Haematol 1979; 42:207.

134. Brenner B, Nagler A, Tatarsky I, et al: Splenectomy in agnogenic myeloid metaplasia and postpolycythemic myeloid metaplasia. Arch Intern Med 1988; 108:2501.

135. Benbassat J, Gilon D, Penchas S: The choice between splenectomy and medical treatment in patients with advanced agnogenic myeloid metaplasia. Am J Hematol 1990; 33:128.

136. Barosi G, Ambrosetti A, Buratti A, et al: Splenectomy for patients with myelofibrosis and myeloid metaplasia: Pretreatment variables and outcome prediction. Leukemia 1993; 7:200.

137. Towel BL, Levine SP: Massive hepatomegaly following splenectomy for myeloid metaplasia. Am J Med 1987; 82:371.

138. Lopez-Guillermo A, Cervantes F, Bruguera M, et al: Liver dysfunction following splenectomy in idiopathic myelofibrosis: A study of 10 patients. Acta Haematol 1991; 85:184.

139. Petroianu A: Subtotal splenectomy for treatment of patients with myelofibrosis and myeloid metaplasia. Internal Surg 1996; 81:177.

140. Parmeggiani L, Ferrant A, Rodhain J, et al: Alpha interferon in the treatment of symptomatic myelofibrosis with myeloid metaplasia. Eur J Haematol 1987; 39:228.

141. Gilbert HS: Persistence of remission of myeloid metaplasia after treatment with recombinant interferon alpha 2B. Blood 1987; 72:771.

142. Barosi G, Liberato LN, Costa A, et al: Cytoreductive effect of recombinant alpha interferon in patients with myelofibrosis with myeloid metaplasia. Blut 1989; 58:271.

143. Martyre M-C, Magdelenat H, Calvo F: Interferon-γ in vivo reverses increased platelet levels of platelet-derived growth factor and transforming growth factor-B in patients with myelofibrosis with myeloid metaplasia. Br J Haematol 1991; 77:431.

144. Silverstein MN, Brown AL, Linman JW: Idiopathic myeloid metaplasia: Its evolution into acute leukemia. Arch Intern Med 1973; 132:709.

145. Polliack A, Prokocimer M, Matzner Y: Lymphoblastic leukemic transformation (lymphoblastic crisis) in myelofibrosis and myeloid metaplasia. J Hematol 1980; 9:211.

146. Choate JJ, Domenico DR, McGraw TD, et al: Diagnosis of acute megakaryoblastic leukemia by flow cytometry and immunoalkaline phosphatase techniques: Utilization of new monoclonal antibodies. Am J Clin Pathol 1988; 89:247.

147. Garcia S, Miguel A, Zinares M, et al: Idiopathic myelofibrosis terminating in erythroleukemia. Am J Hematol 1989; 32:70.

148. Cervantes F, Tassies D, Salgado C, et al: Acute transformation in nonleukemic chronic myeloproliferative disorders: Actuarial probability and main characteristics in a series of 218 patients. Acta Haematol 1991; 85:124.

149. Hernandez JM, San Miguel JF, Gonzalez M, et al: Development of acute leukemia after idiopathic myelofibrosis. J Clin Pathol 1992; 45:427.

150. Bently SA, Murray KH, Lewis SM, et al: Erythroid hypoplasia myelofibrosis: A feature associated with blastic transformation. Br J Haematol 1977; 36:41.

151. Garcia S, Miguel A, Miguel A, et al: Idiopathic myelofibrosis terminating in erythroleukemia. Am J Hematol 1989; 32:70.

152. Choate JJ, Domenico DR, McGraw TD, et al: Diagnosis of acute megakaryoblastic leukemia by flow cytometry and immunoalkaline phosphatase techniques. Am J Clin Pathol 1988; 89:247.

153. Polliack A, Prokocimer M, Matzner Y: Lymphoblastic leukemia transformation (lymphoblastic crisis) in myelofibrosis and myeloid metaplasia. Am J Hematol 1989; 9:211.

154. Hasselbach H: Idiopathic myelofibrosis: A clinical study of 80 patients. Am J Hematol 1988; 29:174.

155. Garcia S, Miguel A, Zinarea M, et al: Idiopathic myelofibrosis terminating in erythroleukemia. Am J Hematol 1989; 32:70.

156. Hernandez JM, Miguel S, Gonzalez M, et al: Development of acute leukemia after idiopathic myelofibrosis. J Clin Pathol 1992; 45:427.

157. Wolf BC, Luevano E, Neiman RS: Evidence to suggest that the human fetal spleen is not a hematopoietic organ. Am J Clin Pathol 1983; 80:140.

158. Calhoun DA, Li Y, Braylan RC, et al: Assessment of the contribution of the spleen to granulocytopoiesis and erythropoiesis of the mid-gestation human fetus. Early Hum Dev 1996; 46:217.

159. Chervenic PA: Increase in circulating stem cells in patients with myelofibrosis. Blood 1973; 41:67.

160. Wang JC, Cheung CP, Fakhiuddin A, et al: Circulating granulocyte and macrophage progenitor cells in primary and secondary myelofibrosis. Br J Haematol 1983; 54:301.

161. Hibbin JA, Njoku OS, Matutes E, et al: Myeloid progenitor cells in the circulation of patients with myelofibrosis and other myeloproliferative disorders. Br J Haematol 1984; 57:495.

162. Carlo-Stella C, Cazzola M, Gasner A, et al: Effects of recombinant α and γ interferons on in vitro growth of circulating hematopoietic progenitor cells (CFU-GEMM, CFU-Mk, BFU-E and CFU-GM) from patients with myelofibrosis with myeloid metaplasia. Blood 1987; 70:1014.

163. Juvonen E: Megakaryocyte colony formation in chronic myeloid leukemia and myelofibrosis. Leuk Res 1988; 12:751.

164. Gilbert HS, Prolaran V, Stanley ER: Increased circulating CSF-1 (M-CSF) in myeloproliferative disease: Association with myeloid metaplasia and peripheral bone marrow extension. Blood 1989; 74:1231.

165. Wang JC, Tobin MS: Mechanism of extramedullary haematopoiesis in rabbits with saponin-induced myelofibrosis and myeloid metaplasia. Br J Haematol 1982; 51:277.

166. O'Keane JC, Wolf BC, Neiman RS: The pathogenesis of splenic extramedullary hematopoiesis in metastatic carcinoma. Cancer 1989; 63:1539.

167. Freedman MH, Saunders EF: Hematopoiesis in the human spleen. Am J Hematol 1981; 11:271.

168. Lewis SM, Szur L: Malignant myelosclerosis. Br Med J 1963; 2:472.

169. Bergsman ML, Van Slyck EJ: Acute myelofibrosis: An accelerated variant of agnogenic myeloid metaplasia. Ann Intern Med 1971; 74:232.

170. Estevez JM, Urueta EE, Moran TJ: Acute megakaryocytic myelofibrosis: Case report of an unusual myeloproliferative syndrome. Am J Clin Pathol 1974; 62:52.

171. Fabich DR, Raich PC: Acute myelofibrosis: A report of three cases. Am J Clin Pathol 1977; 67:334.

172. Bearman RM, Pangalis GA, Rappaport H: Acute ("malignant") myelosclerosis. Cancer 1979; 4:279.

173. Weisenburger DD: Acute myelofibrosis terminating as acute myeloblastic leukemia. Am J Clin Pathol 1980; 73:128.

174. Dunphy CH, Kitchen S, Saravia O, et al: Acute myelofibrosis terminating in acute lymphoblastic leukemia: Case report and review of the literature. Am J Hematol 1996; 51:85.

175. Bain BJ, Catovsky D, O'Brien M, et al: Megakaryoblastic leukemia presenting as acute myelofibrosis: A study of four cases with the platelet-peroxidase reaction. Blood 1981; 58:206.

176. Maj JS, Roslan K, Fic-Sikorska B: Acute myelofibrosis in children: Report on two cases. Acta Haematol Pol 1996; 27:79.

177. Mitus WF, Coleman N, Kiossoglou KA: Abnormal (marker) chromosomes in two patients with acute myelofibrosis. Arch Intern Med 1969; 123:192.

178. Van Slyck EJ, Weiss L, Dully M: Chromosomal evidence for the secondary role of fibroblastic proliferation in acute myelofibrosis. Blood 1970; 36:729.

179. Nowell P, Jensen J, Gardner F, et al: Chromosome studies in "preleukemia." III. Myelofibrosis. Cancer 1976; 38:1873.

180. Shah I, Mayeda K, Koppitch F, et al: Karyotypic polymorphism in acute myelofibrosis. Blood 1982; 60:841.

181. Hruban RH, Kuhajda FP, Mann RB: Acute myelofibrosis: Immunohistochemical study of four cases and comparison with acute megakaryocytic leukemia. Am J Clin Pathol 1987; 88:578.

182. den Ottolander GJ, teVelde J, Brederoo P, et al: Megakaryoblastic leukaemia (acute myelofibrosis): A report of three cases. Br J Haematol 1979; 42:9.

183. Amberger DM, Saleem A, Kemp BL, et al: Acute myelofibrosis: A leukemia of pluripotent stem cell. Ann Clin Lab Sci 1990; 20:409.

184. Bird T, Proctor SJ: Malignant myelosclerosis: Myeloproliferative disorder or leukemia? Am J Clin Pathol 1977; 67:512.

185. Sultan C, Sigaux F, Imbert M, et al: Acute myelodysplasia with myelofibrosis: A report of eight cases. Br J Haematol 1981; 49:11.

186. Imbert M, Nguyen D, Sultan C: Myelodysplastic syndromes (MDS) and acute myeloid leukemias (AML) with myelofibrosis. Leuk Res 1992; 16:51.

187. Allen EF, Lunde JH, McNally R, et al: A case of acute myelofibrosis with complex karyotypic changes: A type of myelodysplastic syndrome. Cancer Genet Cytogenet 1996; 90:24.

188. Lambertenghi-Deliliers G, Orazi A, Luksch R, et al: Myelodysplastic syndrome with increased marrow fibrosis: A distinct clinicopathological entity. Br J Haematol 1991; 78:161.

189. Najean Y, Dresch C, Rain JD: The very-long-term course of polycythaemia: A complement to the previously published data of the polycythaemia vera study group. Br J Haematol 1994; 86:233.

190. Fruchtman SM, Wasserman LR: Therapeutic recommendations for polycythemia vera, in Wasserman LR, Berck PD, Berlin NI (eds): Polycythemia Vera and the Myeloproliferative Disorders, p 337. Philadelphia, WB Saunders, 1995.

191. Furgerson JL, Vukelja SJ, Baker WJ, et al: Acute myeloid leukemia evolving from essential thrombocythemia in two patients treated with hydroxyurea. Am J Hematol 1996; 51:137.

192. Najean Y, Rain J-D: Treatment of polycythemia vera: The use of hydroxyurea and pipobroman in 292 patient under the age of 65 years. Blood 1997; 90:3370.

193. Weinfeld A, Swolin B, Westin J: Acute leukaemia after hydroxyurea therapy in polycythaemia vera and allied disorders: Prospective study of efficacy and leukaemogenicity with therapeutic implications. Eur J Haematol 1994; 52:134.

194. Brandt L, Schnell CR: Granulopoiesis in bone marrow and spleen in chronic myeloid leukaemia. Scand J Haematol 1969; 6:65.

195. Stroll C, Oberling F, Flori E: Chromosome analysis of spleen and/or lymph nodes of patients with chronic myeloid leukaemia. Blood 1978; 52:328.

14

NON-NEOPLASTIC VASCULAR LESIONS

SPLENIC INFARCTS

Generally, splenic infarcts may be divided into two types: those caused by embolization of splenic vessels and those caused by a variety of pathologic processes within the spleen or splenic vessels. All splenic infarcts are initially hemorrhagic (Color Plate 21), but with the passage of time they become pale with hyperemic borders (Color Plate 22), and eventually they become fibrotic. Acute splenic infarction may cause left upper quadrant abdominal pain and mild splenomegaly. On occasion, after infarction, Howell-Jolly bodies may appear transiently in the peripheral blood, particularly if the infarction is massive (Color Plate 23).[1, 2] In a patient with hypersplenism, the spontaneous disappearance of hypersplenic signs and symptoms may indicate splenic infarction.[3]

The spleen is a frequent site of systemic emboli, and splenic infarction is a common result.[4] The emboli arise most commonly from valvular lesions or from mural thrombi in the left side of the heart. They lodge in the splenic artery or one of its tributaries. The majority of these infarcts are wedge-shaped, with the base abutting the capsular surface, following the distribution of the occluded vessel (Fig. 14–1).[5] Septic infarcts in the spleen are often observed in patients with infective endocarditis.[6–10] Splenomegaly caused by such infarcts is common in patients with subacute bacterial endocarditis, and its presence may be an important diagnostic feature in a patient with a cardiac murmur.[11] These infarcts may lead to splenic rupture.[7, 10] Occasionally, acute infectious diseases with bacteremia may cause an infectious vasculitis resulting in splenic throm-

bosis. This may produce a miliary distribution of small infarcts, resulting in the so-called spotted spleen, or fleckmilz.

Splenic infarction may also be associated with a wide variety of intrinsic disease processes within the spleen, both hematopoietic and nonhematopoietic. Infarcts in these conditions do not have a wedge-shaped configuration. They may assume any shape and occur anywhere within the parenchyma of the organ, depending on the location of the pathologic process in question.

Primary vascular lesions, such as splenic vein thrombosis or splenic vasculitides, may be a contributing factor leading to splenic infarction.[12] Although the majority of the systemic vasculitides do not involve the spleen, occasional involvement of splenic vessels may cause thrombosis and infarction.[13–15] In patients with leukemia, particularly chronic myeloid leukemia, subendothelial infiltration of splenic vessels by tumor cells may lead to vascular thrombosis with resultant splenic infarcts.[5, 16] Splenic infarcts may also occur in the myeloproliferative disorders,[17, 18] most notably in essential thrombocythemia (ET) and chronic idiopathic myelofibrosis (CIMF). The pooling of large masses of platelets in ET may cause multiple splenic infarcts, which lead to splenic atrophy.[5, 19, 20] Splenic infarcts have also been reported to occur in patients with paroxysmal nocturnal hemoglobinuria,[21] aplastic anemia after erythropoietin treatment,[22] and autoimmune diseases.[23, 24] Splenic infarcts are common in patients with sickle cell disease (SCD), eventually resulting in an atrophic, fibrotic organ in which the encrustation of calcium and iron produces the characteristic

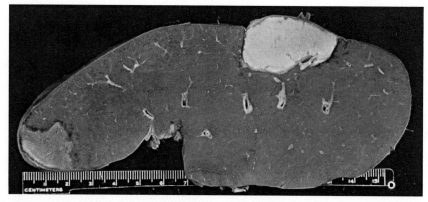

Figure 14–1. Two organizing infarcts of the spleen. The one at the left pole of the organ still has a hyperemic margin, and the one to the upper right appears uniformly pale.

Gamna-Gandy bodies.[5] Infarcts may also be precipitated by high-altitude flying in patients with sickle cell trait because of the lower oxygen tension that results in sickling.[25–27] Splenic abscess and infected splenic infarcts are also described in patients with SCD.[28] SCD predisposes to splenic infections because of progressive splenic atrophy causing functional hyposplenism and defective phagocyte function.[28] Splenic infarction is also common in vascular tumors of the spleen and, in particular, in hemangiosarcomas. In these latter tumors, necrosis may be so prominent as to mask the presence of the tumor itself. Splenic infarcts have also been described as a complication in both *Plasmodium falciparum* and *P. vivax* malaria.[29]

CHRONIC PASSIVE CONGESTION

Congestive splenomegaly results from persistent venous congestion. Systemic venous congestion appearing in patients with right-sided heart failure, usually secondary to tricuspid or pulmonic valve lesions or constrictive pericarditis, may occasionally result in congestive splenomegaly.[30, 31] However, this condition occurs more commonly in patients with congestion of the portal venous system, usually secondary to cirrhosis of the liver.

The term "Banti syndrome" was often used in the past synonymously with "fibrocongestive splenomegaly."[32] However, Banti's original description referred specifically to examples of splenomegaly with cytopenias in patients with cirrhosis, ascites, and esophageal varices.[33] Banti believed that splenomegaly preceded the cirrhosis and postulated that the enlarged spleen produced a noxious factor that caused the liver damage; however, this has never been confirmed. Banti syndrome, now more appropriately termed "noncirrhotic" or "idiopathic portal hypertension," is currently believed to arise following subclinical occlusion of the portal vein, usually many years after the original occlusive event.[34] Postulated causes include neonatal omphalitis, dehydration, sepsis, or previous umbilical vein catheterization. Other causes include hypercoagulable myeloproliferative disorders, biliary tract surgery, peritonitis, and exposure to arsenicals.[34] However, recent evidence has been presented to suggest that proliferation of splenic endothelial cells possibly induced by an immunologic mechanism may play an important pathogenetic role in idiopathic portal hypertension.[35–37]

Any disorder that results in intrahepatic congestion may cause congestive splenomegaly, including cirrhosis of any cause, hepatic veno-occlusive disease, and congenital hepatic fibrosis. Schistosomiasis mansoni may cause occlusion of the intrahepatic portal venous radicles, sometimes resulting in cirrhosis with moderate congestive splenomegaly.[38] Portal hypertension with resultant fibrocongestive splenomegaly may also occur in the Budd-Chiari syndrome due to hepatic venous occlusion and in patients with portal vein obstruction due to thrombosis, stenosis, or compression. Splenic vein thrombosis may occasionally cause acute congestive splenomegaly. This phenomenon usually occurs as a result of systemic venous thromboses in patients with myeloproliferative disorders, paroxysmal nocturnal hemoglobinuria,[21] or certain nonhematopoietic tumors. Less commonly, splenic vein thrombosis may result from pancreatitis, retroperitoneal fibro-

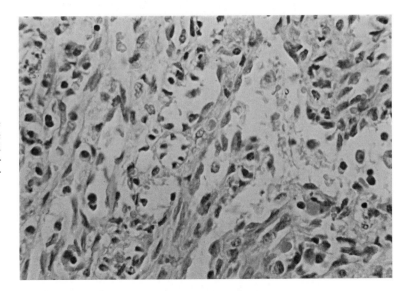

Figure 14–2. Fibrocongestive splenomegaly. Fibroblasts in the cords of Billroth stiffen the red pulp, creating a morphologic picture that resembles a hemangioma.

sis, or trauma. Idiopathic (noncirrhotic) portal hypertension has been described in renal transplant recipients. These patients present with splenomegaly and dilated splenic artery and vein, portal hypertension, and esophageal varices.[39] The condition is usually cured by splenectomy. It is postulated that the increased blood flow to the spleen plays an important role in the development of portal hypertension in these patients.[39]

The spleen in cases of fibrocongestive splenomegaly is usually moderately enlarged, rarely weighing more than 1000 g. The capsule is often thickened, and the cut surface appears firm and dry. The color ranges from salmon to deep red, depending on the degree of fibrosis, and the white pulp markings are usually indistinct. There may be extensive hemosiderin deposition due to increased red cell breakdown. Early in the course of the disease the cords may show increased cellularity due to a proliferation of macrophages and endothelial cells.[35, 36] There is hyperplasia of sinus lining cells, and there may also be an inflammatory infiltrate. However, as the fibrosis increases, the red pulp appears hypocellular. Over time, the cords of Billroth become rigid due to collagen deposition, and the sinuses are often dilated. The result is a morphologic change that may superficially resemble a hemangioma (Fig. 14–2). Nodules of fibrous tissue may become encrusted, with iron and calcium producing Gamna-Gandy bodies.[40]

Fibrotic thickening of the splenic capsule—hyaline perisplenitis—may occur in patients with long-standing ascites. The thickening may be focal or diffuse and results in acellular plaques, sometimes termed "sugarcoated spleen" (Fig. 14–3).[40]

VASCULITIDES

A number of conditions may affect the splenic vasculature. Hyalinosis of the arterioles is a common change in adult spleens. Although its frequency appears to increase with age, it may commonly occur in the pediatric age group.[41] It is not associated with hypertension.[3] The hyaline deposition begins between the intima and media of the vessel and may later involve the entire wall (Fig. 14–4). The hyaline material is composed of plasma proteins, fibrin, and lipids[42] and may frequently stain positively with fibrin stains. Occasionally, such hyalinosis may be found in the spleens of young persons with hereditary spherocytosis or idiopathic thrombocytopenic purpura. Because of its location in small arterioles and its homogeneous appearance, it may be mistaken for amyloid or for the hyaline subendothelial deposits in thrombotic thrombocytopenic purpura (TTP). However, the lesion does not stain for amyloid, and it is unassociated with the normoblasts in the red pulp that occur in TTP. We have gained the impression from a number of cases that hyalinosis is unusually frequent in spleens that have undergone rupture with questionably significant trauma. That hyalinosis of splenic vessels predisposes the spleen to rupture is a conjecture we suspect may be true but for which we have no proof.

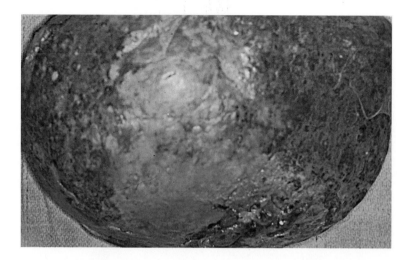

Figure 14–3. Hyaline perisplenitis showing focal capsular thickening.

The noninfectious systemic vasculitides do not commonly involve the splenic vessels. Occasionally, however, the typical lesions of polyarteritis nodosa may involve splenic vessels, which display fibrinoid necrosis of the vascular wall and an inflammatory infiltrate that may include neutrophils and eosinophils (Fig. 14–5).[43] The individual lesions occur as sharply localized swellings, usually at arteriolar bifurcations, which may lead to small aneurysmal dilatations. Vascular thromboses may lead to multiple splenic infarcts, resulting in extensive confluent splenic necrosis (Fig. 14–6). Splenic rupture has also been associated with periarteritis nodosa[44] as well as with Wegener granulomatosis.[15] Lesions histologically similar to those in polyarteritis nodosa have been described in spleens of patients with the allergic granulomatosis and angiitis of Churg-Strauss (Fig. 14–7).[45, 46] Hypersensitivity, or leukocytoclastic, angiitis, a necrotizing vasculitis that involves smaller vessels than those affected by polyarteritis nodosa, may involve the spleen (Fig. 14–8).[47] Hypersensitivity angiitis is believed to result from immune complex deposition. In some cases an antigenic stimulus such as a drug or certain microorganisms may be identified.[48] In other cases, however, disseminated vascular lesions may occur in association with such conditions as autoimmune disorders and malignancies. In particular, systemic lupus erythematosus (SLE) and rheumatoid arthritis may be associated with a systemic vasculitis with fibrinoid necrosis and an inflammatory infiltrate.[43, 48] In addition to leukocytoclastic vasculitis, other characteristic vascular lesions

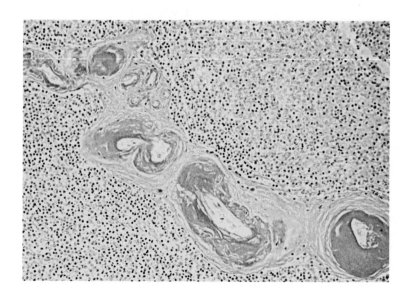

Figure 14–4. Splenic hyalinosis. The morphologic picture simulates thrombotic thrombocytopenic purpura. Special stains can rule out amyloidosis in such cases.

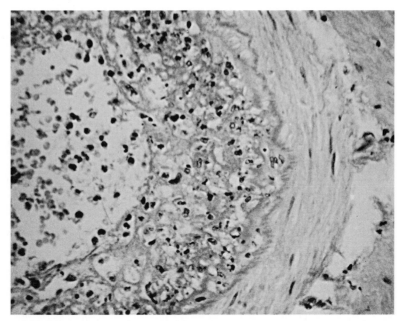

Figure 14–5. Polyarteritis nodosa. The intima and media of the arteriole show fibrinoid necrosis with an acute inflammatory infiltrate.

are seen in the spleen of patients with SLE.[49–52] They are concentric perivascular fibrosis of the penicilliary arterioles, resulting in the characteristic "onion skin" lesions (Fig. 14–9).[50] The vascular involvement is patchy and does not affect the arterioles uniformly. SLE is a multisystem disease that may affect any organ in the body. It is associated with circulating autoantibodies, particularly antinuclear antibodies.[53–55] Immunoglobulin, DNA, and the third component of complement have been identified in the vessel walls, and it has been postulated that the vascular lesions may result from immune complex deposition (DNA-anti-DNA complexes), the antigen being DNA.[56] Occasionally, onion skin lesions are found in patients with polyarteritis nodosa and idiopathic thrombocytopenic purpura.

Platelet-fibrin thrombi may be found in the penicilliary arterioles of the white pulp in the

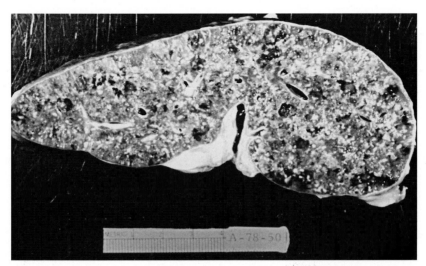

Figure 14–6. Confluent splenic necrosis in a case of polyarteritis nodosa with prominent splenic involvement. Such extensive splenic involvement may result in hyposplenism.

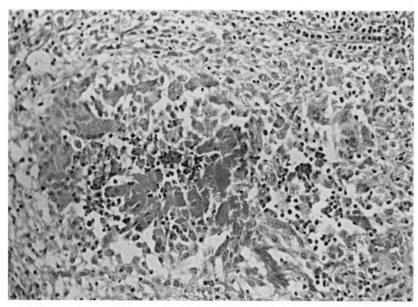

Figure 14–7. Churg-Strauss disease (allergic granulomatosis). There is an eosinophilic abscess with necrotic material present in this area of the red pulp of the spleen. The lesion, not visible in this section, likely originated in a penicilliary arteriole.

spleens of patients with TTP (Fig. 14–10).[5,] [57, 58] TTP is typically characterized by fever, thrombocytopenia, microangiopathic hemolytic anemia, transient neurologic deficits, and renal failure.[59–61] The incidence of TTP is about 1 in 500,000 per year. Women are affected about twice as often as men. The incidence is increasing. This may be at least partially related to the increase in frequency of TTP observed in patients with human immunodeficiency virus type 1 infection.[62] TTP is

believed to be caused by the intrusion into the circulation of one or more platelet aggregating agents. The aggregating substance has been reported to be a calcium-activated protein (calpain) of 37,000 or 59,000 daltons,[63, 64] with the capacity to cleave von Willebrand factor (vWF) multimers into fragments with increased platelet-binding capacity,[65] or "unusually large" (UL) vWF multimeric forms[66, 67] that may be released into the circulation from endothelial cells damaged or stimulated by the

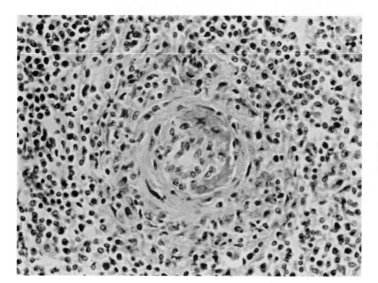

Figure 14–8. Involvement of a penicilliary arteriole by hypersensitivity angiitis in a patient with systemic lupus erythematosus.

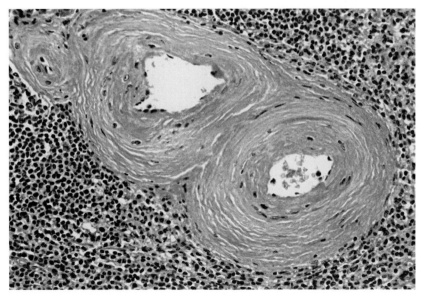

Figure 14–9. The typical onion-skin lesions in arterioles of the spleen in a patient with systemic lupus erythematosus.

contact with autoantibodies, immune complexes, or toxins. In most patients with TTP, vWF multimers have been found in plasma during the acute episode.[67] If a patient survives and suffers no relapse, ULvWF multimeric forms in recovery samples quickly normalize. If, however, ULvWF remains detectable after recovery, then the likelihood is considerable that the patient will have recurrent episodes of TTP. Most patients can be successfully treated with emergency plasma exchanges.[68, 69]

Splenectomy is occasionally performed in cases of TTP refractory to medical therapies.[70–73] The possible beneficial role of splenectomy in TTP is, however, still controversial.[74, 75] In contrast to immune thrombocytopenic purpura, the rationale for splenectomy and its mechanism of action remain unclear in TTP.[74] Several authors have suggested that splenic extravascular platelet destruction may be a predominant factor in the pathogenesis of at least some cases of TTP.[76–78]

Pathologically, TTP is characterized by microthrombi in arterioles, capillaries, and venules of many organs. The thrombi are composed of aggregates of platelets with some

Figure 14–10. Fibrin thrombi in a small arteriole of the spleen in a case of thrombotic thrombocytopenic purpura.

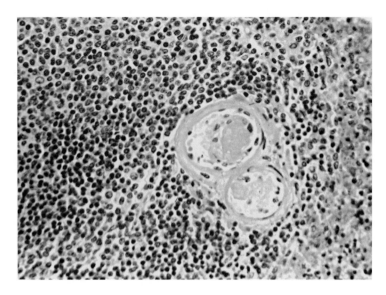

fibrin and an abundance of von Willebrand factor.[57] There is no inflammatory infiltrate. In addition, TTP spleens show hyaline subendothelial deposits, occasional onion-skin periarteriolar fibrosis, increased hemophagocytosis, foci of extramedullary erythropoiesis, and a variable degree of follicular hyperplasia.[57]

PELIOSIS

Splenic peliosis is much less common than hepatic peliosis.[79–81] Involved spleens are usually only mildly to moderately enlarged, although Lacson and colleagues[81] reported a case in which the organ weighed 1150 grams. The cut surface of the spleen shows blood-filled cystic spaces of variable sizes and with varying degrees of organization that may involve the spleen diffusely or may be patchy, scattered irregularly throughout the red pulp (Color Plate 24). In early stages the cystic cavities may be detectable only microscopically.[81, 82] Histologically, the cystic spaces are round or irregular and seem to preferentially involve the parafollicular areas, including the marginal zones at the interface of the white and red pulp (Fig. 14–11).[81, 82] In some cases the cysts may surround the white pulp so that the arterial vessels and their associated periarterial lymphoid sheaths appear to project into the lumen. The parafollicular location is useful in differentiating peliosis from dilatation of splenic sinuses secondary to chronic passive congestion, which is a diffuse red pulp process.[83] The smaller cysts may be recognized as focal dilatations of the red pulp sinuses with intact sinus lining cells and ring fibers (Fig. 14–12). Sinus lining cells appear flattened in the larger cysts, and in some areas the lining cells cannot be identified. The cystic spaces contain erythrocytes as well as histiocytes and other inflammatory cells. Spleens with numerous cysts usually show atrophy of the white pulp. Earlier reports of splenic peliosis suggested that this lesion occurred only in association with hepatic involvement.[81] However, in the series of Tada et al,[83] eight out of ten cases occurred in patients without peliosis hepatitis.

The pathogenesis of splenic peliosis is unclear. Most cases of hepatic peliosis have been reported in patients who had received either anabolic steroids[84–86] or, less commonly, oral contraceptives.[87] One case occurred in the puerperium after normal pregnancy.[88] There is also an apparent association with tuberculosis and malignancies.[89, 90] Rare cases have occurred in the absence of previous steroid administration, tuberculosis, or malignancy. Most of these "idiopathic" cases occurred in males, and it has been postulated that androgens might play an etiologic role.

Splenic peliosis has also been reported to

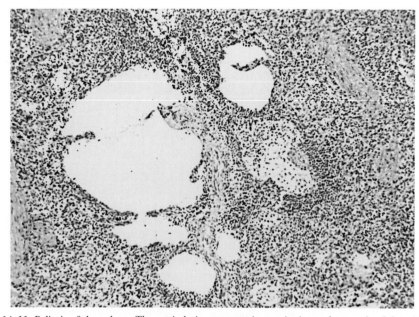

Figure 14–11. Peliosis of the spleen. The cystic lesions appear in contiguity to the vessels of the white pulp.

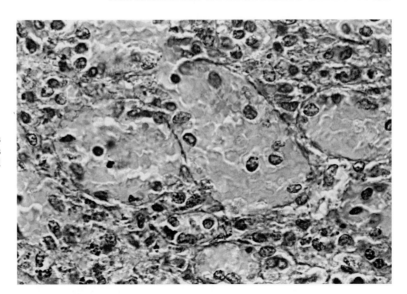

Figure 14–12. In the early stages of splenic peliosis the small cysts appear as dilatations of the red pulp sinuses.

occur in immunocompromised patients as part of the spectrum of extracutaneous bacillary angiomatosis.[91–93] Bacillary angiomatosis is an opportunistic infection most often seen in HIV-infected patients whose reported manifestations have largely been cutaneous vascular lesions that can be mistaken for Kaposi sarcoma.[91, 94] In disseminated cases other sites, including lymph nodes, liver, spleen, and bone marrow, may be involved.[94] Macroscopically, the cut surface of the spleen presents multiple coalescent nodules. Histologically, the nodules are composed of ectatic vessels lined by plump endothelium. The vessels are surrounded by neutrophils and abundant eosinophilic to amphophilic interstitial material that, on Warthin-Starry or Giemsa staining, proves to be aggregated bacilli of *Rochalimaea henselae (Bartonella henselae)*.[94] The bacilli can also be demonstrated by immunohistochemistry using an antibody reactive to *R. quintana*, a closely related rickettsia.[93, 94] Splenic peliosis in immunocompromised patients may occur alone or be associated with bacillary angiomatosis.[92–95] In these patients, the peliotic cavities are surrounded by amorphous stroma harboring bacilli.[91]

Isolated splenic peliosis is usually an incidental finding with few complications. Occasionally, however, a larger cyst may rupture with intraperitoneal hemorrhage.[81, 90, 96–98] Hypersplenism with thrombocytopenia may also occur.[80, 81] Peliotic lesions associated with hormonal therapy usually disappear after cessation of the drug treatment. Therapy with erythromycin or doxycycline is effective in cases due to *R. hensalae*.[95]

SPLENIC ARTERY ANEURYSMS

The widespread use of computed tomography has led to increased detection of asymptomatic visceral artery aneurysms, such as those of the splenic artery.[99] However, aneurysms of the splenic artery may cause splenomegaly, splenic infarctions and, occasionally, splenic rupture.[100, 101] There is an unexplained increased incidence of splenic artery aneurysms in pregnant women.[101–103] These aneurysms have multiple causes; some are probably congenital. However, mycotic aneurysms may result from endocarditis.[103, 104] Inflammatory aneurysms similar to those occurring in the aorta have also been reported to occur in the splenic artery.[105] Splenic artery aneurysms may rupture or penetrate into surrounding structures, occasionally forming arteriovenous fistulas due to erosion into the splenic vein. Splenic artery dissection can also rarely occur.[106] It usually presents in a dramatic fashion and is often fatal if surgical treatment is not undertaken promptly.[106]

REFERENCES

1. DeBartolo HM Jr, Van Heerden JA, Lynn HB, et al: Torsion of the spleen: A case report. Mayo Clin Proc 1973; 48:783.

2. Larrimer JH, Mendelson DS, Metz EN: Howell-Jolly bodies: A clue to splenic infarction. Arch Intern Med 1975; 135:857.

3. Capron JP, Chivrac D, Dupas JL, et al: Massive splenic infarction in cirrhosis: Report of a case with spontaneous disappearance of hypersplenism. Gastroenterology 1976; 71:308.

4. O'Keefe JH, Holmes DR, Schaff HV, et al: Thromboembolic splenic infarction. Mayo Clin Proc 1986; 61:967.

5. Neiman RS, Orazi O: Spleen, in Damjanov I, Linder J (eds): Anderson's Pathology, 10th ed, vol 1, p 1201. St. Louis, Mosby–Year Book, 1996.

6. Pelletier LL Jr, Petersdorf RG: Infective endocarditis: A review of 125 cases from the University of Washington hospitals, 1963. Medicine 1977; 56:287.

7. Baron JM, Weinshelbaum EI, Block GE: Splenic rupture associated with bacterial endocarditis and sickle cell trait. JAMA 1968; 205:102.

8. Chase RM Jr: Infective endocarditis today. Med Clin North Am 1973; 57:1383.

9. Lingeman CJ, Smith EB, Battersby JS, et al: Subacute bacterial endocarditis: Splenectomy in cases refractory to antibiotic therapy. Arch Intern Med 1956; 97:309.

10. Vergne R, Selland B, Gobel FL, et al: Rupture of the spleen in infective endocarditis. Arch Intern Med 1975; 135:1265.

11. Buchbinder NA, Roberts WC: Left-sided valvular active infective endocarditis: A study of forty-five necropsy patients. Am J Med 1973; 53:20.

12. Rosenblum AL, Bonner H Jr, Milder MS, et al: Cavitating splenic infarction. Am J Med 1974; 56:720.

13. Fonner BT, Nemcek AA Jr, Boschman C: CT appearance of splenic infarction in Wegener's granulomatosis. Am J Roentgenol 1995; 164:353.

14. Harten P, Müller-Huelsbeck S, Regensburger D, et al: Multiple organ manifestations in thromboangiitis obliterans (Buerger's disease): A case report. Angiology 1996; 47:419.

15. Franssen CF, Ter Maaten JC, Hoorntje SJ: Spontaneous splenic rupture in Wegener's vasculitis. Ann Rheum Dis 1993; 53:314.

16. Wolf BC, Neiman RS: The histopathologic manifestations of the lymphoproliferative and myeloproliferative disorders involving the spleen, in Knowles DM (ed): Neoplastic Hematopathology. Baltimore, Williams & Wilkins, 1992.

17. Shaldon S, Sherlock S: Portal hypertension in the myeloproliferative syndrome and the reticuloses. Am J Med 1962; 32:758.

18. Downer WR, Peterson MS: Massive splenic infarction and liquefactive necrosis complicating polycythemia vera. Am J Roentgenol 1993; 161:79.

19. Hardisty RM, Wolff HH: Haemorrhagic thrombocythaemia: A clinical and laboratory study. Br J Haematol 1955; 1:390.

20. Marsh GW, Lewis SM, Szur L: The use of ^{51}Cr-labeled heat-damaged red cells to study splenic function. II. Splenic atrophy in thrombocythaemia. Br J Haematol 1966; 12:167.

21. Mathieu D, Rahmouni A, Villeneuve P, et al: Impact of magnetic resonance imaging on the diagnosis of abdominal complications of paroxysmal nocturnal hemoglobinuria. Blood 1995; 85:3283.

22. Imashuku S, Nakagawa Y, Hibi S: Splenic infarction after erythropoietin therapy. Lancet 1993; 342:182.

23. Jaroch MT, Broughan TA, Hermann RE: The natural history of splenic infarction. Surgery 1986; 100:743.

24. Georg C, Schwerk WB: Splenic infarction: Sonographic patterns, diagnosis, follow-up, and complications. Radiology 1990; 174:803.

25. Conn HO: Sickle-cell trait and splenic infarction associated with high-altitude flying. N Engl J Med 1954; 251:417.

26. Cooley JC, Peterson WL, Engle CE, et al: Clinical triad of massive splenic infarction, sickle cell trait and high altitude flying. JAMA 1954; 154:111.

27. Stock AE: Splenic infarction associated with high altitude flying and sickle cell trait. Ann Intern Med 1956; 44:554.

28. Cavenagh JD, Joseph AE, Dilly S, et al: Splenic sepsis in sickle cell disease. Br J Haematol 1994; 86:187.

29. Hovette P, Lecoules S, Boete F, et al: Splenic infarction during P. falciparum and P. vivax malaria. Presse Medicale 1994; 23:1226.

30. Cremer J, Schleiblinger W: Klinik der Milzkrankheiten, p 52. Stuttgart, Ferdinand Enke Verlag, 1967.

31. Videbaek A, Christensen BE, Jonsson V: The Spleen in Health and Disease, p 178. Chicago, Year Book Medical Publishers.

32. Ravenna P: Banti syndrome (fibrocongestive splenomegaly). Arch Intern Med 1943; 72:786.

33. Banti G: La splenomegalie avec cirrhose du foie. La Semaine Medicale 1894; 14:318.

34. Ohnishi K, Saito M, Sata S, et al: Portal hemodynamics in idiopathic portal hypertension (Banti's syndrome): Comparison with chronic persistent hepatitis and normal subjects. Gastroenterology 1987; 92:751.

35. Maesawa C, Sakuma T, Sato T, et al: Structural characteristics of splenic sinuses in idiopathic portal hypertension. Pathol Intern 1995; 45:642.

36. Chen S: Effects of spleen on inducing portal hypertension and liver cirrhosis in rats. Chin Med J 1992; 72:338.

37. Umeyama KK, Yamashita T, Yoshikawa K: Etiology of idiopathic portal hypertension (IPH): The role of immunological mechanism in IPH. J Jpn Surg Soc 1992; 93:400.

38. Stone PWM, MacKay M, Pellish P, et al: Surgical therapy in schistosomal cirrhosis of the liver. Ann Surg 1956; 144:79.

39. Yoshimura N, Oka T, Ohmori Y, et al: Idiopathic portal hypertension in renal transplant recipients: Report of two cases. Surg Today 1994; 24:1111.

40. Carr I, Henry L, Murari PJ: Lymph nodes and spleen, in Silverberg SG (ed): Principles and Practice of Surgical Pathology, p 335. New York, John Wiley & Sons, 1983.

41. Lindley RP: Splenic arteriolar hyalin in children. J Pathol 1986; 148:321.

42. Crawford T, Woolf N: Hyaline arteriosclerosis in the spleen: An immunohisto-chemical study. J Pathol Bacteriol 1960; 79:221.

43. Fauci AS, Haynes BF, Katz P: The spectrum of vasculitis: Clinical, pathologic, immunologic and therapeutic considerations. Ann Intern Med 1978; 89:660.

44. Fallingborg J, Laustsen J, Jakobsen J, et al: A traumatic rupture of the spleen in periarteritis nodosa. Acta Chir Scand 1985; 151:85.

45. Churg J, Strauss L: Allergic granulomatosis, allergic angiitis, and periarteritis nodosa. Am J Pathol 1947; 33:251.

46. Tai PC, Holt ME, Denny P, et al: Deposition of eosinophil cationic protein in granulomas in allergic granulomatosis and vasculitis: The Churg-Strauss syndrome. Br Med J 1984; 289:400.

47. Alarcon-Segovia D: The necrotizing vasculitides: A new pathogenetic classification. Med Clin North Am 1977; 61:241.
48. Sokoloff L, Bunim JJ: Vascular lesions in rheumatoid arthritis. J Chron Dis 1957; 5:668.
49. Kaiser IH: Pathology of disseminated lupus erythematosus. Bull Johns Hopkins Hosp 1942; 71:31.
50. Klemperer P, Pollack AD, Baehr G: Pathology of disseminated lupus erythematosus. Arch Pathol 1941; 32:569.
51. Alarcon-Segovia D: Systemic lupus erythematosus—pathology and pathogenesis, in Schumacher HR Jr, Klippel JH, Robinson DR (eds): Primer on the Rheumatic Disease. Atlanta, The Arthritis Foundation, 1993.
52. Ansari A, Larson PH, Bates HD: Vascular manifestations of systemic lupus erythematosus. Angiology 1986; 37:423.
53. Lorincz LL, Soltani K, Bernstein JE: Antinuclear antibodies. Int J Dermatol 1981; 20:401.
54. Schwartz RS: Immunologic and genetic aspects of systemic lupus erythematosus. N Engl J Med 1979; 30:803.
55. Tan EM: Antinuclear antibodies in diagnosis and management. Hosp Pract 1983; 18:79.
56. McCluskey RT: Evidence for an immune complex disorder in systemic lupus erythematosus. Am J Kid Dis 1982; 2:199.
57. Saracco SM, Farhi DC: Splenic pathology in thrombotic thrombocytopenia purpura. Am J Surg Pathol 1990; 14:223.
58. Distenfeld A, Oppenheim E: The treatment of acute thrombotic thrombocytopenic purpura with corticosteroids and splenectomy: Report of 3 cases. Ann Intern Med 1966; 65:245.
59. Amorosi EL, Ultmann JE: Thrombotic thrombocytopenic purpura: Report of 16 cases and review of the literature. Medicine 1966; 45:139.
60. Byrnes JJ, Moake JL: Thrombotic thrombocytopenic purpura and the hemolytic-uremic syndrome: Evolving concepts of pathogenesis and therapy. Clin Haematol 1986; 15:413.
61. Umlas J, Kaiser J: Thrombohemolytic thrombocytopenic purpura (TTP): A disease or a syndrome? Am J Med 1970; 40:723.
62. Laurence J, Mitra D, Steiner M, et al: Plasma from patients with idiopathic and human immunodeficiency virus–associated thrombotic thrombocytopenic purpura induces apoptosis in microvascular endothelial cells. Blood 1996; 87:3245.
63. Siddiqui FA, Lian EC-Y: Novel platelet-agglutinating protein from a thrombotic thrombocytopenic purpura plasma. J Clin Invest 1985; 76:1330.
64. Cheng SH, Lian EC-Y: Purification and some properties of a 59 *kda* platelet-aggregating protein from the plasma of a patient with thrombotic thrombocytopenic purpura. Thromb Haemost 1989; 62:568.
65. Moore JC, Murphy WG, Kelton JG: Calpain proteolysis of von Willebrand factor enhances its binding to platelet membrane glycoprotein IIb/IIa: An explanation for platelet aggregation in thrombotic thrombocytopenic purpura. Br J Haematol 1990; 74:457.
66. Moake JL, Rudy CK, Troll JH, et al: Unusually large plasma factor VIII: von Willebrand factor multimers in chronic relapsing thrombotic thrombocytopenic purpura. N Engl J Med 1982; 307:1432.
67. Moake JL, McPherson PD: Abnormalities of von Willebrand factor multimers in thrombotic thrombocy-

topenic purpura and the hemolytic-uremic syndrome. Am J Med 1989; 87:3.
68. McLeod BC, Wu KK, Knospe WH: Plasmapheresis in thrombotic thrombocytopenic purpura. Arch Int Med 1980; 140:1059.
69. Moake JL: Thrombotic thrombocytopenic purpura and the hemolytic uremic syndrome, in Hoffman R, Bena EJ, Shattie SJ, et al (eds): Hematology, Basic Principles and Practice, p 1879. New York, Churchill Livingstone, 1995.
70. Bernard RP, Bauman AW, Schwartz SI: Splenectomy for thrombotic thrombocytopenic purpura. Ann Surg 1969; 169:616.
71. Reynolds PM, Jackson JM, Brine JAS, et al: Thrombotic thrombocytopenic purpura: Remission following splenectomy—report of a case and review of the literature. Am J Med 1976; 61:439.
72. Rodriguez HF, Babb DR, Perez-Santiago E, et al: Thrombotic thrombocytopenic purpura: Remission after splenectomy. N Engl J Med 1957; 257:983.
73. Shapiro HD, Doktor D, Chung J: Thrombotic thrombocytopenic purpura (Moschcowitz's disease): Report of a case with remission after splenectomy and steroid therapy. Ann Intern Med 1957; 47:582.
74. Thompson CE, Damon LE, Ries CA, et al: Thrombotic microangiopathies in the 1980s: Clinical features, response to treatment, and the impact of the human immunodeficiency virus epidemic. Blood 1992; 80:1890.
75. Bell WR, Braine HG, Ness PM, et al: Improved survival in thrombotic thrombocytopenic purpura/hemolytic uremic syndrome: Clinical experience in 108 patients. New Engl J Med 1991; 325:398.
76. Kadri A, Moinuddin M, de Leeuw NKM: Phagocytosis of blood cells by splenic macrophages in thrombotic thrombocytopenic purpura. Ann Int Med 1975; 82:799.
77. Rosove MH, Bhuta S: Splenectomy and extravascular platelet destruction in thrombotic thrombocytopenic purpura. Arch Intern Med 1985; 145:937.
78. Talarico L, Grapski R, Lutz CK, et al: Late postsplenectomy recurrence of thrombotic thrombocytopenic purpura responding to removal of accessory spleen. Am J Med 1987; 82:845.
79. Kent G, Thompson JR: Peliosis hepatis: Involvement of the reticuloendothelial system. Arch Pathol 1961; 72:658.
80. Taxy JB: Peliosis: A morphologic curiosity becomes an iatrogenic problem. Hum Pathol 1978; 9:331.
81. Lacson A, Berman LD, Neiman RS: Peliosis of the spleen. Am J Clin Pathol 1979; 71:586.
82. Chopra S, Edelstein A, Koff RS, et al: Peliosis hepatis in hematologic disease: Report of two cases. JAMA 1978; 240:1153.
83. Tada T, Wakabayashi T, Kishimoto H: Peliosis of the spleen. Am J Clin Pathol 1983; 79:708.
84. Bagheri SA, Boyer JL: Peliosis hepatis associated with androgenic anabolic steroid therapy. Ann Intern Med 1974; 81:610.
85. Naeim F, Cooper PH, Semion AA: Peliosis hepatitis: Possible etiologic role of anabolic steroids. Arch Pathol 1973; 95:284.
86. Wadell J, Kaiser J: Peliosis hepatis: Twelve cases associated with oral androgen therapy. Arch Pathol 1977; 101:405.
87. O'Sullivan JP, Wilding RP: Liver hamartomas in patients on oral contraceptives. Br Med J 1974; 3:7.
88. Patrioct LM, Dumont M, Duvernois JP, et al: [A

case of hepatic and splenic peliosis occurring in the puerperium after normal pregnancy] [French]. Journal de Gynecologie, Obstetrique et Biologie de la Reproduction 1986; 15:321.

89. Zak PG: Peliosis hepatis. Am J Pathol 1950; 26:1.

90. Diebold J, Audouin J: Peliosis of the spleen: Report of a case associated with chronic myelomonocytic leukemia, presenting with spontaneous splenic rupture. Am J Surg Pathol 1983; 7:197.

91. Perkocha LA, Ferrell L, Yen TSB, et al: Extracutaneous manifestations of bacillary angiomatosis. Mod Pathol 1991; 4:88A.

92. Slater LN, Welch DF, Min KW: *Rochalimaea henselae* causes bacillary angiomatosis and peliosis hepatic. Arch Intern Med 1992; 152:602.

93. Reed JA, Brigati DJ, Flynn SD, et al: Immunocytochemical identification of *Rochalimaea henselae* in bacillary (epithelioid) angiomatosis, parenchymal bacillary peliosis, and persistent fever with bacteremia. Am J Surg Pathol 1992; 16:650.

94. Warnke RA, Weiss LM, Chan JKC, et al (eds): Atlas of Tumor Pathology: Tumors of the Lymph Nodes and Spleen, 3rd series, fascicle 14, p 468. Washington, DC, Armed Forces Institute of Pathology, 1995.

95. Cotell SL, Noskin GA: Bacillary angiomatosis: Clinical and histologic features, diagnosis, and treatment. Arch Intern Med 1994; 154:524.

96. Benjamin DR, Shink B: A fatal case of peliosis of the liver and spleen. Am J Dis Child 1978; 132:207.

97. Kohr RM, Haendiges M, Taube RR: Peliosis of the spleen: A rare cause of spontaneous splenic rupture with surgical implications. Am Surg 1993; 59:197.

98. Garcia RL, Khan MK, Berlin RB: Peliosis of the spleen with rupture. Hum Pathol 1982; 13:177.

99. Carr SC, Pearce WH, Vogelzang RL, et al: Current management of visceral artery aneurysms. Surgery 1996; 120:627.

100. Jacobson IV, Crowe PJ: Splenic infarction: A complication of splenic artery aneurysm. Aust N Z J Surg 1994; 64:53.

101. Bedford PD, Lodge B: Aneurysm of the splenic artery. Gut 1960; 1:312.

102. MacFarlane JR, Thorbjarnarson B: Rupture of splenic artery during pregnancy. Am J Obstet 1966; 95:1023.

103. Owens JC, Coffey RJ: Aneurysm of the splenic artery including a report of six additional cases. Int Abstr Surg 1953; 97:313.

104. Stengel A, Wolferth CC: Mycotic (bacterial) aneurysms of intravascular origin. Arch Intern Med 1923; 31:527.

105. Billeter M, Franzeck UK, won Segesser L, et al: Inflammatory aneurysm of the splenic artery. Intern Angiol 1994; 13:160.

106. Merrell SW, Gloviczki P: Splenic artery dissection: A case report and review of the literature. J Vas Surg 1992; 15:221.

SPLENIC CYSTS, NONHEMATOPOIETIC TUMORS, AND TUMORLIKE LESIONS

SPLENIC CYSTS

Cystic lesions of the spleen are rare.[1–5] These lesions are usually classified as parasitic or nonparasitic, based on their etiology, and true (primary) or pseudo (false, secondary), based on the presence or absence of a lining epithelium.

Nonparasitic Cysts

Pseudocysts

The most common nonparasitic cyst, constituting 80 percent of the total, is the pseudocyst (Color Plate 25). Pseudocyst formation is generally believed to be the result of degradation of a posttraumatic splenic hematoma.[5–8] However, a history of previous trauma is often not obtained.[9] Other possible causes include cystic degeneration of a splenic infarct, hamartoma, angioma, or a degenerated healed histoplasmic granuloma (Color Plate 26). Most pseudocysts are incidental findings, but some are large and cause symptoms. Abdominal ultrasonography and computerized tomography are useful in the identification of cystic lesions of the spleen, as is angiography, which often delineates an avascular mass.[10–14]

Although most pseudocysts are unilocular, rare cases of multiloculated false cysts have been reported (Fig. 15–1).[15] Pseudocysts differ from epithelial cysts in that the luminal surfaces in the former are often smooth rather than trabeculated. They are often filled with opaque or cloudy fluid. The pseudocyst wall is formed by fibrous tissue with a central calcified zone, often containing cholesterol crystals. Hemosiderin is often present in the fibrous wall. By definition, an epithelial lining is absent. Once diagnosed, a splenic pseudocyst should be treated if it is symptomatic or larger than 10 cm.[16] Risks of unremoved splenic pseudocysts include spontaneous rupture with hemoperitoneum and infection with abscess formation. Traditionally, splenectomy has been the treatment of choice. Currently, many authors advocate splenic preservation to avoid the possibility of severe infections associated with the postsplenectomy state.[16, 17] This is particularly important in children and in tropical countries where post-traumatic cysts are relatively common and splenectomy may be fatal in patients with malaria.[18] Spleen-sparing procedures include cyst excision and splenorrhaphy or, alternatively, partial cyst excision and marsupialization.[16, 17] Despite a high incidence of recurrences, radiographically assisted percutaneous drainage can be successfully employed in selected cases.[19]

True Cysts

True cysts, also termed "epithelial," "epidermoid," and "mesothelial" cysts, account for the remaining 20 percent of splenic non-

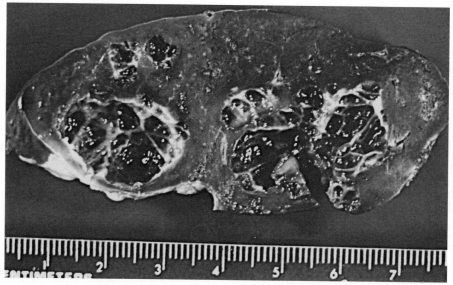

Figure 15–1. Splenic pseudocyst. This example is unusual because most pseudocysts are unilocular.

parasitic cysts.[10, 20–22] They usually occur in children or in young adults, and most series report no gender predominance.[23] They may be congenital, and a few familial cases have been reported.[24, 25] They are usually asymptomatic but may cause pressure symptoms due to their mass effect or, less commonly, cause left upper quadrant abdominal pain.[11] The cysts sometimes adhere to adjacent viscera or to the diaphragm. They may be quite large, the average size in one series being 10 cm.[6] True cysts are mostly single and unilocular, although occasionally there may be satellites in the wall of the main cyst. However, multiple as well as multilocular cysts have been reported.[6, 11–14, 24–26]

The lining of a true cyst is usually shiny and trabeculated (Color Plate 27).[27] It may contain either clear fluid or turbid fluid with cholesterol and blood.[22] The wall is composed of fibrous tissue with an interior epithelial lining. Occasionally the wall of the cyst may be focally calcified.[10, 28–31] Because the epithelial lining is often partially denuded, numerous histologic sections may be required to identify the epithelium.[10, 32] The cyst is most commonly lined by stratified squamous epithelium that may show keratinization (Fig. 15–2). Rete ridges and skin appendages are absent. Transitional epithelium as well as foci of intraepithelial glandlike structures containing mucin have been reported.[9] The cyst lining may occasionally be composed partially or wholly of columnar, cuboidal, or flattened epithelium (Fig.

15–3).[11] The presence of flattened to hobnail cells in the cyst lining is generally interpreted as evidence of mesothelial differentiation. When lined by transitional epithelium-containing mucinous cells, these small satellite cysts may closely resemble cystitis cystica.

The etiology and histogenesis of splenic epidermoid cysts are controversial. Several authors have postulated that they are congenital, representing embryonic inclusions of splenic capsular mesothelium,[33, 34] fetal squamous epithelium,[35] or mesoderm.[36, 37] Others have postulated they represent invaginations of either endoderm or ectoderm[38, 39] or of mesonephric tissue.[40] A teratomatous origin has also been proposed.[35] However, a mesothelial derivation is favored by most investigators. It has been suggested that intrasplenic entrapment of splenic capsular mesothelium may occur as a consequence of trauma. True cysts have been reported in patients with a history of abdominal trauma, raising the possibility that a subclinical tear in the splenic capsule with subsequent mesothelial entrapment may be the etiologic factor in "spontaneous" cases as well. Electron microscopic studies have provided supportive evidence of a mesothelial origin of the cyst epithelium.[34] Immunohistochemical studies have also generally confirmed a mesothelial origin by demonstrating reactivity with keratin and vimentin as well as the mesothelial-associated marker HBME-1.[41, 42]

True dermoid cysts, similar to benign cystic teratomas of the ovary, with hair follicles and

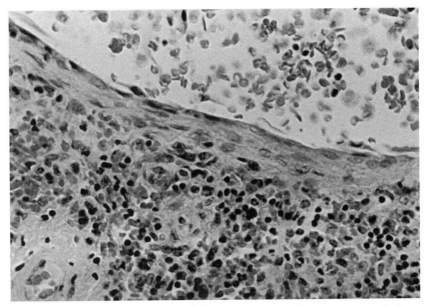

Figure 15–2. Epidermoid cyst. The lining is composed of stratified squamous epithelium.

sebaceous glands, have been reported rarely.[1] Primary splenic lymphoma may occasionally present as a splenic cyst.[43] Complications of splenic cysts include hemorrhage, rupture, and secondary bacterial infection.[44, 45] Rarely, rupture of a cyst may cause symptoms of an acute abdomen.[38, 45, 46] Although cysts may lead to marked splenomegaly, hypersplenism is unusual. Patients with true cysts are treated in the same way as patients with false cysts.[47]

Parasitic Cysts

The most common parasitic cyst is caused by larvae of the tapeworm of the genus *Echinococcus*, resulting from ingestion of tapeworm eggs (Fig. 15–4).[48] The larvae invade the tributaries of the portal vein and encyst in the viscera. Two thirds of echinococcal (hydatid) cysts are found in the liver; isolated splenic infection is exceptionally rare.[49] The most

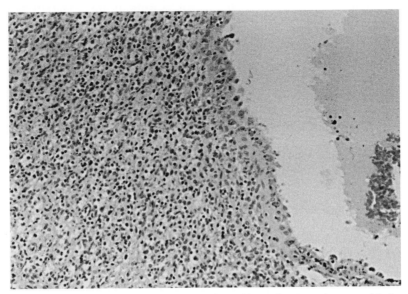

Figure 15–3. A portion of the lining of an epidermoid cyst showing columnar epithelium.

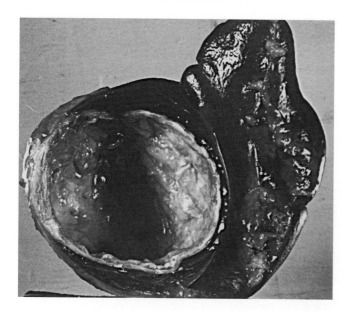

Figure 15–4. Ecchinococcal cyst of the spleen.

prevalent species is *E. granulosus*, which forms unilocular cysts. Although infection may occur anywhere in the world, it is most common in the western United States, New Zealand, Australia, and the Near East. Dogs and sheep are the definitive hosts. *E. multilocularis* is also found in central and eastern Europe, and *E. volegi* is found in northern Latin America. The latter species forms multilocular cysts. Echinococcal cysts are rare in the United States, constituting only 2 percent of the Armed Forces Institute of Pathology series of 102 splenic cysts.[11, 48, 50]

Whenever echinococcal cysts form, the larvae incite an inflammatory response. The outer cyst is composed of a laminated fibrous layer, which is lined by an inner germinative layer made up of daughter cysts, termed "brood capsules."[48, 50] The cyst may be surrounded by inflammatory cells, predominantly mononuclear cells and eosinophils. Scolices develop on the inner aspect of the brood capsules, which separate from the cyst wall and form a sandlike material that becomes suspended in the cyst fluid. Using the acid-fast stain (Fig. 15–5),[6] the scolices can be recognized in imprints of the cyst wall. Complications of echinococcal cysts include leakage into the abdomen of cholesterol-rich fluid, which is allergenic, and bacterial superinfection. Large cysts may cause pressure symptoms owing to compression of other viscera. If the parasite dies, the cyst may undergo fibrosis and calcify. Treatment is surgical removal of the cyst. Care must be taken to avoid rupture

at surgery, which may result in an anaphylactic reaction or the spread of multiple cysts throughout the abdomen.

BENIGN MESENCHYMAL TUMORS

Vascular Tumors

Hemangiomas

Hemangiomas are the most common benign neoplasms of the spleen.[51–53] They occur most frequently in young to middle-aged adults without any apparent gender or racial predilection.[54] The majority are incidental findings. Larger hemangiomas, however, may be associated with symptomatic splenomegaly, cytopenias related to hypersplenism, or microangiopathic hemolytic anemia.[6] A consumption coagulopathy has been reported secondary to the sequestration of clotting factors.[55, 56] Patients with large hemangiomas may report symptoms of several years' duration, indicating the slow growth of the lesion. Occasionally, large hemangiomas may rupture, resulting in shock from acute hemorrhage.[57]

Hemangiomas are usually solitary lesions, although occasionally they may be multiple.[52] Garvin and King[6] reported an average size of 5 to 8 cm, with an average splenic weight of 300 to 400 g. Grossly, hemangiomas usually appear blue-red and spongy. They are usually well circumscribed, although occasionally they may blend imperceptibly with the surrounding

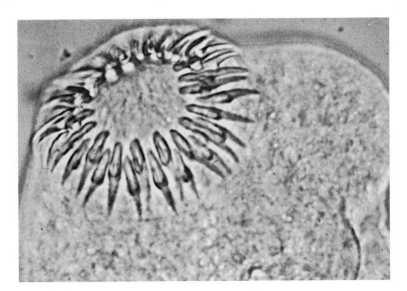

Figure 15–5. Ecchinococcal scolex from imprint of the wall of an ecchinococcal cyst.

parenchyma. Larger lesions may undergo regressive changes, including infarction, fibrosis, and cystic degeneration.[52] Microscopically, hemangiomas may be either capillary or cavernous, although the latter is more common (Fig. 15–6). Cavernous hemangiomas are composed of interconnected dilated vascular spaces lined by plump endothelial cells with little intervening fibrous tissue (Fig. 15–7).

Within any given lesion the vascular channels may vary in size. As a result, the lesion may contain both capillary and cavernous features. Clusters of normoblasts and megakaryocytes may occur in the stroma and in the vascular spaces of both types of hemangioma (Fig. 15–8). Cavernous hemangiomas are easily distinguished from splenic hamartomas by their gross and microscopic appearance, and capillary hemangiomas may resemble hamartomas. Some investigators have even suggested that splenic hamartomas may be identical to capillary hemangiomas.[58–61] This is not likely, for there are immunohistochemical differences between the two lesions. Hamartomas contain

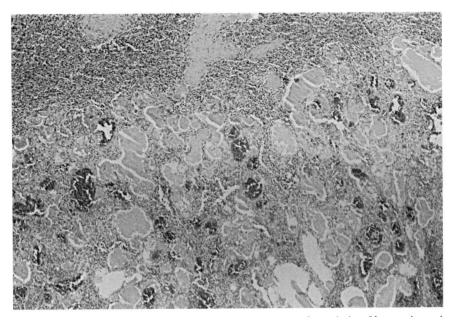

Figure 15–6. Hemangioma of the spleen. This example is cavernous, as are the majority of hemangiomas in the spleen.

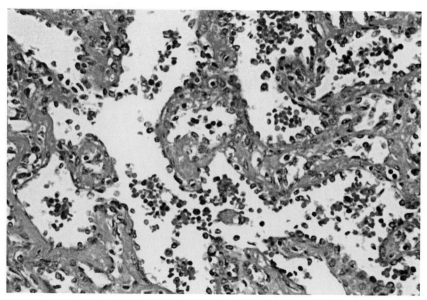

Figure 15–7. Splenic hemangioma. The lesion displays a single lining of plump endothelial cells.

vascular channels lined by sinus endothelial cells that are CD8-positive, CD68-positive and CD34-negative. Hemangiomas are CD8-negative and CD68-negative and usually express CD34, an endothelial marker strongly expressed by pulp cord capillaries and postsinusoidal veins but not found in normal littoral cells or sinus endothelium within hamartomas.[62]

Diffuse hemangiomatosis of the spleen is a rare benign neoplastic condition in which the whole spleen is diffusely permeated by neoplastic blood vessels (Fig. 15–9). The vessels are of varying caliber and often appear ectatic. Most of these cases have been reported in association with generalized angiomatosis involving skin, bones, and liver.[63–69] A case associated with hereditary telangiectasia has also been reported.[68] Ruck et al[70] described a case of isolated splenic hemangiomatosis in which immunohistochemical stains showed a splenic sinus endothelial (littoral cell) derivation.

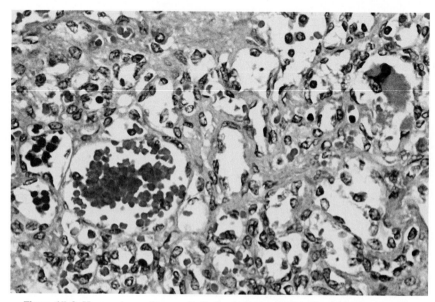

Figure 15–8. Hemangiomas frequently display hematopoietic cells within their lumens.

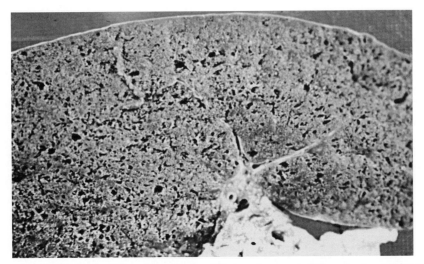

Figure 15–9. Angiomatosis of the spleen showing diffuse replacement of the organ by vascular spaces.

Splenic hemangioma may be confused with the diffuse sinusoidal hyperplasia that occurs in patients with congestive splenomegaly and history of repeated blood transfusion (see Chapter 11). The origin of splenic hemangiomas is unclear. Because of their resemblance to hamartomas, some believe that they are of developmental origin.[52] Others have postulated that they are true neoplasms and cite reports of malignant degeneration within benign hemangiomas with resulting metastases.[71] We believe that such cases were probably angiosarcomas from their inception and were considered benign because of the relatively high degree of differentiation in the lesions. It has been our experience that hemangiomas in children may be characterized by more hyperplastic endothelial cells and more frequent papillary growth (Fig. 15–10). This is not associated with an aggressive clinical behavior and should not prompt a diagnosis of low grade hemangiosarcoma.

Littoral Cell Angiomas

Littoral cell angioma (LCA) is a rare benign splenic vascular tumor derived from the sinus lining cells, or littoral cells, of the red pulp (Fig. 15–11).[72–76] As discussed in Chapter 1, these cells show immunophenotypic evidence of endothelial and histiocytic differentiation.[77] LCAs may occur both in adults and children, and have a median age incidence of 49.[72] There is no gender predilection. In most cases splenectomy is performed for splenomegaly of unknown origin, often associated with evidence of hypersplenism (thrombocytopenia and/or anemia). Fever of unknown origin, which abated after splenectomy, has been documented in a few patients. Although the tumor is benign, a malignant variant has recently been reported.[78–80]

Macroscopically, spleens involved by LCA show multiple dark, spongy, cystic nodules that are indistinguishable from hemangiomas. Less frequently, cases present as a solitary nodule. In rare cases the splenic tissue is completely replaced by vaguely nodular spongy lesions.[72, 74] Microscopically, the lesion is found within red pulp, appears well circumscribed, and compresses the adjacent splenic parenchyma. The tumor may appear subdivided into lobules by areas of sclerosis. Multifocal confluent lesions may surround splenic follicles. The vascular spaces have variable width, some showing only slitlike lumina, others appearing dilated or cystic. The vascular channels are lined by a single layer of endothelial cells, which may be either tall or flat. In the majority of cases the lining consists entirely of tall endothelial cells (Fig. 15–12) that possess large vesicular nuclei with open chromatin and small nucleoli. Occasionally the lumina are filled by proliferations of tall endothelial cells with variable amounts of fibrous stroma. In a minority of cases a second component of flat cells with small indented nuclei, coarse chromatin, and scant cytoplasm is also observed. The latter cells are virtually indistinguishable from normal splenic littoral cells. Cytoplasmic globules that are periodic acid–Schiff–positive may be present in the proliferating cells. These glob-

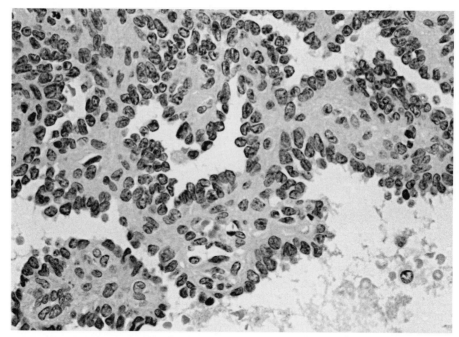

Figure 15–10. Hemangioma in a 5-year-old child. The endothelial cells are hyperplastic, and papillary growth is present. These findings in children should not be interpreted as evidence of malignancy.

ules may be detected by light microscopy and ultrastructurally.[81] Incomplete annular reticulin fibers can be demonstrated focally around the vascular spaces. Mitoses are very rare. Exfoliated cells are frequently observed within the vascular lumina, some of which may demonstrate evidence of phagocytosis of red cells or other cellular material. Immunohistochemically, LCA cells express vimentin and the endothelium-associated markers factor VIII an-

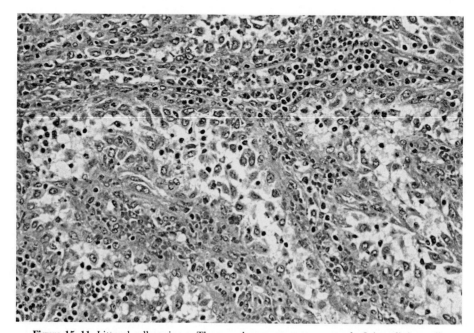

Figure 15–11. Littoral cell angioma. The vascular spaces are composed of sinus lining cells.

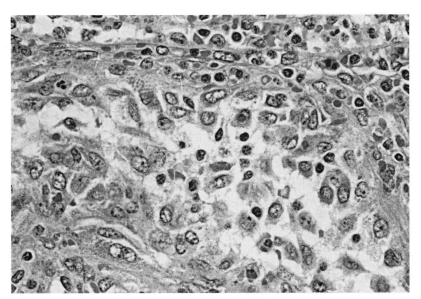

Figure 15–12. Littoral cell angioma. Sinus lining cells desquamate into the lumen.

tigen and Ulex europaeus lectin[72]; CD34 is negative. [73] In addition, the cells express the histiocytic markers alpha$_1$-antichymotryspin, lysozyme, and CD68 (KP-1).[72–74, 76] CD21 and, less frequently, S-100 expression have been observed.[72, 73] The CD8 antigen, which is normally expressed by splenic sinus lining cells, was found to be negative in a recent series of six cases of LCA.[73] This result is at variance with an earlier report.[79]

The differential diagnosis of LCA includes other benign and malignant vascular tumors of the spleen. The combination of distinctive morphologic features and characteristic immunohistochemical findings usually allows an easy separation of LCA from other benign splenic lesions. Difficulties can, however, be experienced in the distinction from angiosarcomas, especially when LCAs contain numerous papillary projections and more solid areas. However, the absence of cytologic atypia, irregular anastomosing vascular channels, or necrosis argues against malignancy. In addition, the immunohistochemical reactivity of LCA for histiocytic markers as well as for CD21 can be helpful in excluding an angiosarcoma. However, rare cases of angiosarcoma of presumed littoral cell derivation (littoral cell angiosarcoma) have been described (Fig. 15–13).[78–80] Littoral cell angiosarcoma is composed of poorly circumscribed nodules that lack a lobular pattern and presents, at least focally, prominent intravascular papillary fronds lined by tall cells displaying obvious malignant features.

Necrosis is absent. The presence of solid nests composed of malignant cells displaying mitotic activity also distinguishes this rare tumor from the benign LCA.[78]

Lymphangiomas

Lymphangiomas of the spleen are less common than hemangiomas. They may occur as part of disseminated lymphangiomatosis in children.[82–86] Rare cases of nonsystemic lymphangiomatosis of the spleen associated with massive splenomegaly have also been reported.[87–90] In these cases the splenic involvement is usually in the form of large multicentric nodules. An association of splenic lymphangioma and the Klippel-Trénaunay-Weber syndrome has also been described.[91] Lymphangiomas may also be observed as an incidental finding in spleens removed for various reasons. These tumors are usually small subcapsular multicystic proliferations.[42, 85] Grossly, distinction of lymphangiomas from hemangiomas is not always possible.[6] Unlike the random localization of hemangiomas, lymphangiomas often involve the large trabeculae and capsule, where lymphatic structures are normally present.[92] Histologically, lymphangiomas are composed of thin-walled cysts of varying sizes and contain watery, pink proteinaceous material instead of blood. Scattered foamy histiocytes are usually present within the cyst cavities, and cholesterol crystals may be noted (Fig. 15–14). The lining endothelium

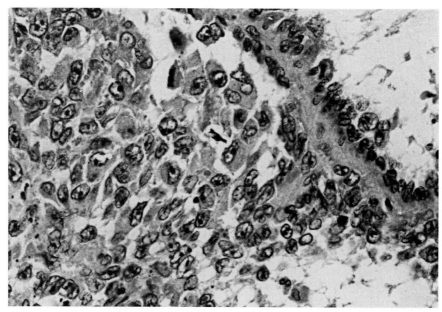

Figure 15–13. Littoral cell angiosarcoma. Littoral cells display hypercellularity and cellular atypia.

is predominantly flat (Fig. 15–15). However, plump cells with occasional foamy cytoplasm as well as small papillary projections into the cyst lumen occasionally occur.[92] Although these changes have been interpreted as indicative of malignancy in two published cases,[93, 94] in neither case was the tumor known to have metastasized.

The lining cells of lymphangiomas usually express CD31 and factor VIII-related antigen. CD34 and CD8 are negative.[42, 70] A recent immunohistochemical study by Arber et al[42] of six cases of solitary subcapsular splenic lymphangiomas suggested a mesothelial derivation of these lesions rather than a lymphatic origin. The authors postulated that these lesions are

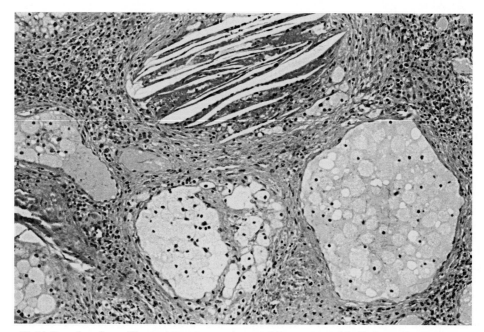

Figure 15–14. Lymphangioma. The cystic spaces contain proteinaceous material. Cholesterol crystals are present.

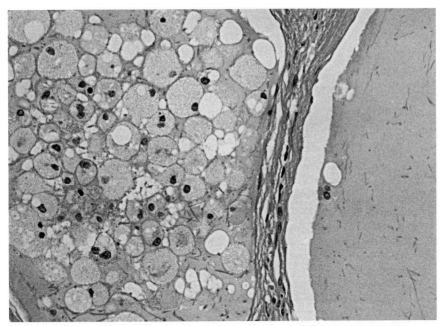

Figure 15–15. Lymphangioma. The endothelium lining the cystic cavities is flat. Numerous foamy macrophages are present.

similar to the larger true cysts of the spleen because both share immunoreactivity with mesothelium. The larger true cysts, however, are usually unilocular and are often lined by squamous or transitional cell epithelium, features not seen in these small subcapsular lymphangiomas. Further immunohistochemical analysis of a larger number of cases is needed to clarify whether solitary splenic lymphangiomas represent an unusual morphologic variant of true splenic cysts or if they are a distinct tumor.

Hemangiopericytomas

Hemangiopericytomas are rare vascular tumors, most frequently occurring in the soft tissues of the lower extremities and retroperitoneum.[95] Visceral involvement is uncommon. Only two cases have been reported in the spleen.[96, 97] Histologically, hemangiopericytoma is characterized by spindle-shaped, uniform tumor cells grouped around dilated vascular channels, appearing as if the cells were originating from the vessel walls.[95] The relationship of hemangiopericytoma to normal pericytes, however, has never been confirmed.[97, 98] In particular, questions exist regarding the diagnostic specificity of the histologic pattern.[98] It has been shown repeatedly that these same histologic features may be ob-

served in a diversity of neoplasms, including a variety of sarcomas.[98] Hemangiopericytomas must therefore be distinguished from other neoplasms by immunohistochemical and ultrastructural analysis. Immunohistochemically, hemangiopericytoma is defined by its reactivity with vimentin, with or without CD57 and CD34, and its negativity with antigens is associated with epithelial, neural, and myogenic differentiation.[98] Ultrastructurally, hemangiopericytomas show the presence of a well-formed basement membrane around tumor cells and the presence of myogenic-type intermediate filaments, features considered typical although not completely specific.[99]

The splenic hemangiopericytoma reported by Neill and Park[97] occurred in a 44-year-old woman as an incidental finding. No follow-up information is provided in the report. The lesion was a solitary well-circumscribed nodule with light microscopic and ultrastructural features typical of hemangiopericytoma. The reactivity with desmin in this case, which is not seen in hemangiopericytomas,[98] was interpreted by the authors as indicative of a possible derivation from red pulp stromal myoid cells. These cells, a specialized subset of splenic reticular cells,[100] contain smooth-muscle antigens. In the red pulp, stromal myoid cells express only desmin, an intermediate filament also expressed by pericytes in various organs.

A second case, reported by Jurado et al,[96] is much less well characterized and could represent an angiosarcoma. The lesion occurred in a symptomatic 38-year-old with a large spleen weighing 2300 g and containing numerous large necrotic and hemorrhagic tumor nodules. Follow-up at 6 months showed evidence of generalized metastatic disease. In this case the typical histologic features seen in hemangiopericytoma are not identifiable in Jurado's figures, and there are no immunohistochemical and ultrastructural studies of the lesion.

Nonvascular Tumors

Nonvascular mesenchymal tumors of the spleen are rare. Easler and Dowlin[101] reported a primary splenic lipoma composed of mature adipocytes, which was not associated with hematologic abnormalities. Angiomyolipoma is an uncommon hamartomatous lesion of the kidney that can be seen as a component of the tuberous sclerosis complex.[92] In one case, splenic involvement was also reported.[102] In spite of the extrarenal involvement, the behavior of this tumor was benign. The consensus in the literature suggests that this nonaggressive behavior is a manifestation of multicentricity rather than of metastasis.[102–106] The lesion is characterized by an irregular proliferation of smooth muscle, adipose cells, and vascular channels with thickened walls. The smooth muscle cells may focally exhibit epithelioid features and considerable nuclear pleomorphism. The cells express smooth muscle antigens as well as the melanoma-associated antigen HMB-45.[91] There have also been occasional case reports of splenic fibromas.[54] Rare cases of primary splenic leiomyoma have been reported. These have occurred in immunodeficient patients. One was observed in a child with ataxia telangiectasia, a genetic disease predisposing to cancer,[107] and another occurred in a patient after kidney transplant.[108] Smooth muscle tumors have also been reported with increased frequency in patients, especially children, with AIDS.[109–115] In one case, a child presented with abdominal leiomyomas and a peculiar calcification of the intima of intrasplenic arteries.[115] Epstein-Barr virus has recently been implicated in the pathogenesis of smooth muscle tumors such as these, which occur in transplant and AIDS patients.[116, 117] Morel et al[108] reported one case of a post-transplant splenic leiomyoma in which the presence of Epstein-Barr virus transcripts in the nuclei of the tumor cells was identified by in situ hybridization.

Grossly, splenic leiomyomas are well-circumscribed nodules with a whitish whorled surface and no evidence of necrosis. Histologically, the lesions consist of a spindle-cell proliferation of relative cellular density arranged in fascicles with absence of mitosis. The nuclei are cigar-shaped with round or blunt extremities.[107, 108] Smooth muscle cell tumors must be distinguished from other conditions that may also occur in the spleens of immunocompromised patients: mycobacterial spindle cell pseudotumor and Kaposi sarcoma. In addition, inflammatory pseudotumors may enter the differential diagnosis because of their prominent spindle cell component.

MALIGNANT MESENCHYMAL TUMORS

Early reports of mesenchymal tumors of the spleen are difficult to interpret because of the use of confusing or outdated terminology. Part of the confusion in terminology resulted from controversy concerning the origin of these tumors. Smith and Rusk[71] divided all splenic tumors into derivatives of the capsule and trabeculae, lymphoid elements, or vascular elements. Rousselot and Stein[118] classified two types of nonhematopoietic splenic tumors into two groups: those arising from connective tissue elements (spindle cell sarcomas and fibrosarcoma) and those arising from the sinus endothelium (endotheliomas and angiosarcomas). Weichselbaum[119] distinguished three types of splenic sarcomas based on morphologic features: spindle cell, endothelial cell, and lymphosarcoma. It is now known that the majority of primary sarcomas of the spleen are of vascular origin.[50]

Vascular Sarcomas

Hemangioendotheliomas

The term "hemangioendothelioma" has been used historically to define a vascular tumor distinct from hemangiosarcoma and intermediate in cytologic and clinical characteristics between hemangioma and hemangiosarcoma. Hemangioendothelioma is characterized by vascular lesions demonstrating well-formed vascular channels, mild atypia, absence of necrosis, a low mitotic rate, and borderline malignant potential. We believe that most cases of hemangioendotheliomas are examples of well-differentiated splenic angiosarcoma and that the term "hemangioendothelioma" should not be used to define these lesions. However, certain variants of hemangioendothelioma, such as epithelioid,[120–122] spindle cell,[123–125] and endovascular papillary angioendothelioma (Dabska tumor),[126–128] are now generally accepted as specific pathologic entities that should be distinguished from angiosarcoma. Epithelioid hemangioendothelioma includes lesions previously termed "histiocytoid hemangiomas."[129] It is a tumor composed of endothelial cells with ample eosinophilic cytoplasm that resemble histiocytes. Most cases arise in superficial or deep soft tissue, but similar tumors have been described in the lungs, liver, and bone.[120, 121, 130] They rarely occur in children.[118, 130] Although most lesions behave in a benign fashion, as many as a third eventually metastasize.[121] Spindle cell hemangioendothelioma[123–125] is a rare tumor known to occur at all ages; most cases have, however, been reported in young adults.[121] The tumor is restricted to the soft tissue of distal extremities, particularly the hands.[123–125] We are unaware of any cases involving the spleen.

True hemangioendotheliomas of the spleen are very rare. However, several cases have been reported. Kaw et al[131] described a hemangioendothelioma in the spleen of a 48-year-old man. The tumor was a well-circumscribed 7-cm lesion that was divided into lobules of variable size by intersecting dense fibrous bands. Some of the lobules contained vascular spaces lined by atypical large, plump, spindle-shaped cells with hyperchromatic nuclei. There was a proliferation of spindle stromal cells with eosinophilic cytoplasm between the vascular spaces. There was no necrosis, and mitotic figures were rare. Suster[132] reported a well-circumscribed 4.5-cm splenic lesion in a 3-year-old boy. The tumor was characterized histologically by a biphasic growth pattern with nodular areas composed of epithelioid endothelial cells and areas showing a proliferation of vascular channels lined by elongated spindle cells. Due to the lack of mitoses, infiltrative margins, or necrosis, the lesion was not considered to be an angiosarcoma but a previously undescribed type of splenic vascular tumor; it was termed "epithelioid and spindle-cell

splenic hemangioendothelioma." These two cases of splenic hemangioendothelioma did not metastasize, and both patients remained well after surgery. Two other cases of epithelioid hemangioendothelioma have been reported in which synchronous metastatic involvement was present at laparotomy. The first[133] occurred in a 29-year-old woman. The splenic lesion was associated with intrasplenic as well as liver metastasis. No follow-up information was provided. The second case, reported by our group,[134] was observed in a 9-year-old girl with a history of acute lymphoblastic leukemia, who presented with a multinodular lesion diffusely involving the spleen. An accessory spleen, two regional lymph nodes and the liver were also involved. In spite of the multiple organ involvement, the splenic lesion showed little cellular atypia, rare mitoses, and absence of necrosis. The patient has not received any therapy and is alive with no evidence of disease after more than 4 years.

Katz et al[135] reported a case of endovascular papillary angioendothelioma of the spleen in a 5-year-old boy. The spleen weighed 346 g and contained multiple well-circumscribed brown nodules. Histologically, the lesion was composed of cystic vascular spaces into which papillary projections lined by plump endothelial cells protruded. Factor VIII and Ulex europaeus antigens were detected in the endothelial cell tufts as well as in the flattened endothelial cells lining the cyst walls. No evidence of tumor outside the spleen was found in this patient.

From these data it appears that splenic hemangioendothelioma is a rare vascular tumor occupying an intermediate position, in terms of histology and clinical behavior, between hemangioma and angiosarcoma. It can be distinguished from the latter mainly by the absence of dissecting growth, lack of significant cellular atypia, low-to-absent mitotic activity, and absence of necrosis. No metastatic spread has been reported in the cases characterized by well-circumscribed lesions.[131, 132] In our case,[134] the benign clinical course in spite of the occurrence of the lesion in multiple extrasplenic sites may suggest multifocality and not metastasis, as is the case with infantile hemangioendothelioma of the liver, a pediatric vascular tumor that is typically locally aggressive but devoid of significant metastatic potential.[136, 137]

Angiosarcomas

True angiosarcomas of the spleen are uncommon (Color Plate 28). Slightly more than

100 cases have been reported since the first description by Langhans in 1879.[54, 138-144] A variety of terms have been used in the literature, such as "angioblastoma," "hemangiosarcoma," "malignant hemangioendothelioma," and "endothelial sarcoma." Most of the cases are single-case reports in which stringent morphologic criteria were not employed. Angiosarcoma is usually a disease of older individuals, with a peak incidence in the 6th decade of life,[140, 142] although it can affect a wide age range, including children.[144] There is no gender predominance.[140-142]

Although angiosarcoma of the liver has been associated with previous exposure to thorium dioxide (Thorotrast),[145, 146] vinyl chloride,[147, 148] or arsenic,[149] these associations have not been documented with splenic angiosarcoma. However, sporadic splenic cases have been associated with previous chemotherapy for malignant lymphoma[142, 150] or radiotherapy for breast cancer.[151] The Kaposi sarcoma–associated herpes virus (KSHV), or human herpes virus 8 (HHV8),[152] has been identified by molecular analysis in biopsy specimens with angiolymphoid hyperplasia[153] and angiosarcomas in immunocompromised patients.[154-156]

The majority of patients with splenic angiosarcomas present with splenomegaly and with abdominal pain, most frequently localized to the upper left quadrant. Fatigue, fever, and weight loss also commonly occur.[140, 142] Abnormal laboratory findings include normochromic/normocytic anemia, thrombocyto-penia and, less commonly, pancytopenia.[139, 142] Rare cases present with leukocytosis and thrombocytosis.[142] Occasionally patients may present with a microangiopathic hemolytic anemia and/or coagulation abnormalities.[6, 157] Hemolytic anemia is most likely secondary to erythrocyte damage by irregularly lined vascular channels in the tumor.[155, 158]

Splenic weights in cases of angiosarcoma may range widely, with many being over 1000 g. Grossly, splenic angiosarcomas appear as poorly delimited nodular masses blending imperceptibly with the remaining red pulp, or they may involve the spleen diffusely.[53, 143] Large areas of hemorrhage and necrosis are typical (Fig. 15–16). The microscopic appearance is often quite variable. The degree of differentiation may vary significantly within the same tumor.[92, 142] Some areas consist of well-formed vascular channels lined by plump endothelial cells with rare mitoses and little nuclear atypia (Fig. 15–17). Even in these well-differentiated cases, however, significant nuclear pleomorphism is at least focally present. Proliferation of the endothelial cells may result in a papillary appearance (Fig. 15–18). Anastomosing vascular channels are often noted. Other areas may be solid, resembling an undifferentiated spindle cell sarcoma (Fig. 15–19). Tumor cells may be quite pleomorphic, with better differentiated tumors showing coffee bean–shaped nuclei and scant cytoplasm, typical of endothelial cells; others display spindled, polygonal, epithelioid, or

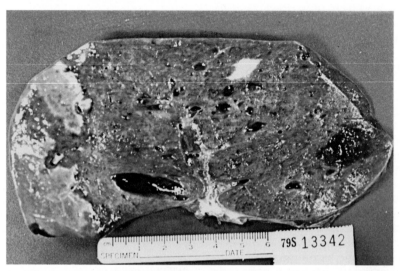

Figure 15–16. Angiosarcoma of the spleen. Virtually the entire organ is involved. There is fresh hemorrhage at the right pole of the specimen and an old organized infarct at the upper right. The left end of the specimen shows a recent infarct.

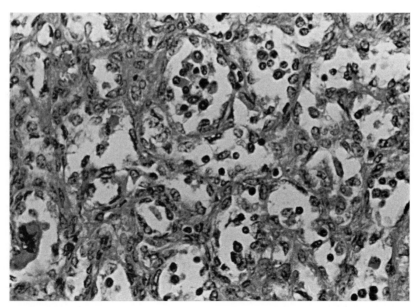

Figure 15–17. The microscopic appearance of some hemangiosarcomas may be deceptively bland. In this photomicrograph the vascular channels appear well-formed, and the endothelial cells display little nuclear atypia or evidence of mitotic activity. Such examples of low-grade hemangiosarcoma were once termed "hemangioendothelioma." Note the clusters of normoblasts.

primitive round cell morphologic features. The reticulin stain may be useful in delineating small vascular spaces hidden within the solid areas. In some cases the pattern may be subtle, resembling the appearance of some hepatic angiosarcomas, with architecture of the sinuses apparently intact although lined by atypical endothelial cells (Fig. 15–20). The tumors frequently contain foci of extramedullary hematopoiesis (see Fig. 15–17). In some

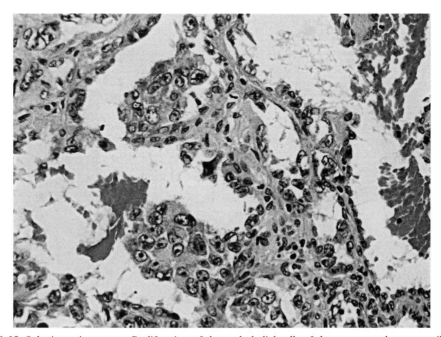

Figure 15–18. Splenic angiosarcoma. Proliferation of the endothelial cells of the tumor produces a papillary appearance.

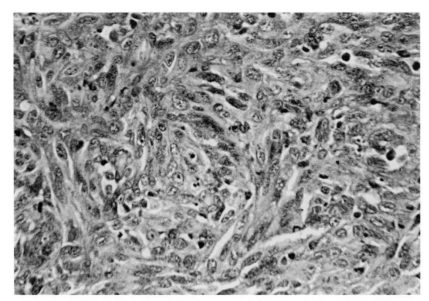

Figure 15–19. Example of splenic hemangiosarcoma resembling an undifferentiated spindle cell tumor.

cases, erythrophagocytosis by the neoplastic cells has been observed. Immunoperoxidase techniques using an antibody for factor VIII–related antigen, which is normally present in endothelial cells, is generally used to confirm the vascular origin of an angiosarcoma.[159] However, this antigen is more likely to be expressed in well-differentiated tumors, and the absence of staining in sarcomatous areas does not rule out a vascular origin.[160] CD31 is a highly specific and sensitive marker that can be used to confirm the endothelial nature of poorly differentiated tumors.[161–163] Ulex europaeus lectin type I, although a sensitive marker,[161, 162] is not very specific. CD34 is positive only in well-differentiated cases.[161, 162] An-

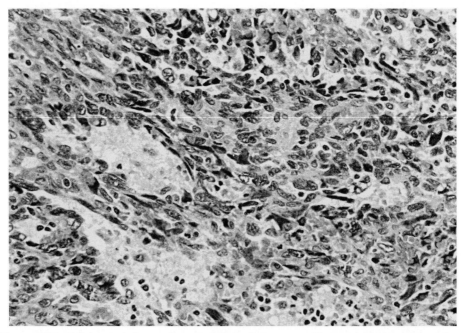

Figure 15–20. Cellular atypia in vascular endothelial cells in a case of hemangiosarcoma of the spleen.

giosarcomas express cytokeratin rarely.[73, 163] HMB-45[163] and S-100[142] are generally reported as negative. The expression of CD68[142] and other histiocytic markers (as well as CD8 reactivity[78, 79]) that are occasionally observed suggest that some angiosarcomas may be of sinus endothelial cell (littoral cell) derivation.

Angiosarcomas can be distinguished from benign vascular tumors by the presence of cellular atypia, nuclear pleomorphism, mitoses, necrosis, anastomosing vascular channels, and frequent solid areas.[91] These histologic findings can also help in distinguishing angiosarcomas from hemangioendotheliomas and littoral cell angiomas. In the past, several cases of this latter benign lesion were mistaken for angiosarcomas of the spleen. In immunodeficient patients, splenic involvement by Kaposi sarcoma may closely simulate angiosarcoma because both may exhibit spindle cell differentiation, little cytologic atypia in endothelial cells, iron deposits, and hyalin globules.[142] However, Kaposi sarcoma usually presents as multiple small foci, often with sclerosis and without associated hemorrhage or necrosis. This presentation is in contrast to that of splenic angiosarcoma, which characteristically shows massive involvement, extensive hemorrhage and necrosis, and lacks significant sclerosis. Hemangiosarcoma must also be distinguished from splenic bacillary angiomatosis,[91] a reactive vasoproliferative lesion in immunodepressed patients. Grossly, bacillary angiomatosis is composed of fleshy whitish nodules lacking the hemorrhagic quality of angiosarcoma. Distinctive features in bacillary angiomatosis include abundant interstitial material that, on Warthin-Starry stain, proves to be aggregated bacilli; numerous neutrophils; and the absence of anastomosing vascular channels.[91] Poorly differentiated angiosarcoma with a predominantly spindle cell component may resemble malignant fibrous histiocytoma or fibrosarcoma. However, the presence of an unequivocal vasoformative component is indicative of angiosarcoma.[142] Its identification can be greatly helped by the detection of endothelial antigens such as factor VIII and CD31.

Ultrastructural examination can also be useful in confirming the diagnosis of angiosarcoma in selected cases, for electron microscopy has confirmed the endothelial origin of splenic angiosarcoma. Chen and associates[139] reported ultrastructural findings consistent with a blood vessel origin, including partial basement membranes, pinocytotic vesicles,

and intercellular junctions. Silverman and colleagues[143] reported the ultrastructural findings in a case that they termed "malignant hemangioendothelioma." These authors found evidence for two tumor cell types. The more well-formed vascular spaces were lined by cells with features of endothelial cells, whereas in the more solid areas the tumor cells had irregular cytoplasmic processes. Weibel-Palade bodies, found in normal endothelial cells and in some vascular tumors, have only rarely been observed in splenic angiosarcomas.

Rappaport[53] postulated that angiosarcomas did not derive from sinus lining cells, which he believed were modified histiocytes rather than true endothelial cells. He suggested that these tumors arose from preexisting hemangiomas, from endothelium of splenic veins, or from primitive pluripotential mesenchymal cells. On the basis of our examination of a number of splenic angiosarcomas in which we have noted in situ cytologic atypia of sinus lining cells, we believe that at least some angiosarcomas arise from these cells. Two cases of splenic angiosarcoma showing histochemical and immunohistochemical evidence of splenic sinus endothelial cell (littoral cell) derivation have been reported, in support of our contention.[78, 80]

The prognosis of splenic angiosarcoma is poor.[142] Metastases are usually hematogenous, most often to liver and lung,[138, 142, 151] although Autrey and Weitzner[138] reported lymph node metastases in 13 of 50 previously reported cases. Metastases occur early in the course of the disease, and survival is usually less than 1 year. In a recent series, 79 percent of the patients were dead 6 months after diagnosis.[142] Pathologic rupture is a known ominous complication of splenic angiosarcomas that is not related to patient age, hematologic profile, or size of the tumor.[138, 164] Several investigators have reported a better prognosis in cases in which splenectomy is performed before rupture.[138, 165] Splenectomy is the treatment of choice; the benefit of irradiation and chemotherapy remains to be demonstrated.[141, 166] A partial response in an advanced case with metastatic liver involvement was obtained by the combination of splenic artery embolization and intravenous chemotherapy.[167]

Kaposi Sarcoma

Kaposi sarcoma (KS) is a vascular tumor that may occur in a variety of clinical settings.[92, 168]

The classic form occurs mostly in elderly men of Mediterranean or eastern European (especially Ashkenazic) descent,[169] but it is uncommon in the United States. Clinically, KS consists of multiple skin plaques or nodules in the lower extremities and has an indolent course for 10 to 15 years. Systemic lesions may eventually develop in various organs, including lymph nodes.[92] One third of the patients with KS present with or subsequently develop a second malignancy, most often a lymphoproliferative disorder.[170] Another type of KS, the so-called African or endemic type, occurs in young male adults in equatorial Africa and presents with cutaneous and regional lymph node involvement. Clinically quiescent visceral lesions may be observed.[92] KS is also known to occur in organ transplant recipients on immunosuppressive therapy[171, 172] and, less frequently, in patients receiving immunosuppressive therapy for malignancies and autoimmune disorders.[92, 171, 173] The lesions may be localized or widespread with systemic involvement but often regress when immunosuppressive therapy is discontinued.

In contrast, epidemic KS, a subtype in approximately one third of AIDS patients, especially homosexual men,[92, 174] is generally highly aggressive, with widespread organ involvement and a fulminant course with less than 20 percent survival at 2 years if associated with opportunistic infections.[92] At autopsy, KS is reported to occur in 23 to 94 percent of patients with AIDS.[175–178] The incidence of splenic involvement in patients with disseminated KS varies from 12.5 to 73 percent in different series.[175–178] Although solitary splenic involvement by KS has not been reported, Sarode et al[179] reported a case of KS in an immunocompetent 40-year-old woman that presented as a single 5-cm splenic mass. The patient was later found to have disseminated intra-abdominal and pleural involvement without cutaneous lesions. The authors postulated that the spleen represented the primary site of disease in this patient. This type of clinical presentation must be considered truly exceptional for KS.

Involvement of the spleen by KS manifests either as multiple dark nodules or as a diffusely infiltrative process without a mass effect.[175, 176, 178] The involvement is mainly in the fibrous trabeculae and around small arteries in the white pulp (Fig. 15–21).[92, 175, 176] The lesions show ill-defined margins and freely invade into the surrounding red pulp.[177] Well-developed lesions are characterized by curved fascicles of spindle cells with intertwined short slits containing extravasated red blood cells. Nuclear pleomorphism in both spindle and endothelial cells is slight, and the mitotic count is low (Fig. 15–22). Distinctive cytoplasmic eosinophilic hyaline globules that can be detected using periodic acid–Schiff stain occur in most KS cases. Extensively fibrotic lesions with abundant hemosiderin deposition are frequently observed in involved spleens.[175, 176] Such cases with a predominant fibrotic pattern have been termed "sclerosing KS."[175] An association between KS and splenic infarcts has also been reported.[175]

Immunohistochemically, the spindle cells of Kaposi sarcoma stain strongly with CD31 and CD34, show inconsistent staining with factor VIII–related antigen and Ulex europaeus lectin, and do not stain for actin.[92] Although the precise histogenesis of KS is still controversial, recent immunohistochemical studies have provided evidence for a vascular endothelial cell origin.[180, 181] Sequences of a new herpes virus were recently isolated from a KS lesion in an HIV-positive individual by Chang et al.[152] This virus, known as KSHV or HHV8, has been identified in more than 95 percent of HIV-associated, classic, African, and transplant-related KS.[182] In situ polymerase chain reaction studies have demonstrated KSHV in the spindle cells and endothelial cells of KS lesions, suggesting that this virus may be directly involved in the pathogenesis of the tumor.[183]

Lymphangiosarcomas

Well-documented cases of lymphangiosarcomas of the spleen are rare.[93, 94, 184, 185] Gordon and Paley,[185] in a review of the literature in 1951, found 42 cases of lymphangiosarcomas. There have been only a few cases reported since. Hamoudi and associates[93] reported a tumor in a 13-year-old girl; they termed the tumor "malignant lymphangioendothelioma." It weighed 850 g, was multinodular, and was composed of cystic spaces containing watery pink fluid with rare erythrocytes. The endothelial cells lining the cyst were flattened but proliferated focally to form solid intraluminal masses. Large cystic spaces alternated with more sarcomatous areas. The nuclei were variably pleomorphic and hypochromatic, and occasional mitotic figures were found. Feigenberg et al[94] reported a case of primary malignant lymphangioma of the spleen in a 66-year-old man. The spleen weighed 3640 g. The

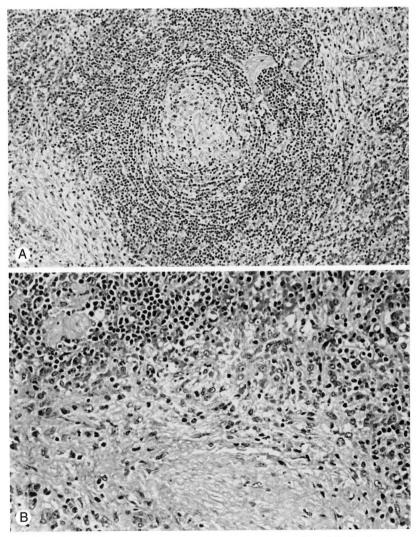

Figure 15–21. Kaposi sarcoma involving the spleen. The lesions appear preferentially in the areas surrounding the white pulp (A) and also occur contiguous to trabecular structures (B).

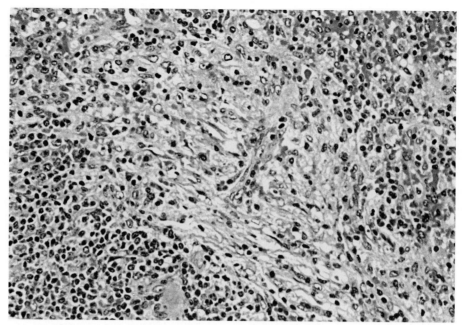

Figure 15–22. Kaposi sarcoma of the spleen. The lesions display typical spindle cells with erythrocytes occurring in vascular slits.

splenic parenchyma was almost totally replaced by cystic spaces of various sizes containing a homogeneous eosinophilic fluid, interspersed with solid areas composed of proliferating endothelial cells. In these solid areas the endothelial cells showed nuclear pleomorphism with nucleoli and numerous mitosis. The patient, who did not receive any systemic therapy, was reported to be disease-free at a 12-month follow-up.

OTHER PRIMARY MALIGNANT TUMORS

Malignant Fibrous and Fibrohistiocytic Tumors

Primary nonvascular sarcomas of the spleen are exceedingly uncommon. Rare splenic fibrosarcomas have been reported, probably arising from the capsule or fibrous trabeculae. Because malignant fibrous histiocytoma was not distinguished pathologically from fibrosarcoma until recently, it is likely that some previous reports of fibrosarcoma of the spleen may represent examples of malignant fibrous histiocytoma.[140] Five cases of primary splenic malignant fibrous histiocytoma have been reported,[140, 186–188] and we have seen a single additional case. The patients are usually middle-aged and present with splenomegaly that is

often massive.[140] Abdominal pain, weight loss, fever, and anemia are also frequently reported clinical findings.[92] The tumor is aggressive; both peritoneal recurrences and distant metastases have been reported.[140, 187, 188] In the series reported by Wick et al,[140] the tumors ranged in size from 8.0 to 27 cm. As in the case we have studied, they were lobulated and yellow-tan, with foci of cavitary necrosis. Histologically, these tumors are variable. Most are composed of spindle cells in a storiform pattern with numerous mitotic figures. However, myxoid and giant cell types also occur (Fig. 15–23). Inflammation in the form of necrosis with numerous polymorphonuclear leukocytes, histiocytes, and xanthoma cells is common. Malignant fibrous histiocytoma is characterized immunohistochemically by vimentin positivity but may also be desmin- or cytokeratin-immunoreactive as well. [189] Electron microscopy reveals fibroblastic and histiocytic cells as well as intermediate forms of both types.[140] A single case of rhabdomyosarcoma of the spleen has been reported.[190] The occurrence of leiomyosarcoma in the human spleen has also been suggested but not well documented.[191]

PRIMARY EPITHELIAL MALIGNANCIES

Primary malignant epithelial neoplasms of the spleen are extremely rare.[140] Nearly all

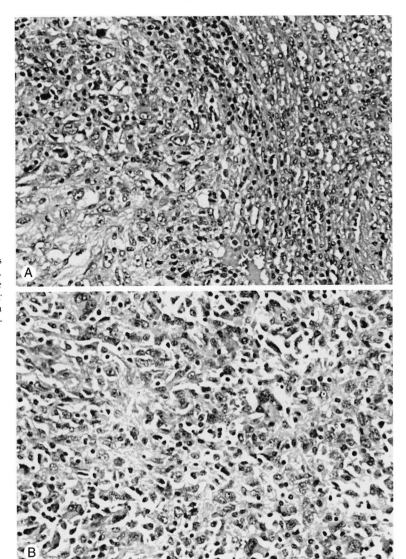

Figure 15–23. Malignant fibrous histiocytoma involving the spleen. (A) The tumor extends into the red pulp. Histologically, the tumor is composed of spindle cells with a myxoid component. (B) Numerous giant cells are also present.

cases of primary carcinoma of the spleen were reported in the medical literature before 1923, when precise morphologic criteria and reliable ancillary techniques to distinguish between uncommon malignant neoplasms were not available. We agree with Bostick[54] that these so-called primary splenic epithelial tumors were probably all sarcomas, erroneously diagnosed as primary carcinoma. It is likely that the majority of these tumors were examples of poorly differentiated angiosarcoma. However, during the last decade two well-documented cases of primary splenic carcinoma have been described. Elit and Aylward[192] reported a case of squamous cell carcinoma arising from an epithelial cyst (true cyst) of the spleen in a

pregnant woman, and Morinaga et al[193] described a case of splenic low-grade mucinous cystadenocarcinoma in a 69-year-old man. Surface mesothelium has been proposed as the histogenetic origin of these epithelial malignancies.[192, 193] Invagination of surface mesothelial cells with subsequent squamous metaplasia may represent the pathogenetic mechanism in the formation of an epithelial cyst.[33, 34] Its malignant transformation into a splenic squamous cell carcinoma would explain the case reported by Elit and Aylward.[192] The metaplastic capacity of the peritoneal mesothelium as well as the occasional presence of focal or complete mucinous cell metaplasia within true splenic cysts suggests that a similar pathogenetic mechanism may also apply to the case of Morinaga et al.[193]

A case of carcinosarcoma of the spleen was reported by Westra et al[194] in a 55-year-old woman. In this case, the authors suggested a derivation from entrapped mesothelium that underwent müllerian differentiation as a pathogenetic mechanism. A case of malignant splenic teratoma was reported by Daftary and Barnett[195] in a 69-year-old woman. Abnormal migration of the spleen and the left ovary during gestation were thought to result in abnormal connections between the two organs.[196, 197] A possible origin from the gonadal element of a splenic-gonadal fusion was therefore postulated in this case.[195] However, because no anatomic continuity between the spleen and ovary was observed, it is conceivable that this case may represent a malignant transformation of a true dermoid cyst.[198] Heterotopic displacement of an embryonal rest has also been suggested as an alternative cause of splenic teratoma.[194]

A case of adenocarcinoma arising in the spleen from heterotopic pancreatic tissue has been reported.[200] In a large series of cases of pancreatic tissue heterotopia, Barbosa et al[201] found that the spleen was involved in 1 percent of cases. Heterotopic pancreatic tissue is believed to be at greater risk of neoplastic transformation than its normally located counterpart.[201] Among the various neoplasms known to arise in these heterotopic foci, pancreatic adenocarcinoma and islet cell tumors are by far the commonest.[194] These rare cases must be differentiated from neoplasms of the tail of the pancreas involving the splenic hilum and adjacent splenic parenchyma, which can be clinically mistaken for primary splenic tumors.[202] Invasion of the spleen by other tumors arising in the vicinity (such as stomach, kidney, and adrenal gland) has also been reported[92] and also must not be mistakenly considered to be primary in the spleen.

METASTATIC TUMORS

Although epithelial tumors may invade the spleen from contiguous viscera, true tumor metastases to the spleen are relatively uncommon and usually occur only in patients with disseminated tumors (Color Plate 29).[190] Several theories have been proposed to explain the relative scarcity of splenic metastases.[203] Early investigators postulated that the spleen

might produce antineoplastic factors that inhibited tumor growth.[204, 205] However, there has been no clear-cut evidence indicating any factor within the spleen that would make the spleen an unsuitable environment for tumor growth. Others have suggested that contractions of the organ might dislodge tumor cells, preventing their implantation.[206-208] However, in contrast to some animal species, the human splenic capsule does not contain smooth muscle, and the spleen does not undergo contractions.[209] Another theory suggested that the anatomy of the splenic vascular system, possibly the sharp angle made by the splenic artery leaving the celiac axis, might play a role in limiting tumor metastasis.[210] However, the most reasonable and widely held theory attempting to explain the relative rarity of splenic metastatic disease is that the spleen lacks afferent lymphatic vessels.[210, 211] Tumor metastasis to the spleen would therefore have to occur through hematogenous dissemination.[207, 208, 212] The frequency of splenic metastasis detected at autopsy in patients with cancer is indeed comparable to that of the kidney and brain, both of which are organs involved typically by blood-borne metastasis.[212, 213]

The majority of tumors metastatic to the spleen are carcinomas. Marymount and Gross[203] reported one case each of neuroblastoma, mediastinal teratoma, and "meningeal sarcoma," and we have seen two cases of metastasis of choriocarcinoma to the spleen, confirmed by the presence of human chorionic gonadotropin in the tumor cells (Fig. 15–24). We are unaware of any soft tissue sarcomas that have been reported metastatic to the spleen. The incidence of metastases of epithelial tumors at autopsy is stated to vary from 16 to 30 percent.[214] Several large series have indicated that carcinomas of the lung, breast, melanoma, and ovary have the highest incidence of splenic metastases.[215-221] Warren and Davis,[210] in their autopsy review of 1140 cases of carcinoma excluding malignant melanoma, found splenic metastases in 42 cases (3.7 percent). Fifteen percent of breast carcinomas and 23 percent of lung carcinomas involved the spleen in their series. In all cases, the tumors were disseminated, with metastases to three or more organs other than the spleen and lymph nodes. Other investigators substantiated the observation that splenic metastases occur only late in the course of a disease when tumors are widely disseminated.[212] However, Klein and colleagues[214] reported four cases

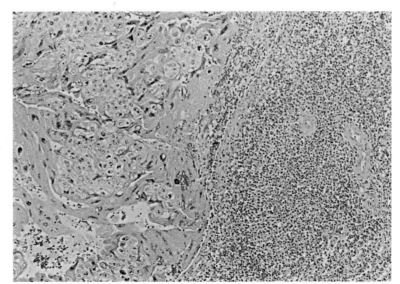

Figure 15–24. Choriocarcinoma metastatic to the spleen.

with solitary spleen metastasis, in all of which splenectomy resulted in survival of at least 1 year. Although uncommon, splenomegaly resulting from metastatic involvement may be the first manifestation of recurrent carcinoma, a phenomenon more frequently observed with gynecologic malignancies.[214, 222–224] On rare occasions, splenic metastasis is detected simultaneously with the primary carcinoma.[225, 226] In one case, the spleen was the sole site of distant metastasis from a primary lung adenocarcinoma.[225] In another, metastatic adenocarcinoma compatible with prostatic origin was reported in which the spleen was both the presenting finding and the sole site of metastasis.[227]

In recent years ultrasound examination of the spleen and ultrasound-guided fine-needle aspiration biopsy has been successfully used for detection and histological confirmation of splenic metastatic involvement.[228–230] Although palpable splenomegaly may result from metastatic disease, hypersplenism is rare.[231] Spontaneous rupture of the spleen secondary to metastatic involvement has been observed as a rare complication in patients with carcinoma,[232–237] melanoma,[238–241] and teratoma.[242] Refractory thrombocytopenia may be another complication.[243] In a review of 93 cases of tumors with splenic metastasis, Marymount and Gross[203] found that 67 percent were evident grossly, and tumor metastases were found only on histologic examination in 33 percent of cases. The majority of spleens with only microscopic metastases weighed less than 200 g, and

the average weight of those with grossly evident metastases was 235 g. Most metastatic tumors form solitary or multiple nodules in the spleen (Fig. 15–25 and Color Plate 29), although occasionally the involvement is miliary (Fig. 15–26). We have seen two cases of metastatic carcinoma to the spleen, one breast adenocarcinoma and one small cell carcinoma of the lung, which resulted in homogeneous enlargement secondary to diffuse neoplastic infiltration of the red pulp (Fig. 15–27). Cummings and Mazur[243] have recently reported two patients with breast carcinoma metastatic to the spleen that showed a similar diffuse pattern.

Rarely, metastatic involvement is confined to the trabecular lymphatic vessels. Goldberg[244] reported two such cases in which he demonstrated tumor cells within the adventitial trabecular veins and in the lymphatics surrounding follicular arteries. This phenomenon has been interpreted as retrograde permeation of splenic lymphatics, usually from tumor deposits in the splenic hilum.[244] In exceptional circumstances, carcinomatous infiltration in the spleen can cause a nodular transformation of the splenic red pulp, simulating a lymphoma.[245]

TUMORLIKE LESIONS

Hamartomas

Splenic hamartoma (splenoma) is a tumorlike lesion composed of structurally disor-

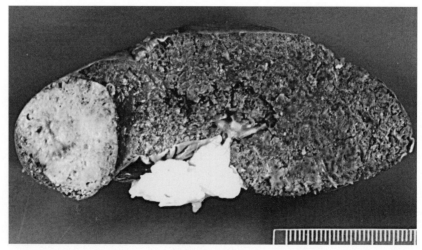

Figure 15–25. Metastatic carcinoma. Metastatic epithelial tumors most frequently cause single or a few grossly visible nodules.

ganized, mature splenic red pulp elements. Splenic hamartomas are usually noted incidentally either at autopsy or in spleens removed for unrelated causes.[58, 190, 246–248] They are most commonly found in adults but may occur in spleens of patients of younger ages. There is no apparent gender predilection. The majority of patients with splenic hamartomas are asymptomatic. However, larger lesions may result in symptoms related to an abdominal mass[249–251] and may be associated with cytopenias due to sequestration of hematopoietic cells, particularly platelets, within the substance of the hamartoma.[246, 252–254] The cytopenias in these cases usually reverse following

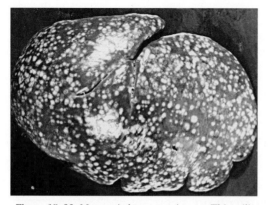

Figure 15–26. Metastatic breast carcinoma. This miliary pattern of involvement by metastatic carcinoma is unusual and mimics malignant lymphoma. However, examination of a cross section of the spleen in cases such as this demonstrates that the lesions are not necessarily associated with the white pulp, as are malignant lymphomas.

splenectomy.[253–255] Splenic rupture has been reported in rare cases.[256, 257]

Splenic hamartomas are well-circumscribed, bulging nodules that compress the surrounding splenic parenchyma (Color Plate 30). They vary from less than 1.0 cm in diameter to large lesions weighing up to 2 kg.[252] The majority of hamartomas are solitary, although multiple hamartomas have been reported.[190, 258–260] Microscopically, they appear less obviously demarcated than they seem grossly, for they do not have true capsules. The nodule is surrounded by a rim of compressed red pulp usually without associated fibrosis (Fig. 15–28), a phenomenon best demonstrated by reticulin stains. Histologically, hamartomas resemble normal red pulp, with slitlike vascular spaces that are lined by plump endothelial cells containing erythrocytes (Fig. 15–29).[246] Normal white pulp is usually absent, with trabecular structures devoid of normal lymphoid cuffs (Fig. 15–30). These features may make hamartomas difficult to distinguish from hemangiomas. However, hamartomas can be recognized by the presence of two elements: sinuslike structures mixed with pulp cord–like elements. The endothelial lining cells of hamartomas show immunohistochemical evidence of sinus-type derivation (e.g., CD8 expression), whereas capillary hemangiomas do not.[62] Sclerosing hemangiomas can be distinguished by their prominent fibrosis, a feature not observed in hamartomas. Hamartomas may contain areas of hemorrhage and infarction with hemosiderin deposition, hyalinization, or cal-

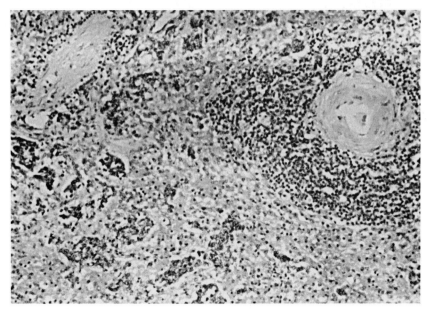

Figure 15–27. Metastatic undifferentiated carcinoma, small-cell type. The tumor infiltrates the sinuses of the red pulp, sparing the white pulp.

cification.[261] Normal splenic trabeculae and white pulp are usually absent in hamartomas, but lymphoid cells are usually present either in the form of scattered lymphocytes or small aggregates of lymphoid cells. The reticulin framework is disorganized, and the annular fibers typical of normal red pulp may be ab-

sent. The hamartoma and/or surrounding normal spleen may contain immature hematopoietic cells and eosinophils.[261]

The origin of splenic hamartomas is controversial. Although considered by most authors to represent a focal developmental disturbance, others have referred to these lesions as

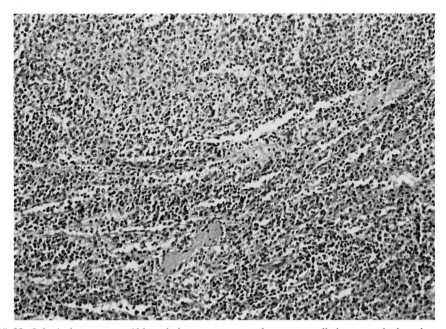

Figure 15–28. Splenic hamartoma. Although hamartomas grossly appear well demarcated, they do not contain a capsule and only display a compressed rim of tissue separating them from the normal spleen.

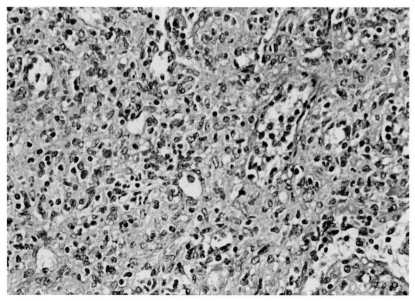

Figure 15–29. Splenic hamartoma. Cords and sinuses are evident. The amorphous material in the cords is composed largely of trapped platelets.

benign neoplasms (splenomas) and grouped them with hemangiomas.[6, 59, 258] In fact, some hamartomas with a distinctive lobular pattern and immunohistochemical reactivity have been reclassified as red pulp capillary hemangiomas.[262] Other hypotheses are that hamartomas are congenital anomalies[58] or, less likely, the result of trauma.[248] Splenic hamartomas have been reported in patients with tuberous sclerosis.[263, 264] This association provides additional support to the hypothesis of the hamartomatous nature of this splenic lesion. An association of splenic hamartomas with neoplastic hematologic diseases has been suggested.[259, 265] Diebold and Audouin[266] reported multiple splenic hamartomas, peliosis, and sea-

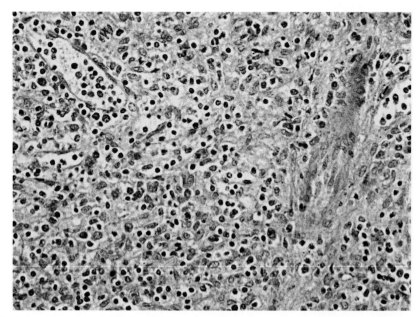

Figure 15–30. Splenic hamartoma. The lymphoid tissue normally associated with the trabecular structures is absent.

blue histiocytosis in two patients with idiopathic thrombocytopenia purpura (ITP) after long-term treatment with steroids. Although the spleen in ITP is associated with an increased number of cordal macrophages and ITP has been reported in association with hepatosplenic peliosis,[267-269] no other such association has been described for hamartoma. However, a direct effect of prolonged corticosteroid treatment has been hypothesized to be responsible for the association.[266]

Inflammatory Pseudotumors

Inflammatory pseudotumor (IPT) is a benign tumorlike lesion composed of proliferating spindle cells admixed with an inflammatory infiltrate usually rich in reactive plasma cells.[92] Although the lung is the most common location,[270-273] IPTs have been observed in other sites including the orbit,[274, 275] the liver,[276-279] and the lymph nodes [280-282] as well as the spleen (Color Plate 31).[283-297] Other terms used to described this lesion are "plasma cell granuloma," "plasma cell pseudotumor," "xanthomatous pseudotumor," "pseudosarcomatous myofibroblastic proliferation," "inflammatory myofibroblastic tumor," and "inflammatory myofibrohistiocytic proliferation."[298] Although the origin of IPT is not known, it is generally accepted that IPT may be an unusual tissue response to injury.[92, 297-299] Rare cases have been associated with prior systemic bacterial or fungal infections.[290] Other suggested causes include vascular obstruction and autoimmune disorders.[290] IPT is considered by some to be a localized fibroproliferative lesion related the myofibromatoses/fibromatoses.[298] The spindle cell population has been variously thought to be fibroblastic,[280, 300, 301] myofibroblastic,[280, 301] or histiocytic[299, 300] by ultrastructural and/or immunohistochemical criteria. The uncertainty concerning the cellular origin of IPT explains why so many different terms have been used to define IPT.

Splenic IPT occurs at an older age than IPTs of other sites.[92, 296, 298] In a large series of splenic IPTs, the patients averaged 53 years of age, with a range of 19 to 87 years. Rare cases have been reported in young patients.[283, 296, 297] No gender predilection has been noted.[92] Some lesions are found incidentally, whereas other patients are symptomatic, primarily with leukocytosis, fever, weight loss, abdominal pain, and vomiting. Other patients have signs of immune thrombocytopenic purpura.

Splenic IPT can mimic malignant lymphoma clinically, radiologically, and grossly. The lesion is solitary in 85 percent of cases, its size ranging from 0.5 to more than 10 cm.[92, 296] Multiple lesions are usually smaller (1.5 cm or less), suggesting that the larger single tumors may arise, at least in some cases, from coalescence of small lesions.[296] The lesions are usually well circumscribed, firm, tan-white, vaguely lobulated, and bulging.[92] However, some may appear infiltrative (Fig. 15–31).

Histologically, splenic IPT is characterized by a mixture of spindle-shaped, fibroblastlike cells with bland-looking oval nuclei; chronic inflammatory cells; and variable number of neutrophils (Fig. 15–32).[92] Plasma cells are often the predominant cell type, and they are present as small aggregates among the spindle cells or more uniformly dispersed in the background. Occasionally this infiltrate may be so prominent that plasmacytoma is simulated (plasma cell granuloma), necessitating light-chain immunoglobulin staining to demonstrate its polyclonal nature.[92] Sclerosis may be extensive (Fig. 15–33). Foci of hemorrhage, necrosis, hyalinization, calcification, foamy histiocytes, and foreign body granulomas may also be observed.[283, 284, 286-289, 293] Although the combination of fibroblastlike cells and an inflammatory cellular infiltrate are the principal components in IPT, the microscopic pattern is polymorphous, and striking variation from case to case may be observed.[92, 282] Examples of IPT with prominent myofibroblastic proliferation may resemble fibrous histiocytomas, smooth muscle neoplasms, or fibromatosis.[298] Other cases show a zonal maturational phenomenon similar to other pseudosarcomatous proliferative lesions, such as nodular fasciitis and myositis ossificans, with a central area of coagulative necrosis surrounded by a zone of inflammatory cells that is further surrounded by the spindle cell proliferation.[92]

Immunohistochemically, the spindle cells in IPT show reactivity with vimentin and muscle-specific and smooth muscle actin in most cases.[282, 298, 299, 301] Desmin and cytokeratin reactivity is reported in a minority of cases. The inflammatory cell infiltrate is composed of polyclonal plasma cells, small T lymphocytes, and CD68-positive histiocytes.[92] Follicular dendritic cell immunoreactivity (CD21 positivity) has also been reported in a few IPT cases, including one case involving the spleen.[294, 302, 303]

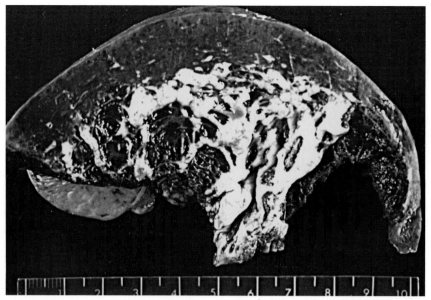

Figure 15–31. Inflammatory pseudotumor. Although most of these lesions are reasonably well circumscribed, some display a diffuse infiltrative appearance, such as this example.

Recently, Arber et al[294] documented the presence of Epstein-Barr virus (EBV) RNA by in situ hybridization in a proportion of cases of IPT occurring in lymph node, spleen, and liver. They found differences in the incidence of EBV infection when extranodal and nodal cases were compared. The highest incidence was found in IPTs in the spleen and liver, the lowest in lymph node. In the extranodal IPT, the EBV-infected cells showed a spindled structure, as well as actin and vimentin expression. In contrast, EBV-positive lymphoid cells, but not spindle cells, were identified in the nodal IPT examined. Shek et al[302, 303] confirmed the presence of EBV in IPT of the liver; lesions in other sites tested by the authors (lung, thyroid,

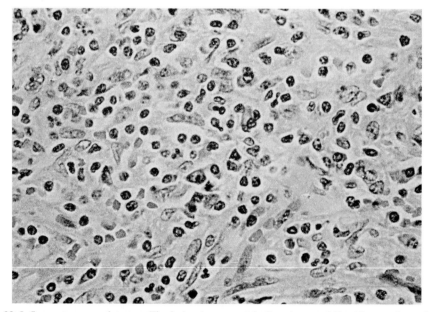

Figure 15–32. Inflammatory pseudotumor. The lesion is composed of a mixture of fibroblasts and a variety of chronic inflammatory cells.

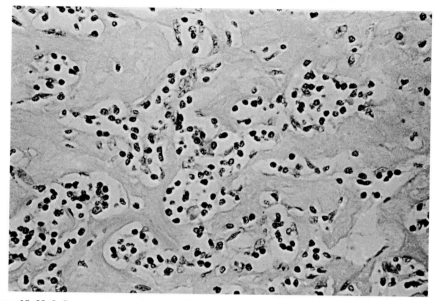

Figure 15–33. Inflammatory pseudotumor. The degree of sclerosis may mimic a sclerosing lymphoma.

epididymis, and peripharyngeal space) did not display evidence of EBV.

The reactive nature of IPT has been challenged by the demonstration of clonal cytogenetic abnormalities in a typical case of pulmonary IPT.[304] Two cases of EBV-positive IPT of the liver have also been reported in which DNA sequencing of the *LMP1* gene showed evidence of clonality. These findings suggest that at least some IPT cases may be true neoplasms.[302, 303, 305]

Mycobacterial Spindle Cell Pseudotumors

Mycobacterial spindle cell pseudotumor (MSCP) of the spleen is a multinodular lesion

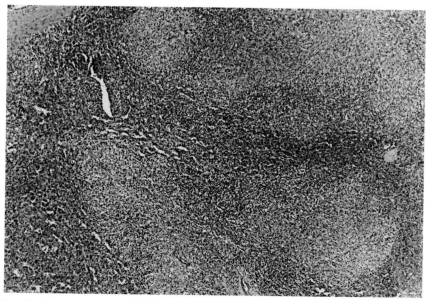

Figure 15–34. Microbacterial spindle cell pseudotumor. The lesion is multinodular. (Courtesy of Dr. J.K.C. Chan, Queen Victoria Hospital, Hong Kong.)

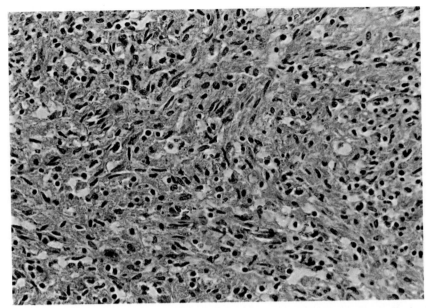

Figure 15–35. Microbacterial spindle cell pseudotumor. The lesion is composed of both spindle-shaped and plump histiocytes that have granular cytoplasm due to the accumulation of acid-fast organisms. (Courtesy of Dr. J.K.C. Chan, Queen Victoria Hospital, Hong Kong.)

(Fig. 15–34) composed of spindle cells growing in fascicles and occasionally adopting a storiform pattern, admixed with capillaries, lymphocytes, and plasma cells.[306–308] The spindle cells have eosinophilic granular cytoplasm and oval nuclei (Fig. 15–35). The cells show positivity for histiocytic markers (e.g., CD68) and contain abundant acid-fast bacilli within the cytoplasm. Bacilli can also be demonstrated lying free in the interstitium. Because of the need for antimycobacterial chemotherapy, MSCP must be distinguished from other morphologically similar lesions. MSCPs may be mistaken for splenic leiomyomas. Both lesions are positive for desmin; however, MSCPs lack actin reactivity.[92, 306] MSCPs must also be distinguished from inflammatory pseudotumors. MSCPs usually occur in the setting of AIDS, lack vasculitis, and do not extend into the splenic hilum.[92] Inflammatory pseudotumor of the spleen, however, in addition to the prominent spindle cell proliferation, shows vasculitis, frequent hilar extension, areas of sclerosis, focal necrosis, granulomatous changes, and polymorphic cellular infiltrates rich in plasma cells and foamy macrophages.[92] A firm diagnosis can be made by demonstrating the presence of acid-fast bacilli in spindle cell pseudotumor and the expression of actin and CD68 in inflammatory pseudotumor.[92] KS also contains fascicles of spindle cells. However, the spindle cells of KS are associated with vascular slits containing red blood cells with hyaline globules and with distinctive perivascular fibrosis surrounding the small arteries of the splenic follicles. Immunohistochemistry can also be used to distinguish KS from the other histologically similar processes (see the earlier section on KS).

REFERENCES

1. Bostick WL, Lucia SP: Nonparasitic noncancerous cystic tumors of the spleen. Arch Pathol 1949; 47:215.
2. Fowler RH: Cystic tumors of the spleen. Int Abstr Surg 1940; 70:213.
3. Fowler RH: Nonparasitic benign cystic tumors of the spleen. Int Abstr Surg 1953; 26:209.
4. Martin JW: Congenital splenic cysts. Am J Surg 1958; 96:302.
5. Qureshi MA, Hafner CD: Clinical manifestations of splenic cysts: Study of 75 cases. Am Surg 1965; 31:605.
6. Garvin DF, King FM: Cysts and nonlymphomatous tumors of the spleen. Pathol Ann 1981; 1:61.
7. Park JY, Song KT: Splenic cysts: A case report and review of literature. Am Surg 1971; 37:544.
8. Sirinek KR, Evans WE: Nonparasitic splenic cysts: Case report of epidermoid cyst with review of the literature. Am J Surg 1973; 126:8.
9. Shousha S: Splenic cysts: A report of six cases and brief review. Postgrad Med J 1978; 54:265.
10. Blank E, Campbell JR: Epidermoid cysts of the spleen. Pediatrics 1973; 51:75.

11. Robbins FG, Yellin AE, Lingua RW, et al: Splenic epidermoid cysts. Ann Surg 1968; 187:231.

12. Clarke JM, Talbert JL: Neoplastic cysts of the spleen in children. Am Surg 1969; 35:488.

13. King MC, Glick BW, Freed A: The diagnosis of splenic cysts. Surg Gynecol Obstet 1968; 127:509.

14. Bron KM, Hoffman WJ: Preoperative diagnosis of splenic cysts. Arch Surg 1971; 102:459.

15. Simmons TC: Traumatic pseudocyst of the spleen. J Nat Med Assoc 1990; 82:727.

16. Woody JD, Craft PR, Fabian TS, et al: Traumatic pseudocyst of the spleen. Tenn Med 1996; 89:372.

17. Williams RJ-LI, Glazer G: Splenic cysts: Changes in diagnosis, treatment and aetiological concepts. Ann R Coll Surg Engl 1993; 75:87.

18. Millar JS: Partial excision and railage of post-traumatic splenic cysts. Br J Surg 1982; 69:477.

19. Smith GW: Tumors, cysts, and abscesses of the spleen, in Cameron JL (ed): Current Surgical Therapy, 5 ed, p 474. St. Louis, Mosby–Year Book, 1995.

20. Allen RP, Condon VR: Epidermoid cysts of the spleen in children. Am J Roentgenol 1961; 86:534.

21. Griscom NT: Huge splenic cysts. Am J Dis Child 1965; 109:224.

22. Talerman A, Hart S: Epithelial cysts of the spleen. Br J Surg 1972; 57:201.

23. Musy PA, Roche B, Belli D, et al: Splenic cysts in pediatric patients: A report on 8 cases and review of the literature. Eur J Ped Surg 1992; 3:137.

24. Gilmartin D: Familial multiple epidermoid cysts of the spleen. Conn Med 1978; 42:297.

25. Iwanaka T, Nakanishi H, Tsuchida Y, et al: Familial multiple mesothelial cysts of the spleen. J Ped Surg 1995; 30:1743.

26. Muaro T, Toda K, Kida T: Multilocular epidermoid cyst of the spleen: Report of a case observed with an electron microscope. Jpn J Cancer Clin 1988; 34:233.

27. Tsakraklides V, Hadley TW: Epidermoid cysts of the spleen: A report of five cases. Arch Pathol 1973; 96:251.

28. Bean LL, Stahlgren LH: Epidermoid cyst of the spleen. US Armed Forces Med J 1953; 4:305.

29. Jameson EM, Smith OF: Calcified cyst of the spleen. US Naval Med Bull 1945; 45:537.

30. Lang VF, Morton SA, Steele JD, et al: Cysts of the spleen. Ann Surg 1948; 127:572.

31. Parnes IH: Nonparasitic cysts of the spleen: A report of two cases. J Mt Sinai Hosp NY 1949; 16:245.

32. Bisceglia M, Nirchio V, Di Mattia A, et al: Primary cysts of the spleen: Review of the literature with report of five cases, four of which not previously published. Pathologica 1994; 86:638.

33. Ough YD, Nash HR, Wood DA: Mesothelial cysts of the spleen with squamous metaplasia. Am J Clin Pathol 1981; 76:666.

34. Burrig K-F: Epithelial (true) splenic cysts: Pathogenesis of the mesothelial and so-called epidermoid cyst of the spleen. Am J Surg Pathol 1988; 12:275.

35. Lifschitz-Mercer B, Open M, Kushnir I, et al: Epidermoid cyst of the spleen: A cytokeratin profile with comparison to other squamous epithelia. Virchows Arch 1994; 424:213.

36. Cave RH, Garvin DR, Doohen DJ: Metaplastic mesodermal cyst of the spleen. Am Surg 1971; 37:97.

37. Linn HJ, Ellias EP: Epidermoid cyst of the spleen: Report of a case. Am J Clin Pathol 1949; 19:558.

38. Lippitt WH, Akhavan T, Caplan GE: Epidermoid cyst of the spleen with rupture and inflammation. Arch Surg 1967; 95:74.

39. Mahour GH, Soule EH, Lynn HB: Multiple epidermoid cysts of the spleen. Arch Surg 1968; 96:394.

40. Santy P: Splenectomie pour un cyste vrai de la rate chez un enfant. Lyon Chir 1930; 27:101.

41. Lee YS, Teh M: Histogenesis of true splenic cysts: A histological and immunohistochemical study. Ann Acad Med 1993; 22:372.

42. Arber DA, Strickler JG, Weiss LM: Splenic mesothelial cysts mimicking lymphangiomas. Am J Surg Pathol 1997; 21:334.

43. Nakashima A, Nakashima K, Seto H, et al: Primary splenic lymphoma presenting as a large cyst. Radiat Med 1994; 12:42.

44. Browne MK: Epidermoid cyst of the spleen. Br J Surg 1963; 50:838.

45. Coleman WO: Epidermoid cyst of the spleen: Report of two cases. Am J Surg 1960; 100:475.

46. Dibble JB, Weigent CE: Epidermoid cyst of the spleen presenting as an abdominal emergency: Report of a case. JAMA 1965; 194:1144.

47. Hoffman E: Nonparasitic splenic cysts. Am J Surg 1957; 93:765.

48. Binford CH, Connor DH (eds): Pathology of Tropical and Extraordinary Diseases, p 530. Washington, DC, Armed Forces Institute of Pathology, 1976.

49. Kellner H, Ziegler L, Fuessl HS, et al: Echinococcus cysticus—rare differential diagnosis of a splenic cyst. Bildgebung 1990; 57:85.

50. Poole JB, Marcial-Rojas RA: Echinococcosis, in Poole JB, Marcial-Rojas RA (eds): Pathology of Protozoal and Helminthic Diseases. Baltimore, Williams & Wilkins, 1971.

51. Neiman RS, Orazi A: Diseases of the spleen, in Damjanov I, Linder J (eds): Anderson's Pathology, 10th ed, p 1201. St. Louis, Mosby–Year Book, 1996.

52. Pines B, Rabinovitch J: Hemangioma of the spleen. Arch Pathol 1942; 33:487.

53. Rappaport H: Tumors of the hematopoietic system, in Atlas of Tumor Pathology, section 3, fascicle 8, p 357. Washington, DC, Armed Forces Institute of Pathology, 1966.

54. Bostick WL: Primary splenic neoplasms. Am J Pathol 1945; 21:1143.

55. Heading RC, McClelland DBL, Stuart AE, et al: Ruptured angiomatous spleen presenting as a severe coagulation defect. Br J Surg 1972; 59:492.

56. Shanberge JN, Tanaka K, Gruhl MC: Chronic consumption coagulopathy due to hemangiomatous transformations of the spleen. Am J Clin Pathol 1971; 56:723.

57. Husni EA: The clinical course of splenic hemangioma: With emphasis on spontaneous rupture. Arch Surg 1961; 33:681.

58. Coe JI, Von Drashek S: Hamartoma of the spleen: A report of four cases. Am J Pathol 1952; 28:663.

59. Berge TH: Splenoma. Acta Pathol Microbiol Scand 1965; 63:333.

60. Benjamin BI, Nohler DN, Sandusky WR: Hemangioma of the spleen. Arch Intern Med 1965; 115:280.

61. Graham JC, Weidner WA, Vinik M: The angiographic features of organizing splenic hematoma. Am J Roentgenol 1969; 107:430.

62. Zukerberg LR, Kaynor BL, Silverman ML, et al: Splenic hamartoma and capillary hemangioma are distinct entities: Immunohistochemical analysis of CD8 expression by endothelial cells. Hum Pathol 1991; 22:1258.

63. Case Records of the Massachusetts General Hospital: Case 23—1971. N Engl J Med 1971; 284:1314.

64. Case Records of the Massachusetts General Hospital: Case 48—1985. N Engl J Med 1985; 313:1405.

65. Florentin P, Chalnot P, Michon P: Angiomatose diffus de la rate avec pancytopenie splenectomie: Resultat favorable. Rev Belge Pathol Med Exp 1955; 24:501.

66. Kellert E: Diffuse hemangioma of the spleen. Am J Cancer 1932; 16:412.

67. Pinkhas J, Djaldetti M, DeVries A, et al: Diffuse angiomatosis of the spleen with hypersplenism: Splenectomy followed by polycythemia. Am J Med 1968; 45:795.

68. Symmers WS: The lymphoreticular system, in Symmers WS (ed): Systemic Pathology, 2nd ed, p 740. Edinburgh, Churchill Livingstone, 1978.

69. O'Brien DM, Ghent WR, Dexter DF: Systemic cystic angiomatosis in a woman with hematuria and splenomegaly. Can J Surg 1987; 30:277.

70. Ruck P, Horny HP, Xioa JC, et al: Diffuse sinusoidal hemangiomatosis of the spleen: A case report with enzyme-histochemical, immunohistochemical, and electron-microscopic findings. Pathol Res Pract 1994; 190:708.

71. Smith CE, Rusk GY: Endothelioma of the spleen: A study of two cases with review of the literature of primary malignancy of the spleen. Arch Surg 1923; 7:371.

72. Falk S, Stutte HJ, Frizzera G: Littoral cell angioma: A novel splenic vascular lesion demonstrating histiocytic differentiation. Am J Surg Pathol 1991; 15:1023.

73. Arber DA, Strickler JG, Chen Y-Y, et al: Splenic vascular tumors: A histologic, immunophenotypic, and virologic study. Am J Surg Pathol 1997; 21:827.

74. Sallah S, Gonzalez P, Maia DM, et al: Littoral cell angioma in a patient with Epstein syndrome. Acta Haematol 1997; 98:113.

75. William YW, Chang T, Chang JKC: Splenic littoral cell angioma, not bacillary angiomatosis. Pathology 1994; 26:347.

76. Michal M, Skalova A, Fakan F, et al: Littoral cell angioma of the spleen: A case report with ultrastructural and immunohistochemical observations. Zentralbl Pathol 1993; 139:361.

77. Buckley PJ, Dickson SA, Walker WS: Human splenic sinusoidal lining cells express antigens associated with monocytes, macrophages, endothelial cells, and T lymphocytes. J Immunol 1985; 134:2310.

78. Rosso R, Paulli M, Gianelli U, et al: Littoral cell angiosarcoma of the spleen: Case report with immunohistochemical and ultrastructural analysis. Am J Surg Pathol 1995; 19:1203.

79. Rosso R, Gianelli U, Chan JKC: Further evidence supporting the sinus lining cell nature of splenic littoral cell angiosarcoma. Am J Surg Pathol 1996; 20:1531.

80. Takato I, Iwamoto H, Ikezu M, et al: Splenic hemangiosarcoma with sinus endothelial differentiation. Acta Pathol Jpn 1993; 43:702.

81. Michal M, Skalova A, Fakan F: Littoral cell angioma of the spleen: A case report with ultrastructural and immunohistochemical observations: Zentralbl Pathol 1993; 139:361.

82. Asch MJ, Cohen AH, Moore TC: Hepatic and splenic lymphangiomatosis with skeletal involvement: Report of a case and review of the literature. Surgery 1974; 76:334.

83. Avigad S, Jaffe R, Frand M, et al: Lymphangiomatosis with splenic involvement. JAMA 1976; 236:2315.

84. Marymont JV, Knight PJ: Splenic lymphangiomatosis: A rare cause of splenomegaly. J Pediatr Surg 1987; 22:461.

85. Morgenstern L, Bello MJ, Fisher BL, et al: The clinical spectrum of lymphangiomas and lymphangiomatosis of the spleen. Am Surg 1992; 58:599.

86. Rappaport H: Tumors of the hematopoietic system, in Atlas of Tumor Pathology, section 3, fascicle 8, p 388. Washington, DC, Armed Forces Institute of Pathology, 1966.

87. Chan KW, Saw D: Distinctive, multiple lymphangiomas of spleen. J Pathol 1980; 131:75.

88. Schmid C, Beham A, Uranus S, et al: Nonsystemic diffuse lymphangiomatosis of spleen and liver. Histopathology 1991; 18:478.

89. Ito K, Murata T, Nakanishi T: Cystic lymphangioma of the spleen: MR findings with pathologic correlation. Abdom Imaging 1995; 20:82.

90. Alerci M, Dore R: Computed tomography of cystic lymphangioma in a wandering spleen. Acta Radiol 1990; 31:589.

91. Nusser CA, Tuggle DW, McLanahan KB, et al: Splenic lymphangioma: An unusual manifestation of the Klippel-Trenaunay-Weber syndrome. Clin Nucl Med 1995; 20:844.

92. Warnke RA, Weiss LM, Chan JKC, et al: Nonhematolymphoid tumors and tumor-like lesions of lymph node and spleen. Atlas of Tumor Pathology, 3rd series, fascicle 14, p 497. Washington, DC, Armed Forces Institute of Pathology, 1995.

93. Hamoudi AB, Vassy LE, Morse TS: Multiple lymphangioendothelioma of the spleen in a 13-year-old girl. Arch Pathol 1975; 99:605.

94. Feigenberg Z, Wysenbeek A, Avidor E, et al: Malignant lymphangioma of the spleen. Isr J Med Sci 1983; 19:202.

95. Miettinen M, Weiss SW: Soft tissue tumors, in Damjanov I, Linder J (eds): Anderson's Pathology, 10th ed, p 2501. St. Louis, Mosby–Year Book, 1996.

96. Jurado JG, Fuentes FT, Menendez CG, et al: Hemangiopericytoma of the spleen. Surgery 1989; 106:575.

97. Neill JSA, Park HK: Hemangiopericytoma of the spleen. Am J Clin Pathol 1991; 95:680.

98. Nappi O, Ritter JH, Pettinato G, et al: Hemangiopericytoma: Histopathological pattern or clinicopathologic entity? Semin Diagn Pathol 1995; 12:221.

99. Dardick I, Hammar SP, Scheithauer BW: Ultrastructural spectrum of hemangiopericytoma: A comparative study of fetal, adult, and neoplastic pericytes. Ultrastruct Pathol 1989; 13:111.

100. Toccanier-Pelte MF: Skalli O, Kapanci Y, Gabbiani G: Characterization of stromal cells with myoid features in lymph nodes and spleen in normal and pathologic conditions. Am J Pathol 1987; 129:109.

101. Easler RE, Dowlin WM: Primary lipoma of the spleen: A case report. Arch Pathol 1969; 88:557.

102. Hulbert JC, Graf R: Involvement of the spleen by renal angiomyolipoma: Metastasis or multicentricity? J Urol 1983; 130:328.

103. Bloom DA, Scardino PT, Ehrlich RM, et al: The significance of lymph nodal involvement in renal angiomyolipoma. J Urol 1982; 128:1292.

104. Brecher ME, Gill WB, Straus FH II: Angiomyolipoma with regional lymph node involvement and long-term follow-up study. Hum Pathol 1986; 17:962.

105. Busch FM, Bark CJ, Clydine HR: Benign renal angiomyolipoma with regional lymph node involvement. J Urol 1976; 116:715.

106. Sant GR, Ucci AA Jr, Meares EM Jr: Multicentric

angiomyolipoma: Renal and lymph node involvement. Urology 1986; 28:111.

107. Coskun M, Aydingoz U, Tacal T, et al: CT and MR imaging of splenic leiomyoma in a child with ataxia telangiectasia. Pediatr Radiol 1995; 25:45.

108. Morel D, Merville P, Le Bail B, et al: Epstein-Barr virus (EBV)–associated hepatic and splenic smooth muscle tumors after kidney transplantation. Nephrol Dial Transplant 1996; 11:1864.

109. Chadwick EG, Connor EJ, Hanson CG, et al: Tumors of smooth muscle origin in HIV-infected children. JAMA 1990; 263:23.

110. Levin TL, Adam HM, van Hoeven KH, et al: Hepatic spindle cell tumors in HIV-positive children. Pediatr Radiol 1994; 24:78.

111. Ha C, Haller JO, Rollins NK, et al: Smooth muscle tumors in immunocompromised (HIV-negative) children. Pediatr Radiol 1993; 23:413.

112. McLoghlin LC, Nord KS, Joshi W, et al: Disseminated leiomyosarcoma in a child with AIDS. Cancer 1990; 67:10.

113. Mueller B, Butler KM, Higham MC, et al: Smooth muscle tumors in children with HIV infection. Pediatrics 1992; 90:3.

114. Balsam D, Segal S: Two smooth muscle tumors in the airway of an HIV-infected child. Pediatr Radiol 1992; 22:552.

115. Toma P, Loy A, Pastorino C, et al: Leiomyomas of the gallbladder and splenic calcifications in an HIV-infected child. Pediatr Radiol 1997; 27:92–94.

116. Lee ES, Locker J, Nalesnik M, et al: The association of Epstein-Barr virus with smooth-muscle tumors occurring after organ transplantation. N Engl J Med 1995; 332:19.

117. McCain KL, Leach CT, Jenson HB, et al: Association of Epstein-Barr virus with leiosarcomas in young people with AIDS. N Engl J Med 1995; 332:12.

118. Rousselot LM, Stein C: Malignant neoplasms of the spleen: Primary and secondary. Surg Clin North Am 1953; 33:493.

119. Weichselbaum A: Beiträge zur Geschwulstlehre. Virchows Arch 1981; 85:554.

120. Weiss SW, Enzinger FM: Epithelioid hemangioendothelioma: A vascular tumor often mistaken for a carcinoma. Cancer 1982; 50:970.

121. Weiss SW, Ishak KG, Dail DH, et al: Epithelioid hemangioendothelioma and related lesions. Semin Diagn Pathol 1986; 3:259.

122. Wick MR, Manivel JC: Epithelioid sarcoma and epithelioid hemangioendothelioma: An immunocytochemical and lectin histochemical comparison. Virchows Arch 1987; 410:309.

123. Weiss SW, Enzinger FM: Spindle cell hemangioendothelioma: A low grade angiosarcoma resembling a cavernous hemangioma and Kaposi's sarcoma. Am J Surg Pathol 1986; 10:521.

124. Scott GA, Rosai J: Spindle cell hemangioendothelioma: Report of seven additional cases of a recently described vascular neoplasm. Am J Dermatopathol 1988; 10:281.

125. Perkins P, Weiss SW: Spindle cell hemangioendothelioma: An analysis of 78 cases with reassessment of its pathogenesis and biologic behavior. Am J Surg Pathol 1996; 20:1196.

126. Dabska M: Malignant endovascular papillary angioendothelioma of the skin in childhood: Clinicopathologic study of 6 cases. Cancer 1969; 24:503.

127. Manivel JC, Wick MR, Swanson PE, et al: Endovascular papillary angioendothelioma of childhood: A vascular lesion possibly characterized by "high" endothelial cell differentiation. Hum Pathol 1986; 17:1240.

128. Quecedo E, Martineq-Escribano JA, Febrer I, et al: Dabska tumor developing within a preexisting vascular malformation. Am J Dermatopathol 1996; 18:302.

129. Rosai J, Gold J, Landy R: The histiocytoid hemangiomas: A unifying concept embracing several previously described entities of skin, soft tissue, large vessels, bone and heart. Hum Pathol 1979; 10:707.

130. Roepke JE, Heifetz SA: Pathological case of the month: Epithelioid hemangioendothelioma (intravascular bronchioloalveolar tumor) of the lung. Arch Pediatr Adolesc Med 1997; 151:317.

131. Kaw YT, Duwaji MS, Knisley RE, et al: Hemangioendothelioma of the spleen. Arch Pathol Lab Med 1992; 916:1079.

132. Suster S: Epithelioid and spindle-cell hemangioendothelioma of the spleen: Report of a distinctive splenic vascular neoplasm of childhood. Am J Surg Pathol 1992; 16:785.

133. Tiu CM, Chou YH, Wang HT, et al: Epithelioid hemangioendothelioma of spleen with intrasplenic metastasis: Ultrasound and computed-tomography appearance. Comput Med Imaging Graph 1992; 16:287.

134. Budke HL, Breitfeld PP, Neiman RS: Functional hyposplenism due to a primary epithelioid hemangioendothelioma of the spleen. Arch Pathol Lab Med 1995; 119:755.

135. Katz JA, Mahoney DH, Shukla LW, et al: Endovascular papillary angioendothelioma in the spleen. Pediatr Pathol 1988; 8:185.

136. Craig JR, Peters RL, Edmondson HA: Tumors of the liver and intrahepatic bile ducts, in Atlas of Tumor Pathology, 2nd series, fascicle 26, p 75. Washington, DC, Armed Forces Institute of Pathology, 1982.

137. Selby DM, Stocker JT, Waclawiw MA, et al: Infantile hemangioendothelioma of the liver. Hepatology 1994; 20:39.

138. Autry JR, Weitzner S: Hemangiosarcoma of spleen with spontaneous rupture. Cancer 1975; 35:534.

139. Chen KTD, Bolles JC, Gilbert EF: Angiosarcoma of the spleen: A report of two cases and review of the literature. Arch Pathol Lab Med 1979; 103:122.

140. Wick MR, Scheithauer BW, Smith SL, et al: Primary nonlymphoreticular malignant neoplasms of the spleen. Am J Surg Pathol 1982; 6:229.

141. Smith VC, Eisenberg BL, McDonald EC: Primary splenic angiosarcoma: Case report and literature review. Cancer 1985; 55:1625.

142. Falk S, Krishnan J, Meis JM: Primary angiosarcoma of the spleen: A clinicopathologic study of 40 cases. Am J Surg Pathol 1993; 17:959.

143. Silverman ML, Federman M, O'Hara CJ: Malignant hemangioendothelioma of the spleen: A case report with ultrasound observation. Arch Pathol Lab Med 1981; 105:300.

144. Alt B, Hafez GR, Trigg M, et al: Angiosarcoma of the liver and spleen in an infant. Pediatr Pathol 1985; 4:331.

145. Dahlgren S: Thorotrast tumors: A review of the literature and report of two cases. Acta Pathol Microbiol Scand 1961; 53:147.

146. MacMahon HE, Murphy AS, Bates ME: Endothelial cell sarcoma of the liver following Thorotrast injection. Am J Pathol 1945; 23:585.

147. Block JB: Angiosarcoma of the liver following vinyl chloride exposure. JAMA 1974; 229:53.

148. Lee FI, Harry DS: Angiosarcoma of the liver in a vinyl-chloride worker. Lancet 1974; 1:1316.

149. Regelson W, Kim U, Ospina J, et al: Hemangioendothelial sarcoma of liver from chronic arsenic intoxication by Fowler's solution. Cancer 1968; 21:514.

150. Zwi LJ, Evans DJ, Wechsler AL, et al: Splenic angiosarcoma following chemotherapy for follicular lymphoma. Hum Pathol 1986; 17:528.

151. Wilkinson HA III, Lucas JC, Foote FW Jr: Primary splenic angiosarcoma: A case report. Arch Pathol 1968; 85:213.

152. Chang Y, Cesarman E, Pessin MS, et al: Identification of herpes-like DNA sequences in AIDS-associated Kaposi's sarcoma. Science 1994; 266:1865.

153. Gyulai R, Kemeny L, Adam E, et al: HHV8 DNA in angiolymphoid hyperplasia of the skin. Lancet 1996; 347:1837.

154. Gyulai R, Kemeny L, Kiss M, et al: Herpes-like DNA sequence in angiosarcoma in a patient without HIV infection. N Engl J Med 1996; 334:540.

155. McDonaugh DP, Liu J, Gaffey MJ, et al: Detection of Kaposi's sarcoma–associated herpesvirus-like DNA sequences in angiosarcoma. Am J Pathol 1996; 149:1363.

156. Kemeny L, Gyulai R, Kiss M, et al: Kaposi's sarcoma–associated herpesvirus/human herpesvirus-8: A new virus in human pathology. J Am Acad Dermatol 1997; 37:107.

157. Donald D, Dawson D: Microangiopathic hemolytic anemia associated with hemangioendothelioma. J Clin Pathol 1971; 24:456.

158. Aranha GV, Gold J, Grage TB: Hemangiosarcoma of the spleen: Report of a case and review of previously reported cases. J Surg Oncol 1976; 8:481.

159. Nadji M, Gonzalez MS, Castro A, et al: Factor VIII–related antigen: An endothelial cell marker. Lab Invest 1980; 42:139A.

160. Burgdorf WHC, Mukai J, Rosai J: Immunohistochemical identification of factor VIII–related antigen in endothelial cells of cutaneous lesions of alleged vascular nature. Am J Clin Pathol 1981; 75:167.

161. Orchard GE, Zelger B, Jones EW, et al: An immunocytochemical assessment of 19 cases of cutaneous angiosarcoma. Histopathology 1996; 28:235.

162. Poblet E, Gonzalez-Palacios F, Jimenez FJ: Different immunoreactivity of endothelial markers in well and poorly differentiated areas of angiosarcomas. Virchows Arch 1996; 428:217.

163. Ohsawa M, Naka N, Tomita Y, et al: Use of immunohistochemical procedures in diagnosing angiosarcoma: Evaluation of 98 cases. Cancer 1995; 75:2867.

164. Stutz FH, Tormey DC, Blom J: Hemangiosarcoma and pathologic rupture of the spleen. Cancer 1973; 31:1213.

165. Montemayor P, Caggiano V: Primary hemangiosarcoma of the spleen associated with leukocytosis and abnormal spleen scan. Intern Surg 1980; 65:369.

166. Mark RJ, Poen JC, Tran LM, et al: Angiosarcoma: A report of 67 patients and a review of the literature. Cancer 1996; 77:2400.

167. Tordjman R, Eugene C, Clouet O, et al: Hepatosplenic angiosarcoma complicated by hemoperitoneum and disseminated intravascular coagulation: Treatment by arterial embolization and chemotherapy. Gastroenterol Clin Biol 1995; 19:625.

168. Templeton AC: Pathology of Kaposi's sarcoma, in Ziegler JL, Dorfman RF (eds): Kaposi's Sarcoma: Pathophysiology and Clinical Management, pp 23–70. New York, Marcel Dekker, 1988.

169. DiGiovanna JJ, Safai B: Kaposi's sarcoma: Retrospective study of 90 cases with particular emphasis on the familial occurrence, ethnic background and prevalence of other diseases. Am J Medicine 1981; 71:779.

170. Safai B, Mike V, Giraldo G, et al: Association of Kaposi's sarcoma with second primary malignancies: Possible etiopathogenic implications. Cancer 1980; 45:1472.

171. Penn I: Etiology: immunodeficiency, in Ziegler JL, Dorfman RF (eds): Kaposi's Sarcoma: Pathophysiology and Clinical Management, pp 129–150. New York: Marcel Dekker, 1988.

172. Penn I: Kaposi's sarcoma in organ transplant recipients: Report of 20 cases. Transplantation 1979; 27:8.

173. Penn I: Kaposi's sarcoma in immunosuppressed patients. J Clin Lab Immunol 1983; 12:1.

174. Safai B, Johnson KG, Myskowski PL, et al: The natural history of Kaposi's sarcoma in the acquired immunodeficiency syndrome. Ann Intern Med 1985; 103:744.

175. Niedt GW, Schinella RA: Acquired immunodeficiency syndrome: Clinicopathologic study of 56 autopsies. Arch Pathol Lab Med 1985; 109:727.

176. Moskowitz LB, Hensley GT, Gould EW, et al: Frequency and anatomic distribution of lymphadenopathic Kaposi's sarcoma in the acquired immunodeficiency syndrome: An autopsy series. Hum Pathol 1985; 16:447.

177. Klatt EC, Meyer PR: Pathology of the spleen in the acquired immunodeficiency syndrome. Arch Pathol Lab Med 1987; 111:1050.

178. Falk S, Muller H, Stutte H-J: The spleen in acquired immunodeficiency syndrome (AIDS). Pathol Res Pract 1988; 183:425.

179. Sarode VR, Datta BN, Savitri K, et al: Kaposi's sarcoma of spleen with unusual clinical and histologic features. Arch Pathol Lab Med 1991; 115:1042.

180. Rutgers JL, Wieczorek R, Bonetti F, et al: The expression of endothelial cell surface antigens by AIDS-associated Kaposi's sarcoma: Evidence for a vascular endothelial cell origin. Am J Pathol 1986; 122:493.

181. Zhang YM, Bachmann S, Hemmer C, et al: Vascular origin of Kaposi's sarcoma: Expression of leukocyte adhesion molecule-1, thrombomodulin, and tissue factor. Am J Pathol 1994; 144:51.

182. Knowles DM, Cesarman E: The Kaposi's sarcoma–associated herpesvirus (human herpesvirus-8) in Kaposi's sarcoma, malignant lymphoma, and other diseases. Ann Oncol 1997; 2:123.

183. Boshoff C, Schulz TF, Kennedy MM, et al: Kaposi's sarcoma–associated herpesvirus infects endothelial and spindle cells. Nat Med 1995; 1:1274.

184. Hausmann PF, Gaarde FW: Malignant neoplasms of the spleen: Review of the literature and report of a case of primary lymphosarcoma (reticulum cell–type). Surgery 1943; 14:246.

185. Gordon JD, Paley DH: Primary malignant tumors of the spleen: Statistical review and report of a case of lymphosarcoma. Surgery 1951; 29:907.

186. Govoni E, Buzzochi F, Pileri S, et al: Primary malignant fibrous histiocytoma of the spleen: An ultrastructural study. Histopathology 1980; 6:351.

187. Sieber SC, Lopez V, Rosai J, et al: Primary tumor of spleen with morphologic features of malignant fibrous histiocytoma: Immunohistochemical evidence

for a macrophage origin. Am J Surg Pathol 1990; 14:1061.

188. Bonilla F, Provencio M, Fernandez E, et al: Malignant fibrous histiocytoma of the spleen and chronic myelogenous leukemia: A case report. Oncol 1994; 51:465.

189. Lawson CW, Fisher C, Gatter KC: An immunohistochemical study of differentiation in malignant fibrous histiocytoma. Histopathology 1987; 11:375.

190. Feakins RM, Norton AJ: Rhabdomyosarcoma of the spleen. Histopathol 1996; 29:577.

191. Morgenstern L, Rosenberg J, Geller SA: Tumors of the spleen. World J Surg 1985; 9:468.

192. Elit L, Aylward B: Splenic cyst carcinoma presenting in pregnancy. Am J Hematol 1989; 32:57.

193. Morinaga S, Ohyama R, Koizumi J: Low-grade mucinous cystadenocarcinoma in the spleen. Am J Surg Pathol 1992; 16:903.

194. Westra WH, Anderson BO, Klimstra DS: Carcinosarcoma of the spleen: An extragenital malignant mixed müllerian tumor? Am J Surg Pathol 1994; 18:309.

195. Daftary M, Barnett RN: Malignant teratoma of the spleen. Yale J Biol Med 1971; 43:283.

196. Meneses MF, Ostrowski ML: Female splenic-gonadal fusion of the discontinuous type. Hum Pathol 1989; 20:486.

197. Putschar WGM, Manion WC: Splenogonadal fusion. Am J Pathol 1956; 32:15.

198. Pantoja E, Noy MA, Axtmayer RW, et al: Ovarian dermoids and their complications: Comprehensive historical review. Obstet Gynecol Surv 1975; 30:1.

199. Symmers WS: The lymphoreticular system, in Symmers WS (ed): Systemic Pathology, 2nd ed, p 738. Edinburgh, Churchill Livingstone, 1978.

200. Shuman RL, Bouterie RL: Cystadenocarcinoma of the pancreas presenting as a splenic cyst. Surgery 1976; 80:652.

201. Barbosa JJ deC, Dockerty MB, Waugh JM: Pancreatic heterotopia: Review of the literature and report of 41 authenticated surgical cases, of which 25 were clinically significant. Surg Gynecol Obstet 1946; 82:527.

202. Lastrapes RG, Parker JR, Kida M: Pancreatic adenocarcinoma presenting as a splenic abscess: Case report and diagnostic approach. J Okla State Med Assoc 1995; 88:333.

203. Marymount JH Jr, Gross S: Patterns of metastatic cancer in the spleen. Am J Clin Pathol 1963; 40:58.

204. Pollard M, Bussel R: Role of the spleen in resistance to experimental tumors. Texas Rep Biol Med 1953; 11:48.

205. Woglom WH: Immunity to transplantable tumors. Cancer Rev 1929; 4:129.

206. Kettle EH: Carcinomatous metastases in the spleen. J Pathol Bacteriol 1913; 17:40.

207. Milton GW: The occurrence of secondary malignant disease in the spleen. Med J Aust 1952; 3:736.

208. Shappington SW: Carcinoma of the spleen: Its macroscopic frequency. JAMA 1922; 78:953.

209. Weiss L: The structure of the normal spleen. Semin Hematol 1965; 2:205.

210. Warren S, Davis H: Studies on tumor metastasis. V. The metastases of carcinoma to the spleen. Am J Cancer 1934; 21:517.

211. Drinker CK, Yoffey JM: Lymphatics, Lymph, and Lymphoid Tissue, p 23. Cambridge, Harvard University Press, 1941.

212. Harman JW, Dacorso P: Spread of carcinoma to the spleen: Its relation to generalized carcinomatous spread. Arch Pathol 1948; 45:179.

213. Berge T: Splenic metastases: Frequencies and patterns. Acta Pathol Microbiol Scand 1974; 82:499.

214. Klein B, Stein M, Kuten A, et al: Splenomegaly and solitary spleen metastasis in solid tumors. Cancer 1987; 60:100.

215. Nathanson L: Biological aspects of human malignant melanoma. Cancer 1967; 20:650.

216. Abrams HL, Spiro R, Goldstein N: Metastases in carcinoma: An analysis of 1000 autopsied cases. Cancer 1950; 3:74.

217. Herbut PA, Gabriel FR: Secondary cancer of the spleen. Arch Pathol 1942; 33:917.

218. Hirst AEJ, Bullock WK: Metastatic carcinoma of the spleen. Am J Med Sci 1952; 223:414.

219. Walther HE: Krebsmetastasen, in Die Blutbildenden Organe, p 240. Basel, Benno, Schwabe and Co, 1948.

220. Matthews MJ: Problems in morphology and behavior of bronchopulmonary malignant disease, in Israel L, Chahanian P (eds): Lung Cancer: Natural History, Prognosis and Therapy, p 23. New York, Academic Press, 1976.

221. Morris M, Gershenson DM, Burke TW, et al: Splenectomy in gynecologic oncology: Indications, complications, and technique. Gynecol Oncol 1991; 43:118.

222. Gilks GB, Acker BD, Clement PB: Recurrent endometrial adenocarcinoma: Presentation as a splenic mass mimicking malignant lymphoma. Gynecol Oncol 1989; 33:209.

223. Jorgensen LN, Chrintz H: Solitary metastatic endometrial carcinoma of the spleen. Acta Obstet Gynecol Scan 1988; 67:91.

224. Nosanchuk JS, Tyler WS, Terepka RH. Fine-needle aspiration of spleen: Diagnosis of a solitary ovarian metastasis. Diagn Cytopathol 1988; 4:159.

225. Edelman AS, Rotterdam H: Solitary splenic metastasis of an adenocarcinoma of the lung. Am J Clin Pathol 1990; 94:326.

226. Falk S, Stutte HJ: Splenic metastasis in an ileal carcinoid tumor. Pathol Res Pract 1989; 185:238.

227. Sharpe RW, Rector JT, Rushin JM, et al: Splenic metastasis in hairy cell leukemia. Cancer 1993; 71:2222.

228. Gorg C, Schwerk WB: Sonographic findings of splenic metastases. Bildgebung 1991; 58:26.

229. Goerg C, Schwerk WB, Goerg K: Splenic lesions: Sonographic patterns, follow-up, differential diagnosis. Eur J Radiol 1991; 13:59.

230. Zeppa P, Vetrani A, Luciano L, et al: Fine needle aspiration biopsy of the spleen: A useful procedure in the diagnosis of splenomegaly. Acta Cytol 1994; 38:299.

231. Dunn MA, Goldwein MI: Hypersplenism in advanced breast cancer: Report of a patient treated with splenectomy. Cancer 1975; 25:1449.

232. Goldstein HS: Spontaneous rupture of the spleen secondary to metastatic carcinoma. South Med J 1966; 59:261.

233. Rydell WB Jr, Ellis R: Spontaneous rupture of the spleen from metastatic carcinoma. JAMA 1978; 240:53.

234. Horie Y, Suou T, Hirayama C, et al: Spontaneous rupture of the spleen secondary to metastatic hepatocellular carcinoma: A report of a case and review of the literature. Am J Gastroenterol 1982; 77:882.

235. Bertolini R, Caselli A, Macarone-Palmieri R, et al: Spontaneous rupture of the spleen, site of metastatic

carcinoma: Presentation of a clinical case. G Chir 1989; 10:323.

236. al-Obaidi SM: Spontaneous rupture of the spleen due to metastatic carcinoma. Br J Clin Pract 1989; 43:385.

237. Gupta PB, Harvey L: Spontaneous rupture of the spleen secondary to metastatic carcinoma. Br J Surg 1993; 80:613.

238. Buzbee TM, Legha SS: Spontaneous rupture of spleen in a patient with splenic metastasis of melanoma: A case report. Tumor 1992; 78:47.

239. Da Gupta T, Brasfield R: Metastatic melanoma: A clinicopathologic study. Cancer 1964; 17:1323.

240. Karakousis CP, Elias EG: Spontaneous (pathologic) rupture of the spleen in malignancies. Surgery 1974; 76:674.

241. Turnbull A, Shah J, Fortner J: Recurrent melanoma of an extremity treated by major amputation. Arch Surg 1973; 106:496.

242. Cook AM, Graham JD: Spontaneous rupture of the spleen secondary to metastatic teratoma. J R Soc Med 1996; 89:710.

243. Cummings OW, Mazur MT: Breast carcinoma diffusely metastatic to the spleen: A report of two cases presenting as idiopathic thrombocytopenic purpura. Am J Clin Pathol 1992; 97:484.

244. Goldberg GM: Metastatic carcinoma of the spleen resulting from lymphogenic spread. Lab Invest 1957; 6:383.

245. Fakan F, Michael M: Nodular transformation of splenic red pulp due to carcinomatous infiltration: A diagnostic pitfall. Histopathology 1994; 25:175.

246. Silverman ML, LiVolsi VA: Splenic hamartoma. Am J Clin Pathol 1978; 70:224.

247. Teates CD, Seale DL, Allen MS: Hamartoma of the spleen. Am J Roentgenol 1972; 116:419.

248. Wallach JB, Nakao N: Hamartoma of the spleen. J Med Soc N J 1962; 59:75.

249. Bhagwat AG, D'Alta DV, Mitra S, et al: Splenoma with portal hypertension. Br Med J 1975; 1:520.

250. Kirkland WG, McDonald J: Hamartoma of the spleen: Report of three surgical cases. Arch Pathol 1948; 45:371.

251. Sweet RH, Warren S: Hamartoma of the spleen: Report of a case. N Engl J Med 1942; 226:757.

252. Ross CF, Schiller KFR: Hamartoma of the spleen associated with thrombocytopenia. J Pathol 1971; 105:62.

253. Beham A, Hermann W, Vennigerholz F, et al: Hamartoma of the spleen with hematological symptoms. Virchows Arch 1989; 414:535.

254. Wirbel RJ, Uhlig U, Futterer KM: Case report: Splenic hamartoma with hematologic disorders. Am J Med Sci 1996; 311:243.

255. Videbaek A: Hypersplenism associated with hamartoma of the spleen. Acta Med Scand 1953; 141:275.

256. Foiada M, Muller W, Conti Rossini B, et al: Case report of spontaneous splenic rupture in splenoma. Helvet Chir Acta 1993; 60:187.

257. Morgenstern L, McCafferty L, Rosenberg J, et al: Hamartomas of the spleen. Arch Surg 1984; 119:1291.

258. Steinberg JJ, Suhrland MJ, Quentin JV: The association of splenoma with disease. Lab Invest 1985; 52:65A.

259. Steinberg JJ, Suhrland M, Valensi Q: The spleen in the spleen syndrome: The association of splenoma with hematopoietic and neoplastic disease—com-

pendium of cases since 1864. J Surg Oncol 1991; 47:193.

260. Falk KKS, Stutte HJ: Hamartomas of the spleen: A study of 20 biopsy cases. Histopathology 1989; 14:603.

261. Iakovidou J, Panayiotides J, Papacharalambous X, et al: Splenic hamartoma: A case report. Eur J Surg Oncol 1995; 21:688.

262. Krishnan J, Danon AD, Frizzera G: Use of anti-factor VIII–related antigen (F8) and QBEND10 (CD34) antibodies helps classify the benign vascular lesions of the spleen. Mod Patholol 1993; 6:94A.

263. Darden JW, Teeslink R, Rarrish A: Hamartoma of the spleen: A manifestation of tuberous sclerosis. Am Surg 1975; 41:564.

264. Van Heerden JA, Longo MF, Cardona F, et al: The abdominal mass in the patient with tuberous sclerosis: Surgical implications and report of a case. Arch Surg 1967; 95:317.

265. Brouland J, Molina T, Delmer A, et al: Splenoma with accumulation of megakaryocytes during the course of an idiopathic myelofibrosis. Ann Pathol 1994; 14:32.

266. Diebold J, Audouin J: Association of splenoma, peliosis and lipid histiocytosis in spleen or accessory spleen removed in two patients with chronic idiopathic thrombocytopenic purpura after long-term treatment with steroids. Pathol Res Pract 1988; 183:445.

267. Lasser A: Diffuse histiocytosis of the spleen and idiopathic thrombocytopenic purpura (ITP): Histochemical and ultrastructural studies. Am J Clin Pathol 1983; 80:529.

268. Luk SC, Musclow E, Simon GT: Platelet phagocytosis in the spleen of patients with idiopathic thrombocytopenic purpura (ITP). Histopathology 1980; 4:127.

269. Nesher G, Dollbert L, Zimran A, et al: Hepatosplenic peliosis after Danazol and glucocorticoids for ITP. New Engl J Med 1985; 312:242.

270. Bahadori M, Liebow AA: Plasma cell granulomas of the lung. Cancer 1973; 31:191.

271. Buell R, Wang NS, Seemayer TA, et al: Endobronchial plasma cell granuloma (xanthomatous pseudotumor): A light and electron microscopic study. Hum Pathol 1976; 7:411.

272. Carter D, Eggleston JC: Tumors of the lower respiratory tract, in Atlas of Tumor Pathology, section 3, fascicle 8, p 300. Washington, DC, Armed Forces Institute of Pathology, 1979.

273. Spencer A: Plasma cell granuloma of the lung, in Pathology of the Lung, 3rd ed, vol 2, p 928. Philadelphia, WB Saunders, 1977.

274. Blodi C, Gass JDM: Inflammatory pseudotumor of the orbit. Br J Ophthalmol 1968; 52:79.

275. Garner A: Pathology of "pseudotumors" of the orbit: A review. J Clin Pathol 1973; 26:639.

276. Shek TW, Ng IO, Chan KW: Inflammatory pseudotumor of the liver: Report of four cases and review of the literature. Am J Surg Pathol 1993; 17:231.

277. Nakanum Y: Nonneoplastic nodular lesions in the liver. Pathol Int 1995; 45:703.

278. Passalides A, Keramidas D, Mavrides G: Inflammatory pseudotumor of the liver in children: A case report and review of the literature. Eur J Pediatr Surg 1996; 6:35.

279. Shek TWH, Ng IOL, Chang KW: Inflammatory pseudotumor of the liver. Am J Surg Pathol 1993; 17:231.

280. Perrone T, De Wolf-Peeters C, Frizzera G: Inflamma-

tory pseudotumor of lymph nodes: A distinctive pattern of nodal reaction. Am J Surg Pathol 1988; 12:351.

281. Davis RE, Warnke RA, Dorfman RF: Inflammatory pseudotumor of lymph nodes: Additional observations and evidence for an inflammatory etiology. Am J Surg Pathol 1991; 15:744.

282. Cotelingam JD, Jaffe ES: Inflammatory pseudotumor of the spleen. Am J Surg Pathol 1984; 81:375.

283. Moran CA, Suster S, Abbondanzo SL: Inflammatory pseudotumor of lymph nodes: A study of 25 cases with emphasis on morphological heterogeneity. Hum Pathol 1997; 28:332.

284. Alper HD, Olson JE, Kozak AJ: Inflammatory pseudotumor of the spleen. J Surg Oncol 1986; 33:46.

285. McMahon RF: Inflammatory pseudotumor of spleen. J Clin Pathol 1988; 41:734.

286. Sheahan K, Wolf BC, Neiman RS: Inflammatory pseudotumor of the spleen: A clinicopathologic study of three cases. Hum Pathol 1988; 19:1024.

287. Fu KH, Liu HW, Leung CY: Inflammatory pseudotumors of the spleen. Histopathol 1990; 16:302.

288. Dalal BI, Greenberg H, Quinonez GE, et al: Inflammatory pseudotumor of the spleen: Morphological, radiological, immunophenotypic, and ultrastructural features. Arch Pathol Lab Med 1991; 115:1062.

289. Monforte-Munoz H, Ro JY, Manning JT, et al: Inflammatory pseudotumor of the spleen: Report of two cases with a review of the literature. Am J Clin Pathol 1991; 96:491.

290. Wiernik PH, Rader M, Becker NH, et al: Inflammatory pseudotumor of the spleen. Cancer 1990; 66:597.

291. Tomita K, Hota G, Iarashi M, et al: A case of splenic inflammatory pseudotumor. Gastroenterol Jpn 1991; 26:783.

292. Inada T, Yano T, Shima S, et al: Inflammatory pseudotumor of the spleen. Int Med 1992; 31:941.

293. Thomas RM, Jaffe ES, Zarate-Osorno A, et al: Inflammatory pseudotumor of the spleen: A clinicopathologic and immunophenotypic study of 8 cases. Arch Pathol Lab Med 1993; 117:921.

294. Arber DA, Kamel OW, van de Rijn M, et al: Frequent presence of the Epstein-Barr virus in inflammatory pseudotumor. Hum Pathol 1995; 26:1093.

295. McHenry CR, Perzy-Gall HB, Mardini G, et al: Inflammatory pseudotumor of the spleen: A rare entity that may mimic hematopoietic malignancy. Am Surg 1995; 61:1067.

296. Herman TE, Shackelford GD, Ternberg JL, et al: Inflammatory myofibroblastic tumor of the spleen: Report of a case in an adolescent. Pediatr Radiol 1994; 24:2890.

297. Aru GM, Abramowsky CR, Ricketts PR: Inflammatory pseudotumor of the spleen in a young child. Pediatr Surg Int 1997; 12:299.

298. Coffin CH, Watterson J, Priest JR, et al: Extrapulmonary inflammatory myofibroblastic tumor (inflammatory pseudotumor): A clinicopathologic and immunohistochemical study of 84 cases. Am J Surg Pathol 1995; 19:895.

299. Davis RE, Warnke RA, Dorfman RF: Inflammatory pseudotumor of lymph nodes: Additional observations and evidence for an inflammatory etiology. Am J Surg Pathol 1991; 15:744.

300. Craig J, Peters R, Edmondson H: Tumors of the liver and intrahepatic bile ducts, in Atlas of Tumor Pathology, 2nd series, fascicle 26, p 94. Washington, DC, Armed Forces Institute of Pathology, 1989.

301. Facchetti F, De Wolf-Peeters C, De Wever I, et al: Inflammatory pseudotumor of lymph nodes: immunohistochemical evidence for its fibrohistiocytic nature. Am J Pathol 1990; 137:281.

302. Shek TWH, Ho FCS, Ng IOL, et al: Follicular dendritic cell tumor of the liver: Evidence for an Epstein-Barr virus-related clonal proliferation of follicular dendritic cells. Am J Surg Pathol 1996; 20:313.

303. Shek TWH, Luk ISC: Letter to the editor. Am J Surg Pathol 1996; 20:990.

304. Snyder CS, Dell'Aquila M, Haghighi P, et al: Clonal changes in inflammatory pseudotumor of the lung: A case report. Cancer 1995; 76:1545.

305. Selves J, Meggetto F, Brousset P, et al: Inflammatory pseudotumor of the liver: Evidence for follicular dendritic reticulum cell proliferation associated with clonal Epstein-Barr virus. Am J Surg Pathol 1996; 20:747.

306. Suster S, Moran CA, Blanco M: Mycobacterial spindle-cell pseudotumor of the spleen. Am J Clin Pathol 1994; 101:529.

307. Kumar S, Kumar D, Cowan DF, et al: Mycobacteria spindle cell pseudotumor of the spleen. Am J Clin Pathol 1994; 102:863.

308. Umlas J, Federman M, Crawford C, et al: Spindle cell pseudotumor due to *Mycobacterium avium-intracellulare* in patients with acquired immunodeficiency syndrome (AIDS): Positive staining of mycobacteria for cytoskeleton filaments. Am J Surg Pathol 1991; 15:1181.

Index